Community rehabilitation
services for people with
disabilities

r'

□ □ □
□ □ □
□ □ □

Community Rehabilitation Services for People with Disabilities

Community Rehabilitation Services for People with Disabilities

Edited by

Orv C. Karan, Ph.D.

Professor and Director
A. J. Pappanikou Center on Special Education
 and Rehabilitation: A University Affiliated Program,
University of Connecticut, Storrs, Connecticut

Stephen Greenspan, Ph.D.

Associate Professor
Department of Educational Psychology,
University of Connecticut, Storrs, Connecticut

WITH THIRTY CONTRIBUTING AUTHORS

Foreword by

Jack Stark, Ph.D.
Creighton/Nebraska Medical School
Omaha, Nebraska

Butterworth–Heinemann
Boston   Oxford   Melbourne   Singapore   Toronto   Munich
New Delhi   Tokyo

Every effort has been made to ensure that the drug dosage schedules within this text are accurate and conform to standards accepted at time of publication. However, as treatment recommendations vary in the light of continuing research and clinical experience, the reader is advised to verify drug dosage schedules herein with information found on product information sheets. This is especially true in cases of new or infrequently used drugs.

Recognizing the importance of preserving what has been written, Butterworth–Heinemann prints its books on acid-free paper whenever possible.

Library of Congress Cataloging-in-Publication Data
Community rehabilitation services for people with disabilities / edited by Orv C.
   Karan, Stephen Greenspan : with thirty contributing authors.
        p.   cm.
   Includes bibliographical references and index.
   ISBN 0-7506-9532-3
   1. Handicapped—Services for—United States. 2. Handicapped—
Rehabilitation—United States. I. Karan, Orv C. II. Greenspan, Stephen.
HV1553.C575   1995
362.4'048-dc20   95-15286
                                                                          CIP

British Library Cataloguing-in-Publication Data
A catalogue record for this book is available from the British Library.

The publisher offers discounts on bulk orders of this book.
For information, please write:

Manager of Special Sales
Butterworth–Heinemann
313 Washington Street
Newton, MA 02158–1626

10 9 8 7 6 5 4 3 2 1

Printed in the United States of America

Dedicated to the memory of
Frank J. Menolascino, M.D. (1930–1992),
a valiant leader in the community revolution
in disability services

Contents

Foreword

Frank Menolascino would have been proud of this book. Proud of its tenets and proud of the book's contributors. The chapter authors, like him, have devoted the bulk of their careers to advocating for community services. To the reader this might seem obvious, but this was not the case 25 years ago when Frank helped to establish one of the first community-based programs that emphasized comprehensive rehabilitation services. Frank, like many of this book's contributors, was criticized for his strong position and the delivery of services in natural settings—close to one's family. Although all of us have paid a price for our beliefs, real leaders seem to get the brunt of the criticism. Frank's favorite quote from Thomas Merton directly applies to this book.

> If a writer is so cautious that he never writes anything that cannot be criticized, he will never write anything that can be read. If you want to help other people, you have to make up your mind to write things that some men will condemn.

This book accomplishes two major goals. First, its "heuristic" research advances the positions the authors developed over their lifetime. Second, it serves as a "cutting edge" blueprint in guiding human service personnel in adapting similar services strategies.

The timing of this book is also critical. Never has there been such a need for specific and practical answers for professionals in a variety of disciplines. There are over 100,000 individuals living in large I.C.F.–M.R. facilities who need to be served in the community along with another 100,000 on waiting lists with no services living at home with their family. In addition, the waiting lists are doubling every 3 to 4 years due to the high "graduation" rates of individuals with disabilities.

It is indeed a sad commentary that on the twentieth anniversary of Public Law 94-142 (1975), record numbers of special education students who have greatly benefited from educational programs are "graduating" at age 21 with no where to go.

What is needed are answers. Specifics on what to do—when, with costs justified and based on sound scientific principles. This book is uniquely qualified to meet this criteria. Hundreds of years of experience in teaching, research, direct services, and public policy efforts are the defining characteristics of this scholarly group of individuals. Seldom has such a gifted group come together to meet this tremendous challenge of the community revolution.

Frank Menolascino worked with many of the authors of this book over the last 25 years. He served as a colleague, friend, and mentor to many of them. He helped to shape their ideas and shared in their devotion. It is fitting that such a book be dedicated to him in that he symbolized the need for community services, for he so clearly identified with the families and understood their need to be with their children. The following quote perhaps best summarizes both what this book and Frank are all about!

> Where there is
> great love
> there are always miracles.
> Miracles rest not so much
> upon faces or voices
> or healing power
> coming to us from afar off
> but on our perceptions
> being made finer,
> so that for a moment
> our eyes can see
> and our ears can hear
> what there is about us
> always.
>
> Willa Cather

The Funeral Liturgy for
Frank Menolascino
Born May 25, 1930
Born to New Life, April 3, 1992

Jack Stark, Ph.D.
Combined Department of Psychiatry
Creighton/Nebraska Medical School
Omaha, Nebraska

Preface

This book deals with the community revolution in disability services that has been occurring in the United States over the past two decades. This revolution involves a fundamental change in the way professionals and agencies relate to individuals with disabilities and their families. In the not-too-distant past, service options were limited, with institutionalization or family sacrifice as the two most likely choices. Although many more options have been created for people with disabilities and their families, until very recently the emphasis was still on fitting individuals into existing slots. The community revolution, on the other hand, is grounded in supporting individuals, empowering them to make choices, and redefining the roles of professionals as facilitators rather than decision makers.

Community Rehabilitation Services for People with Disabilities is intended to serve as an introduction to current thinking about the "paradigm shift" in disability services. The book is divided into three parts. In the first part are several chapters that spell out the principles underlying the community revolution in disability services. The next part contains chapters that discuss problems and issues regarding the implementation of these principles. Finally, the third part details how professional and scientific disciplines have modified their practices and value orientations to reflect this still-evolving paradigm shift.

As with all revolutions, the community revolution in disability services has generated considerable confusion and controversy. Some disciplines have been quicker to adapt to this revolution than others, and within each discipline are practitioners who differ in their willingness to change their values and practices. Financial realities limit the implementation of flexible practices aimed at increasing the quality of life of individuals with disabilities. Nevertheless, the community revolution has brought about—in a comparatively short time—some fundamental changes in the way people with disabilities are viewed and served. It is hoped that this book will help to further this revolution by giving future practitioners an understanding of where the disability field has come from and where it appears to be heading.

Orv Karan

Contributors

Greg Bazinet, Ph.D.c
Coordinator of Vocational Education
University of Southern Maine
Gorham, ME 04038

Valerie Bradley
President
Human Services Research Institute
Cambridge, MA 02140

Stephen N. Calculator, Ph.D.
Professor
Department of Communicative Disorders
PCAC
University of New Hampshire
Durham, NH 03824

Robert E. Cipriano, Ed.D.
Professor
Southern Connecticut State University
New Haven, CT 06515

Bryce Fifield, Ph.D.
Associate Director
Idaho Center on Developmental Disabilities
University of Idaho
Moscow, ID 83841

Marvin Fifield, Ed.D.
Director
Center for Person with Disabilities:
 A University Affiliated Program
Utah State University
Logan, UT 84322-6800

James F. Gardner, Ph.D.
Chief Executive Officer
The Accreditation Council on Services for People
    with Disabilities
Landover, MD 20785-2225

Michael F. Giangreco, Ph.D.
Research Assistant Professor
College of Education
The University Affiliated Program of Vermont
University of Vermont
Burlington, VT 05405-0160

Stephen Greenspan, Ph.D.
Associate Professor
Department of Educational Psychology
University of Connecticut
Storrs, CT 06269-2086

David Hagner, Ph.D.
Research Associate
Training and Research Institute for People
    with Disabilities
Children's Hospital
Boston, MA 02115

Farah A. Ibrahim, Ph.D.
Professor
Department of Educational Psychology
University of Connecticut
Storrs, CT 06269-2086

Ronald K. James, Ph.D.
Assistant Professor and Services Coordinator
Hawaii University Affiliated Program for
    Developmental Disabilities
University of Hawaii at Manoa
Honolulu, HI 96822

Orv C. Karan, Ph.D.
Professor and Director
A. J. Pappanikou Center on Special Education
  and Rehabilitation: A University Affiliated Program
University of Connecticut
Storrs, CT 06269-2086

William E. Kiernan, Ph.D.
Director
Developmental Evaluation Center: A University
  Affiliated Program
Children's Hospital
Boston, MA 02115

James Knoll, Ph.D.
Associate Director
Developmental Disabilities Institute
Wayne State University
Detroit, MI 48202

David Leake, Ph.D.c, M.P.H.
Project Coordinator
Hawaii University Affiliated Program
  for Developmental Disabilities
University of Hawaii at Manoa
Honolulu, HI 96822

Ronnie Leavitt, Ph.D., M.P.H.
Associate Professor
School of Allied Health
University of Connecticut
Storrs, CT 06269-2086

Audrey N. Leviton, M.S.W., L.C.S.W.-C
Program Manager
Child and Family Support Program
Kennedy Krieger Institute
Baltimore, MD 21213

Peter Love, M.P.H.
Executive Director
United Cerebral Palsy of Hartford
Hartford, CT 06105

Frank J. Menolascino, M.D.
Formerly Chairperson (Deceased)
Combined Psychiatry Departments
University of Nebraska and Creighton University
Omaha, NE 68105

Mary H. Mueller, M.S.W., L.C.S.W.-C
Senior Staff Coordinator
Child and Family Support Program
Kennedy Krieger Institute
Baltimore, MD 21213

Mary A. Musholt, R.N., MSN
Public Health Nurse and Clinical Instructor
University of Wisconsin–Madison
School of Nursing
Madison Department of Public Health
Madison, WI 53706

Kay Norlander, Ph.D.
Associate Professor
Department of Educational Psychology
University of Connecticut
Storrs, CT 06269-2086

Beverly Rainforth, Ph.D.
Associate Professor Special Education
School of Education and Human Development
State University of New York at Binghamton
Binghamton, NY 13902-6000

Robert L. Schalock, Ph.D.
Chairman and Professor
Department of Psychology
Hastings College
Hastings, NE 68902-0269

Bonnie Shoultz, M.A.
Associate Director for Information and Training
 at the Research and Training Center on
 Community Integration at the Center on Human Policy
Syracuse, NY 13244-2340

Pamela D. Smith, Ed.D.
Educational Program Specialist
Department of Special Education
University of Georgia
Athens, GA 30602

Patricia McGill Smith
Executive Director of the National Parent Network
 on Disabilities
Alexandria, VA 22314

Robert A. Stodden, Ph.D.
Professor and Director
Hawaii University Affiliated Program
 for Developmental Disabilities
University of Hawaii at Manoa
Honolulu, HI 96822

Harvey N. Switzky, Ph.D., FAAMR
Professor of Educational Psychology
Department of Educational Psychology, Counseling,
 and Special Education
Northern Illinois University
DeKalb, IL 60115

Nancy R. Weiss, M.S.W.
Nancy Weiss Associates
Baltimore, MD 21204

Jennifer York, P.T., Ph.D.
Assistant Professor/Interdisciplinary Coordinator
Institute on Community Integration
University of Minnesota
Minneapolis, MN 55455

Community Rehabilitation Services for People with Disabilities

PART ☐ ☐ ☐
I ☐ ☐ ☐
☐ ☐ ☐

The New Paradigm: Conceptual, Legislative, and Ethical Foundations

The first part of this book provides a conceptual framework and both a historical and ethical perspective on the shifting paradigms, where they came from, the controversies that surround them, the laws that have been shaped by the thinking of the contemporary paradigms, and the ethical implications derived from considerations of the daily decisions and challenges inherent in services built around individual preferences, values, and choices. In Chapter 1 Bradley and Knoll examine the process of change and develop a rationale for the emergence of a new paradigm, identifying its essential characteristics and highlighting the implications for professionals in the field. As they note, the keystones of the emerging paradigm are commitment to community, human relationships, functional teaching, individualization, and flexibility. To these authors, such emerging values are potentially more revolutionary than the values that originally took us as a field out of institutions and into the community. Such changes that have been driven by the new paradigm may cause significant dislocation in existing service structures and complicate the lives of those comfortable with the status quo. However, these shifts will move real services closer to the ultimate goals of normalization and the fulfillment of the dreams of people with disabilities and their families.

In Chapter 2 Leake, James, and Stodden place the concepts of the paradigm shift in historical perspective. They then discuss how commitment to different sets of principles leads to discord within the field over correct policy and practice for services. A primary divide currently appears

1

to be between those guided by empirically supported theories and those guided by philosophical principles. For these authors, the support paradigm is a practical rather than just an ideological response to a crisis that now exists in the service field. The new paradigm from their perspective is capable of bridging differences within the field. In fact, to these authors the support paradigm is the only paradigm that can be used to guide current services into a new era simply because existing paradigms have such serious shortcomings that can be addressed only in terms of more money, more research, and more training of professionals. However, not enough more will be forthcoming from government or private sources.

In Chapter 3 Fifield and Fifield analyze past legislation to identify specific themes that set precedents for current legislation. From these themes they have tried to forecast some of the trends of the future. It is their position that society's attitudes and values and thus its paradigms are codified in the language and provisions of laws and the rules and procedures we follow in meeting the needs of persons with disabilities. They believe it is possible to better understand the legislative provisions through a historical perspective by analyzing legislative trends and thereby anticipating legislation of the future. This second function, forecasting legislative provisions, is particularly important if we are to do more today than fix the problems of yesterday. Their review of the laws impacting on disabilities stretches from those of the seventeenth and eighteenth centuries to the current provisions of the Americans with Disabilities Act.

The final two chapters in this part, both by Greenspan and Love, deal with the ethical challenges involved in supporting people with disabilities and the development of a code of everyday ethics for services. In Chapter 4, Greenspan and Love argue that implicit in the evolving service models is a set of moral judgments about the rightness of making human services more respectful of the individual's preferences, dignity, and personhood. They note that the literature on ethics and disability emphasizes medical issues, and that much less attention has been paid to the ethical aspects of everyday life and services for persons with disabilities. In their first chapter they emphasize the role of ethical theory in guiding the everyday treatment of persons with disabilities. They review the normalization principle because of its central role in providing an ethical framework for changing the way in which people with disabilities are allowed to live their everyday lives. They discuss the new paradigm and note that in spite of its emphasis on individual rights, choice making, and self-expression, there is still the potential for new areas of abuse based on the continuing power differential between consumers and professionals.

In Chapter 5 Greenspan and Love articulate a universal code of conduct to which agencies, professionals, and other workers may subscribe, a code which involves ten universal obligations that support persons and agencies have toward consumers. They believe that the need for a code of conduct in training and supervising professionals has become increasingly pressing. They propose a framework that may help guide professionals through the complex and unpredictable daily decision-making process that the new paradigm, with its emphasis on individual planning and natural supports, has generated.

1

Shifting Paradigms in Services to People with Disabilities

Valerie J. Bradley and James Knoll

INTRODUCTION

For almost a quarter century, services to people with disabilities have been in a seemingly endless state of flux. At the heart of this shift has been the transformation of the system of services from institutions to communities and from segregation to integration. Terms such as *deinstitutionalization, normalization, equal rights, access, least restrictive environment,* and *community-based services* have characterized the direction, and change has been the status quo for the entire career of most workers now in the field.

These changes, however, have been made somewhat haltingly and self-consciously. Though it was relatively easy to critique the shortcomings of institutional services, arriving at the essential components of a system of services in the community has proven somewhat more problematic. Self-scrutiny, rooted in a concern that the abuses of the past not be repeated, has led people with disabilities, parents, advocates, service providers, and researchers to challenge each new approach. While a particular model of service might be hailed at one moment as "the answer" for providing normalized humane services, it is likely in short order to be criticized for embodying some of the limits on individual growth found in earlier modes of service.

Central to this process has been a shift in the dominant theoretical perspective or paradigm that at any one time is shared by the majority of workers in the field. Kuhn (1962) and others, working in the field of philosophy of

5

science, have developed the construct of the dominant paradigm as a way of conceptualizing this higher-order perspective that serves to organize activity in a given field of endeavor. We suggest that this concept is directly applicable to the field of disabilities.

In fact, most people familiar with the history of services to people with disabilities are at least somewhat conversant with the concept of a paradigm, although they have traditionally used other terms to define the concept. People can describe the fundamental shift in the field in the late 1960s and early 1970s, as institutionalization and dependence were de-emphasized in favor of independent living programs and community services. On the "theoretical" level these changes are frequently described as being accompanied by a shift from the "medical model" of care to the "developmental model" or from the "custodial model" to the "rehabilitation model." This transition was the first inkling of what Kuhn has called a paradigm shift. Only now, in the 1990s, can we begin to see the outline of the emerging paradigm that will carry the field into the next century.

This evolutionary process can be broken into three distinct phases. In the first period, the era of institutionalization, dependence, and segregation (roughly ending in the mid-1970s), the governing norms were primarily medical and the impetus was to separate people who were "sick" and vulnerable. This was followed by the era of deinstitutionalization and community development (1976–1986), which was marked by the creation of community services and an emphasis on the provision of specialized services to assist people to grow and learn, and to live in their communities. The third and current period, the era of community membership, is marked by an emphasis on functional supports to enhance community integration, independence, quality of life, and individualization. Only now, as states begin to close and phase down institutions and to redefine their services in terms of supports in homes, schools, and in the workplace, has the community membership model begun to evolve from a theoretical possibility to a governing paradigm.

In this chapter we will examine this process of change, develop our rationale for the emergence of the new paradigm, sketch the essential characteristics of this new perspective, and highlight the implications of this shift for professionals in the field.

INSTITUTIONALIZATION AND SEGREGATION: A MEDICAL MODEL

Until very recently, the locus of services for people with disabilities was out of the home. As a result, the institutional population in the United States peaked in 1968 at more than 200,000, and nursing home populations also soared. The only alternatives to institutions were private facilities and hospitals for families or individuals who could afford such care. Expectations for care in institutional settings were primarily focused on custodial and medical concerns. The first formal expression of concern for the quality of institutional care for people with disabilities, according to Scheerenberger (1983), was the development in 1942 of staffing standards for institutional programs by the American Association on Mental Deficiency (AAMD) (now the American Association on Mental Retardation). By 1953, Scheerenberger adds, the concern for standards led the AAMD to develop "Standards for Public Training Schools" that included programmatic and administrative prescriptions as well as numerical staffing requirements. These initial forays seem rudimentary compared to the complexity of expectations and programmatic issues faced by today's policy makers and practitioners.

The inadequacies of the custodial approach in developmental disabilities, mental health, and physical disabilities became increasingly obvious in the 1960s and 1970s as a parade of plaintiff representatives in a number of key class-action suits around the country began to spell out the woeful shortcomings of institutional care, and as people with disabilities themselves argued eloquently for their independence. Nearly identical accounts of abuse surfaced at Willowbrook in New York, Partlow and Bryce in Alabama, Northampton and Belchertown in Massachusetts, Beatrice State Hospital in Nebraska, Sandhaven in North Dakota, Pennhurst in Pennsylvania, Solomon State Hospital in Maryland, and Cloverbottom in Tennessee.

The response to a nationwide tide of exposés and litigation in the late 1960s and through the 1970s was the simultaneous development of standards to govern services and a wide range of new community-based services that were seen as avoiding the pitfalls of the old isolated institutional model of service. The federal government also responded to the increasingly urgent entreaties of people with physical disabilities for access and independence and developed regulations to implement the nondiscrimination provisions of Section 504 of the Vocational Rehabilitation Act.

In many of the court cases, courts imposed comprehensive minimum standards of care (see, for example, New York State Association for Retarded Children et al. v. Carey et al., 1975; Wyatt v. Stickney, 1972). The standards were an effort to assure that the physical, social, and psychological deprivation in these settings would be corrected (Lottman, 1990). Often the court decrees offered very specific guidelines articulating such things as staffing ratios, daily schedules, professional qualifications, number of residents per toilet, and the nutritional content of meals. While some standards responded to specific issues in a particular court case, most represented an effort to bring custodial facilities into line with minimal care standards as articulated by expert witnesses in the case.

Little consideration, however, was given to how this dominant concern for protection from harm and minimal programmatic standards could facilitate the principles of normalization (Wolfensberger, 1972), maximization of independence, and community access, which were becoming the guiding philosophies of those attempting to reform services to people with disabilities.

DEINSTITUTIONALIZATION AND THE DEVELOPMENTAL MODEL

In the 1970s the appropriateness of institutionalization and segregation—even in newly reformed facilities—began to be questioned and the disabilities field moved into an era that saw the creation of community residential and day programs, outpatient centers, accessible housing, individualized programming, and the consequent ascendancy of the professional (Bradley, 1978). The person with disabilities became an object to be trained, habilitated, socialized, screened, assessed, and assisted through a continuum of educational, vocational, and residential settings.

Instead of custodial care, we moved into the decade of specialized services. Small intermediate-care facilities for people with mental retardation (ICF/MRs), halfway houses, and handicapped housing became the alternatives to institutions. Because they were smaller, we heralded the coming of "homelike" settings. They had to be better than institutions because they were scientifically designed, professionally staffed, and organized according to individual habilitation, rehabilitation, or treatment plan. The basic motivation for these programs was to provide a specialized treatment environment where problems could be worked on, therapies delivered, and skills developed. The underlying assumption was that once people had achieved a higher level of functioning they could move on to a less restrictive setting, typically to a group home or other community facility.

One of the motivating theories that created the paradigm shift from the institutional model to deinstitutionalization and community services was the developmental model. This construct was based on the assumption that all people, regardless of the level of their abilities or severity of their disabilities, could grow and develop. These notions were actively employed in the creation of complex teaching approaches to assist people with disabilities to acquire skills. Teaching curricula were developed and ordinary skills of daily living were broken down into their most minute constituent parts in order to facilitate learning among people with intellectual limitations.

The result was elaborate teaching regimens and lock step progressions through prearticulated learning objectives. Skills were taught without regard to context in many instances and progress through the continuum of living arrangements and day and work training programs became contingent on the acquisition of the appropriate abilities and the mastery of requisite tasks.

Concurrently, in the fields of mental health and physical disabilities, new therapeutic and rehabilitation efforts were being applied by a growing cadre of psychiatrists, social workers, rehabilitation specialists, occupational therapists, speech therapists, mental health nurses, and a vast army of other trained staff.

In addition to the emerging learning and therapeutic technologies, another major underpinning of service development during this period was behaviorism, which assumes that behavior occurs because it is reinforced: change the conditions—eliminate or refocus the reinforcement—and you can change the behavior. This basic insight and its implications radically transformed the lives of many people with severe disabilities because it provided human service practitioners with an alternative to mere custodial care. As experience was gained in using this approach, clinicians realized that with the right interventions they were able to manage or control almost any behavior. The behavior specialist became a surgeon of human behavior: "Show me a maladaptive behavior and I can cut it out." Usually this attitude was guided by the best of human motivations: to improve the quality of life available to people by eliminating those actions that tended to alienate them from other people. Unfortunately this technique was also frequently used for the primary purpose of easing the management of groups of people in large facilities.

Typically, the behaviorist clinician identifies the behavior that interferes with a person living in a community setting and then develops an intervention to remove that behavior from his or her repertoire. The person goes into the "behavioral hospital" or specialized setting to have these treatments applied. Afterwards he or she can move to a less specialized setting where the treatment can be prescriptively reapplied if the symptoms reappear. Unfortunately, as people like Lovett (1985) have shown, this is a basic misdirection of behaviorism since it ignores the total context of behavior and usually does not recognize or respond to the point of view of the "client." When this view is overlooked, little reflection is given to the complex network of factors that influence behavior. The restrictive, unstimulating, and frequently dehumanizing situations that society has forced upon people with severe disabilities are therefore not always credited as primary stimuli for challenging behavior.

Many now believe that "undesirable behavior" has a meaning. In other words, even the most troublesome behavior may serve a function for the person even if its purpose is not initially understood. This suggests that to deal with "problem behaviors," a functional adaptive rather than maladaptive behavior must be found that will fulfill that same need. Lovett and others contend that this type of orientation is more reflective of the promise of behaviorism. This perspective on human behavior is sometimes called an "ecological" or "holistic" approach.

Like the behavioral approach, the traditional developmental and rehabilitation models also assume that skills can be learned in isolation from the ultimate reality of community living. They also presume that true integration is "earned" after multiple hurdles in a therapeutic sequence have been overcome. The recognition that these unintentional barriers have been placed in the way of people with disabilities has spurred the impending paradigm shift described below.

COMMUNITY MEMBERSHIP AND FUNCTIONAL SUPPORTS

In the 1980s doubts began to grow regarding whether the slavish focus on professional services and specialized programs had resulted in changes reflective of the original vision of normalization: Were people with disabilities really any better off in terms of independence, integration, and productivity? Was the notion of a service continuum just a way of denying people full participation in and control over their own lives?

Instead of thinking about how to surround people with services in specially designed and constructed homes, we began to think about moving support to where people lived. Instead of concentrating on how to make the individual adapt to the environment, we began to think about ways of adapting the environment and supports to the individual. We also began to dig deeper into the concept of normalization and to question whether, by surrounding people with professionals, we may have isolated them from friends, family, and community. We also began to wonder whether the skills we were teaching really had any functional meaning and whether the successful acquisition of abilities had any relationship to increased community participation.

The concept of functional supports offers an alternative to the continuum of services and the obsession with "program slots." Rather than focus on putting people into community programs, this developing focus emphasizes the creation of a network of formal and informal supports that a person with a disability needs to meet his or her day-to-day demands

(Ferguson and Olson, 1989; Taylor, 1988; Taylor, Racino, Knoll, and Lutfiyya, 1987).

This shifting focus away from deinstitutionalization and the establishment of "community-based programs" to community membership and meeting the support needs of individuals in their homes presents new challenges to the service planner and policy maker. Providers of disability services are increasingly pressed to consider the degree to which true social integration is taking place and how they can be facilitators. Unfortunately, the literature lags far behind the most advanced thinking in the field (Research and Training Center on Community Integration, 1989). While there have been some efforts to articulate the components of this third phase or program paradigm, they are still very new.

The emerging emphasis is on liberating people with disabilities from the stigma of "clienthood" and providing supports that are in line with typical expectations concerning freedom and control over one's own life (Biklen and Knoll, 1987; McKnight, 1987).

The central idea is to assure people with disabilities a quality of life that is congruent with how that concept is defined by society in general. The concept of quality of life is so pervasive that even individuals who have reservations regarding the "community integration" movement recognize it as a crucial concept to be included in program evaluation (Landesman, 1986, and Robinson, 1987).

People with disabilities themselves are also increasingly making their feelings known regarding what they want in terms of quality of life. As early as 1970, a group of people with developmental disabilities issued a statement of "beliefs, questions, and demands" that was drafted by adults with mental retardation at a conference sponsored by the Swedish Association for Retarded Children. Among the demands made at the national conference in Malmo, Sweden, were the following:

> We wish to have an apartment of our own and not be coddled by personnel; therefore, we want courses in cooking, budgeting, etc.
>
> We want the right to move together with the other sex when we feel ready for it, and we also want the right to marry when we ourselves find the time is right.
>
> We want to have more personal freedom, and not as it is now in certain institutions and boarding homes where you have to ask permission to shop for fruit, newspapers, tobacco, etc.
>
> We who live at home have found that: it is largely good, but one ought to move out when the time is right to a sheltered apartment or hostel; one cannot for his whole life be dependent on his parents. We want, however, to have our own key when we live at home.
>
> We demand more training in a wider range of vocational fields so that we can have larger freedom of choice in determining our vocations.

We want to choose our vocations ourselves and have influence over our education.

We demand more interesting jobs.

We do not want to be used on our jobs by doing the worst and the most boring tasks we do at present.

We demand that our capacity for work should not be underestimated.

We think that we should be present when our situation is discussed by doctors, teachers, welfare workers, floor men, etc. Now it feels as if they talk behind our backs (Wolfensberger, 1972, pp. 190–193).

The message from Malmo was clear. People wanted support to achieve independence, dignity, and personal fulfillment. It has taken more than twenty years, but the developments in the field of services for people with disabilities have come to the point where professional providers and policy makers can hear the testimony of Malmo and can reassess services in terms of the instrumental contribution they make to the achievement of these basic human objectives.

Another way of capturing the spirit of an instrumental or functional approach to services is to think of all interventions as being "holistic." To apply holistic principles is to examine the role people play in their environment, the match between the individual and the demands of the environment, and the complex interplay of forces that influence individual behavior and learning. Rather than see behavior as caused by either some internal drive or the mechanistic response to an external stimuli, the initial formulators of what has become the holistic perspective took their lead from Kurt Lewin's classic statement that behavior is a function of the interaction between a person and the environment ($B = f\{PE\}$) (Lewin, 1935, p. 73). In the years immediately after World War II, a group of researchers used Lewin's earlier work and undertook a social psychological examination of the lives of people with physical disabilities (Dembo, Leviton, and Wright, 1956). This work led to the conclusion that most of the limitations on people with disabilities are imposed by society rather than being intrinsic to an individual's functional deficit. Bronfenbrenner (1979) and his colleagues further developed this theory of behavior by highlighting the need to see individual actions and the definition of that behavior as the product of a series of complex interactions. From this perspective all of the elements that contribute to a behavior are not immediately present in the setting where it occurs.

William Rhodes (1967) was the first to describe the value of a holistic perspective for practitioners in special education and related disciplines. Speaking specifically of students labeled emotionally disturbed, he pointed out that educators had come to see disturbance as something residing in the student. Hence, their interventions were exclusively geared toward remediating the flaw within the person. As a more practical educational alternative, he proposed a holistic view that focused on the interactive nature of the problem behavior and saw disturbance as residing in the tension between the individual and the demands of the environment.

Subsequently, a number of authors have explored the theoretical and programmatic implications of a holistic analysis of people with disabilities in our society (Algozzine, 1977; Apter, 1982; Hobbs, 1975; Hobbs, 1980; Swap, 1974; and Swap, 1978). Following Rhodes's lead, most of these authors have focused almost exclusively on the need to see challenging behavior as resulting "from a discrepancy between . . . skills and abilities and the demands or expectations of . . . [the] environment" (Apter, 1982, p. 2). Similarly, ecological theory has been used as a model for the most innovative programs for individuals with severe disabilities (Brinker, 1985, and Brown, Falvey, Baumgart, Pumpian, Schroeder, and Gruenewald, 1980) and as a framework for viewing issues in community services for people with disabilities (Hitzing, 1987; Lovett, 1985; and Smull, 1987). From this broader view of disability there are three possible areas for intervention: (a) change the person, (b) change the environment, or (c) change societal attitudes and expectations. Many of our efforts in the past have focused on changing the person. Today, we are looking much more at ways to change the environment and attitudes.

Finally, a major implication of a holistic orientation is that we give up searching for a magic answer to the problems of people with disabilities. Instead, we must begin to think about problems in the system and increase our understanding of the interaction between the individual and the environment (Apter, 1982).

The keystones of this emerging paradigm are commitment to community, human relationships, functional teaching and individualization, and flexibility (Taylor, Racino, Knoll, and Lutfiyya, 1987).

Commitment to Community and Families

A key element is a commitment to the community as the place where people should live. From this perspective, the community is not some sort of nirvana, but a place where everyone has a right to live. The job of the practitioner in this framework is to help resolve the barriers that inhibit the individual from participating in his or her chosen community.

Where this perspective has been adopted, people no longer speak of "community-alternatives" or "community-based services" because there is no alternative to the community. A second part of that commitment to community has to do with providing support to people with disabilities in their families. Just as we have begun to recognize that moving people out of their home communities to specialized facilities severs important ties with natural supports, we have also begun to acknowledge that removing people with disabilities from their families—especially when they are children—ignores the commitment of the family, disrupts family connections, and deprives the child of the experience of growing and developing in a family unit.

Human Relationships

Commitment to physical presence in the community must be accompanied by tangible social connections in the community. Being part of a community means that people have enduring relationships with people other than those paid to be with them. With real friendship come natural systems of support that are often able to forestall or prevent relatively minor problems from becoming insurmountable difficulties. Most people have these supports, but for people who have been in the system for years, these relationships have frequently atrophied in favor of professional intervention.

There is no question that finding a "methodology" for linking people is a challenge facing service providers. It has not traditionally been addressed in the course of professional preparation. Indeed, overinvolvement by professionals in this process might lead to the development of a routinized "friendship therapy." The best practices in this area seem to be marked by sensitivity and intuition, and an understanding that any approach to developing community linkages must be idiosyncratic.

Functional Programming and Individualization

The demands of the agency or the nature of the program should not dictate the "individualized" goals for people with disabilities. A functional approach concentrates on developing the skills that are required by the demands of each individual's unique life situation. The mutual interdependence of housemates or workmates and the demands of each individual's daily routine dictate the components of their "functional" program.

Functionality begins by attempting to understand how an array of adaptations can be created to assist a person to gain control over his or her everyday life. Such adaptations may be mechanical, such as an augmentative communication device or specially tailored hearing implements, or may take the form of a personal care attendant. Functional programming does not obviate the need for learning, but does assess the necessity of acquiring skills compared to the role that such skills will play in enhancing community presence and integration.

With respect to controlling or modifying behavior, a truly functional approach is a positive alternative to behavioral interventions that solely attempt to control or eliminate behavior. Service providers and behavioral consultants look to a person's life in an effort to understand his or her behavior. They attempt to identify new, adaptive, functional skills that satisfy the same need as a problem behavior while also serving a real purpose in daily life. Admittedly, all behaviorists will say this is what they do. The difference lies in the fact that most traditional behaviorists take a very narrow focus when they identify the antecedents and consequences of a behavior. From a holistic perspective, the full context of an individual's life is considered.

Individualized planning is key to functional programming. Such planning, to be responsive, brings together all of the people whose cooperation is essential for assuring the future quality of life of the individual of concern. O'Brien (1987) offers a forum for such an approach to planning which he calls "Personal Futures Planning." Some service providers who have implemented this approach have found it particularly useful when the individual of concern is someone who offers the service system a lot of challenges. O'Brien describes five planning perspectives: (1) community presence, (2) choice, (3) competence, (4) respect, and (5) community participation. It is his thesis that these five elements are the way most people define the quality of their lives. Within the framework of these themes the planning process then revolves around eight questions about the person's life:

1. What is the quality of the focal person's present life experience?
2. What is changing for the person or in the surrounding environment that is likely to influence the quality of the focal person's life?
3. What are the most important threats and opportunities to better life experience for the focal person?
4. What is the image of a desirable future for the focal person?
5. What are the most critical barriers to our moving toward the desirable future?
6. How will we most effectively manage these critical barriers and move toward the future we've defined?
7. What are the next steps?
8. Based on our discussions, do we want to make any statements about necessary changes in the capabilities of the service system?

The end result is a shared vision of the unique situation of a specific individual and a plan of action for moving toward that goal. The description of the meeting concludes with a reminder that the nature of the supports available to follow up on the plan will determine if this valuable process really does make a difference.

Flexible and Individualized Supports

With individualized and flexible supports, all natural environments can be open to people with disabilities, even persons with severe disabilities. Community integration means more than just being physically present in the community. It means opportunities and, when necessary, the provision of support to citizens with disabilities in order to make them active participants in the life of the community. Documented best practices in the field have shown that individuals with disabilities can be fellow classmates, good neighbors, contributing coworkers, and involved citizens.

Flexible supports, including individualized housing and work options, encourage persons with disabilities to exercise control and choice. Supported living means that people live where they want and with whom they want, for as long as they want, with the ongoing support needed to sustain that choice (Ferguson and Olson, 1989). Some exemplary supported-living programs include Options in Community Living, in Madison, Wisconsin; Centennial Developmental Services in Evans, Colorado; and the Supported Placements in Community Environments (SPICE) program in Illinois. Features shared by these programs include (1) paid support provided by live-in or on-call staff, roommates or companions, attendants, or neighbors; (2) individualization and flexibility; (3) a focus on the individual; (4) a belief that people live in homes, not facilities; and (5) consumer and family involvement in planning and quality assurance (Nisbet, Clark, and Covert, 1991).

Options, a private nonprofit agency in Madison, Wisconsin, provides residential support services to ninety-five men and women who have developmental disabilities. In operation since 1981, Options provides support and coordinates services to enable adults to live on their own in small, dispersed settings in the community. The agency works with people to help them make their own choices and reach their own goals, with support available to them as often and as long as it is needed. Options is the oldest of such programs in the country and is considered to be the leader of this growing movement.

The state of Colorado has several supported-living programs in operation, successfully assisting adults with disabilities to live in residential settings of their choice. In Illinois, the SPICE Project is actively moving people with disabilities out of nursing facilities into their own one- or two-person homes. SPICE was designed to demonstrate that people with multiple and severe disabilities can live outside of congregate settings if they are provided with appropriate services and supports and to demonstrate a more individualized approach to residential services. Funded through a Medicaid waiver, SPICE serves forty people throughout the state and has targeted people with multiple and severe disabilities who have not traditionally been considered for community placements.

CONCLUSION

The emerging values of individualization, community inclusion, and self-determination are even more subversive and potentially revolutionary than the values that took us out of institutions and into communities—values like maximization of individual potential, placement in the least restrictive environment, and individual rights.

At least the values of the 1970s and 1980s placed the professional very much in charge of the direction and content of services and led to a dramatic expansion of the disability industry in the community. In fact, many of these values increased the preeminence of professionals since they reinforced the virtues of active treatment and enshrined the importance of specialized—and ultimately special—services in the individual education plan and the individualized habilitation plan.

The values that characterize the community membership paradigm, however, are already diminishing the professional hegemony of the past two decades. The changes to come, therefore, may cause significant dislocation in existing service structures and appear incoherent for those comfortable with the routinization of service provision. Far from incoherent, however, these shifts will move the reality of our practice closer to our espoused goal of normalization and to the dreams of people with disabilities and their families.

REFERENCES

Algozzine, B. (1977). The emotionally disturbed child: Disturbed or disturbing? *Journal of Abnormal Child Psychology, 5,* 205–211.

Apter, S.J. (1982). *Troubled children, troubled systems.* New York: Pergamon Press.

Biklen, D., and Knoll, J. (1987). The disabled minority. In S.J. Taylor, D. Biklen, and J. Knoll (Eds.), *Community integration for people with severe disabilities* (pp. 3–24). New York: Teacher's College Press.

Bradley, V.J. (1978). *Deinstitutionalization of developmentally disabled persons. A conceptual analysis and guide.* Baltimore: University Park Press.

Brinker, R.P. (1985). Curricula without recipes: A challenge to teachers and a promise to severely mentally retarded students. In D. Bricker and J. Filler (Eds.), *Severe mental retardation: From theory to practice* (pp. 208-229). Reston, VA: Division on Mental Retardation of the Council for Exceptional Children.

Bronfenbrenner, U. (1979). *The ecology of human development.* Cambridge: Harvard University Press.

Brown, L., Falvey, M., Baumgart, D., Pumpian, I., Schroeder, J., and Gruenewald, L. (1980). *Strategies for teaching chronological age-appropriate skills to adolescents and young adult severely handicapped students* (vol. 9). Madison, WI: Madison Metropolitan School District.

Dembo, T., Leviton, G.L., and Wright, B.A. (1956). Adjustment to misfortune—a problem of social psychological rehabilitation. *Artificial Limbs, 3,* 4–62.

Ferguson, P.M., and Olson, D. (Eds.) (1989). *Supported community life: Connecting policy to practice in disability research.* Eugene, OR: Specialized Training Program, Center on Human Development, University of Oregon.

Hitzing, W. (1987). Community living alternatives for persons with autism and related severe behavior problems. In D.J. Cohen and A.M. Donnellan (Eds.), *Handbook of autism and pervasive developmental disorders.* New York: Wiley.

Hobbs, N. (1975). *The future of children: Categories, labels, and their consequences.* San Francisco: Jossey-Bass.

Hobbs, N. (1980). An ecologically oriented, service-based system for the classification of handicapped children. In S. Salzinger, J. Antrobus, and J. Glick (Eds.), *The ecosystem of the "sick" child* (pp. 271–290). New York: Academic Press.

Kuhn, T. (1962). *The structure of scientific revolutions.* Chicago: University of Chicago Press.

Landesman, S. (1986). Quality of life and personal life satisfaction: Definition and measurement issues. *Mental Retardation, 24,* 141–143.

Lewin, K. (1935). *A dynamic theory of personality.* New York: McGraw-Hill.

Lottman, M.S. (1990). Quality assurance and the courts. In V.J. Bradley and H.A. Bersani (Eds.), *Quality assurance for individuals with developmental disabilities: It's everybody's business.* Baltimore: Paul H. Brookes.

Lovett, H. (1985). *Cognitive counseling and persons with special needs: Adapting behavior to the social context.* New York: Praeger.

McKnight, J. (1987). Regenerating community. *Social Policy,* Winter, 54–58.

New York State Association for Retarded Children et al. v. Carey et al., 393 F. Supp. 715 (E.D. N.Y. 1975).

Nisbet, J., Clark, M., and Covert, S. (1991). Living it up! An analysis of research on community living. In L.H. Meyer, C.A. Peck, and L. Brown (Eds.), *Critical issues in the lives of people with severe disabilities.* Baltimore: Paul H. Brookes.

O'Brien, J. (1987). A guide to life-style planning: Using the activities catalog to integrate services and natural support systems. In G.T. Bellamy and B. Wilcox (Eds.), *A comprehensive guide to the activities catalog: An alternative curriculum for youth and adults with severe disabilities* (pp. 175–189). Baltimore: Paul H. Brookes.

Research and Training Center on Community Integration (1989). *From being in the community to being part of the community.* Center on Human Policy, School of Education, Syracuse University.

Rhodes, W.C. (1967). The disturbing child: A problem of ecological management. *Exceptional Children, 33,* 449–455.

Robinson, N. (1987). Direction for person-environment research in mental retardation. In S. Landesman-Dwyer and P. Vietze (Eds.), *Living environments and mental retardation* (pp. 477–486). Washington, DC: American Association on Mental Deficiency.

Scheerenberger, R.C. (1983). *A history of mental retardation.* Baltimore: Paul H. Brookes.

Smull, M.W. (1987). Systems issues in meeting the mental health needs of persons with mental retardation. In J.A. Stark, F.J. Menolascino, M. Albarelli, and V. Gray (Eds.), *Mental retardation and mental health.* New York: Springer-Verlag.

Swap, S. (1974). Disturbing classroom behavior: A developmental and ecological view. *Exceptional Children, 41,* 162–171.

Swap, S. (1978). The ecological model of emotional disturbance in children: A status report and proposed synthesis. *Behavioral Disorders, 3*(3), 156–186.

Taylor, S.J. (1988). Caught in the continuum: A critical analysis of the principle of the least restrictive environment. *Journal of the Association for Persons with Severe Handicaps, 13,* 41–53.

Taylor, S.J., Racino, J., Knoll, J., and Lutfiyya, Z. (1987). *The nonrestrictive environment: On community integration for people with the most severe disabilities.* Syracuse, NY: Community Integration Project, Center on Human Policy, Syracuse University.

Wolfensberger, W. (1972). *The principle of normalization in human services.* Toronto: National Institute on Mental Retardation.

Wyatt v. Stickney, 344 F. Supp. 387 (M.D. Ala. 1972).

2

Shifting Paradigms to Natural Supports: A Practical Response to a Crisis in Disabilities Services

David W. Leake, Ronald K. James, and Robert A. Stodden

INTRODUCTION

As Bradley and Knoll noted in Chapter 1, services for persons with disabilities have taken on a radically new look over the past twenty-five years as the focus has shifted from segregation to integration within community environments. This revolutionary shift has been driven by a commitment to normalization and associated principles and has become widely institutionalized, largely as the result of legal mandates (Castellani, 1987; Scheerenberger, 1987). The primary service settings have changed from large institutions and special schools to community programs and regular schools.

Now the new status quo is being challenged through the promotion of different sets of guiding principles and concomitant transformations in services. Proposed new approaches stress the principles of (a) self-determination by persons with disabilities and their families and (b) community involvement through the building of relationships (also known as full inclusion). Making these principles primary changes the focus of social welfare services from direct provision of services by professionals to promotion of supports naturally present in the community.

Discussions of this new orientation are often presented in terms of "paradigms" and "paradigm shifts" (e.g., Bradley and Knoll, this book, Chapter 1; Daniels, 1990; McFadden and Burke, 1991; Smull and Bellamy, 1991), although different authors may use the terms in different senses. We will follow Smull and Bellamy (1991) in identifying the prevailing service orientation as the "community program paradigm" and its emerging challenger as the "support paradigm."

One aim of this paper is to place the concepts of paradigms and paradigm shifts in historical context. The way these concepts are currently applied in the disabilities literature is often different from their initial usage in the "hard" sciences (physics, geology, physiology/medicine, chemistry, and so on). Readers unfamiliar with disabilities literature may then gain a better understanding of how paradigms and paradigm shifts relate to values, principles, policies, and practices. In the hard sciences, and often in the social sciences as well, *paradigm* refers to widely shared sets of values and principles that guide the conduct of research. In the realm of social welfare services, on the other hand, *paradigm* tends to be used to refer to service policies and practices, which are guided by higher-order values and principles (such as social equality and normalization) concerning human relations.

We will then discuss how commitment to different sets of principles leads to discord within the disabilities field over correct policy and practice for services. A primary divide appears to be between "empiricists" (those guided by empirically supported theories) and "advocates" (those guided by philosophical principles).

A final primary aim is to show that the support paradigm is a practical (rather than just ideological) response to a crisis in disability services and is therefore capable of bridging differences within the field. Shifting to the support paradigm can increase the impact of limited resources by reorienting those resources away from direct services and toward promotion of community resources through outreach and training activities that help people take greater control of, and responsibility for, their own lives.

CLARIFICATION OF TERMS

We begin by clarifying our use of the term *value*. As one would expect, several dictionaries define *values* as the positive regard of certain customs, behaviors, beliefs, institutions, and so on, by particular groups of people. There are three important corollaries: values guide action, values tend to change over time, and different groups may hold conflicting values (Tropman, 1989). The basic values shared by virtually everyone in the field of disabilities are those underpinning the ideal of egalitarian democratic societies. Interrelated values that are currently stressed, largely due to the impact of the civil rights movement, include social equality, individual dignity, and the inclusion and participation of everyone (Peck, 1991; Scheerenberger, 1983, 1987).

Principles also entail positive regard and guide action. Widely held principles in the field include normalization and a least restrictive environment. However, *value, principle,* and many other terms are commonly used interchangeably. For example, Landesman and Butterfield (1987) refer to "normalization" as not only a principle, but also a concept, a force, a framework, a goal, an ideology, and a movement. For the purposes of this paper, the relationship between values and principles is like that between goals and objectives. Objectives are concrete steps for attaining higher-order goals; principles guide activities so that they conform to higher-order values. The normalization principle, for example, has been used to guide services for persons with developmental disabilities to make the value of universal social equality a reality for them (Peck, 1991).

The guiding values and principles of personnel in the field of disabilities largely determine the policies they help to create and the practices implemented under such policies (Meyer, 1991; Peck, 1991). Obviously, conflict is likely when different individuals or groups are guided by different values or principles (Tropman, 1989), and in fact the field has been described as being in such a state (e.g., Bradley and Knoll, this book, Chapter 1; Landesman and Butterfield, 1987).

The term *paradigm* has become ubiquitous in the social sciences and in political discourse since science historian Thomas Kuhn (1962) first used it to refer to the overarching sets of values, beliefs, and accepted practices that guide the "doing" of hard sciences. Over the years, Kuhn has objected that he has been badly misinterpreted and has expressed serious misgivings (e.g., in Horgan, 1991) about how the concept has been modified in analyses of other fields of human endeavor.

PARADIGMS AND PARADIGM SHIFTS

In this section we use the paradigm concept to discuss differences in how practices are determined and guided in three relatively distinct realms of endeavor. Figure 2-1 schematically summarizes the discussion. It depicts the determinants of practices for the realms of (from left to right) the hard sciences, the social sciences, and social welfare services. Since these realms are not necessarily comparable in terms of

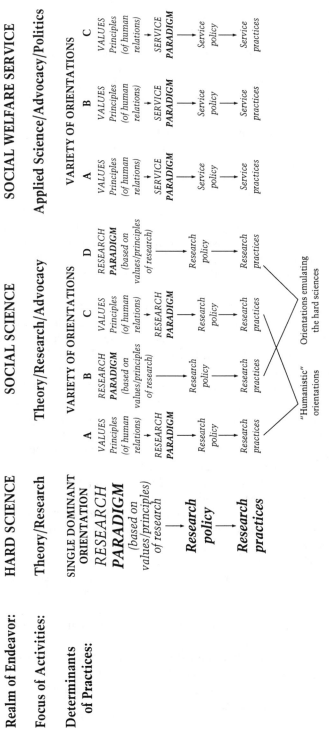

FIGURE 2-1 A comparative representation of the place of "paradigms" within the structures linking principles and values with policies and practices in the hard sciences, social sciences, and social welfare services.

their goals and activities, the concepts of paradigm and paradigm shift tend to take on different ranges of meanings in each of them. It should also be noted that when we refer to "the field of disabilities," it straddles the social science and social welfare service realms, including researchers, policy makers, administrators, and providers.

Kuhn (1962), in assessing historical trends in the hard sciences, asserts that the prevailing paradigm in any particular field implicitly points to critical issues, guides observations and manipulations of the material world, and provides criteria for judging theories. But when anomalous data that cannot be explained within the existing framework reach a critical mass, new paradigms emerge, with each of these eventually coming to prevail in the field. In other words, there is a "paradigm shift," a revolutionary break with past ways. A classic example of such a shift was the "Copernican revolution," which replaced the Ptolemaic view that the Earth is the center of the universe with one that had the planets circling the sun.

For Kuhn (1970), an important aspect of different paradigms is that they are "incommensurate," that is, they define the same terms differently and lack common standards for assessing "progress" in the field. Proponents of different paradigms thus tend to talk past and misunderstand one another. Although sociocultural factors strongly influence how research is targeted, funded, and organized in the modern hard sciences (Cozzens and Gieryn, 1990), differences among hard scientists are expressed mainly in terms of different views of how the physical world works. Some Russian and American physicists, for example, may hold drastically different views of human nature yet form an alliance against other physicists concerning a particular theory of subatomic particle interactions.

In contrast to the hard sciences, the social sciences (psychology, sociology, anthropology, public health, and so on) lack widely accepted paradigms. Rather, there tend to be numerous contesting paradigms, many of which are incommensurate and offer conflicting guidelines for determining which issues are critical, how they are to be addressed, and how research is to be evaluated. The social sciences have therefore been described as "pre-paradigmatic" (Kuhn, 1970) or "multiple paradigmatic" (Masterman, 1970). The primary reason for this state of affairs is, of course, that the social sciences are concerned with the behavior of people rather than matter. Ideology is much more likely to guide practices in the social sciences than in the hard sciences.

A major arena of combat is between those orientations that emulate hard science paradigms with their stress on theory-building through data-based hypothesis testing, and those that are overtly value-driven, rejecting empiricism as inapplicable or too narrow in scope. The former aim to reveal the universal principles of how the human world works, while the latter deny that possibility on the basis that human beings create their own worlds in great variety. Widely recognized oppositions between the two orientations include objectivism versus subjectivism, realism versus nominalism, determination versus voluntarism, and positivism versus anti-positivism (e.g., Burrell and Morgan, 1979). As we will touch on below, this chasm extends to the field of disabilities, since its theory and research are the products of social scientists.

Figure 2-1 indicates that the practitioners of a particular field of social science will tend to be guided either by one of several empirically oriented paradigms or (if they do not take an empirical approach) by one of several sets of values and principles. (Of course, many practitioners are eclectic, appreciating the potential contributions of a variety of approaches.)

Following the hard and social sciences, we come to a third realm of endeavor, that of social welfare services (both public and private). Social welfare services are meant to help persons identified as being in need and include such diverse programs as vocational rehabilitation, special education, food stamps, Head Start, Medicaid, Supplemental Security Income, and so on (Tropman, 1989). The social welfare system is essentially a staging ground for applied science (both hard and social) according to the constraints and demands of politics.

Public officials and even ordinary citizens are much more involved in determining the shape of social welfare services than of hard or social science research. Although social scientists have a significant influence on the creation, design, and implementation of social welfare services, the process is never as "rational" as social scientists would hope since decisions concerning allocations and usage of scarce resources are ultimately political (Tropman, 1989). Social welfare services are far more politicized than the hard or social sciences because they consume a much larger portion of the nation's resources and because they directly impact so many more individuals (many of whom are voters). Clearly, social welfare services (including services for persons with disabilities) do not have prevailing paradigms in the original Kuhnian sense. Such paradigms would provide accepted conceptual frameworks for identifying issues, performing research, translating research results into policy and practice, and evaluating policy and practice effectiveness. Instead of Kuhnian paradigms, the overarching frameworks of social welfare services consist of sets of values (and the goals and objectives they imply) that are necessarily congruent with political trends. Unfortunately, even when ends (values and goals) are agreed upon, the means (policies and practices) of achieving them may be hotly contested (e.g., Republicans and Democrats may claim liberty, justice, and equality as guiding values but battle over the means to achieve them).

What then do writers in the realm of social welfare services mean when they use the term *paradigm*, given that overarching Kuhnian paradigms appear to be absent? In the field of disabilities, *paradigm* is generally used to refer to service paradigms (frameworks that guide the provision of services), such as the old institutional paradigm, the community program paradigm that replaced it, and the emerging support paradigm. Paradigms of this sort are lower-level reflections of overarching guiding values and principles.

However, the same guiding values and principles can be associated with competing service paradigms. The community program paradigm and the support paradigm, for example, are both claimed to be congruent with the principles of normalization, integration, and individualization but lead to different ways of organizing services. The point of contention is the means rather than the ends. In a similar vein, Taylor (1988) notes with regard to the principle of least restrictive environment (a corollary of the normalization principle) that policy debates "assume an aura of philosophical consensus in which the principle is agreed upon but the practical implications are disputed" (p. 46).

THE HISTORICAL CONTEXT OF NORMALIZATION

To set the stage for discussing how the support paradigm might bridge differences in the field, we briefly consider some of the specific values and principles guiding disability services in the past and present. Most readers will be at least passingly familiar with the historical relationships between changing societal contexts and disability services (recent reviews, on which the following brief summary is based, are found in Gleason, 1990; Scheerenberger, 1983, 1987; and Zigler, Hodapp, and Edison, 1990).

During the seventeenth and eighteenth centuries, governments and philanthropists began taking some responsibility for the care of individuals (such as those with serious mental illness) who could not function in industrializing and urbanizing settings. Some persons with disabilities ended up in insane asylums, which generally served as human warehouses without rehabilitative functions. Around the middle of the nineteenth century, however, there was a shift in the service paradigm away from mere warehousing and toward therapy and rehabilitation. A primary stimulus for this shift was increasing acceptance of the value of social equality and the doctrine that the human mind is a "blank slate" at birth and develops through experience via the senses. This vision underlay the pioneering efforts of Itard, Sequin, and others to teach persons with disabilities the skills needed to become functioning members of society.

Another major shift in the service paradigm, this time away from rehabilitation, was associated with the emergence of social Darwinism toward the end of the nineteenth century. During this period the characteristics of persons with disabilities such as mental retardation came to be widely viewed as genetically fixed and therefore impossible to modify significantly. A primary value of the eugenics movement was improvement of the human gene pool, and that meant exclusion of those with behavior and appearances seen as deviant or inferior. The segregation of persons with mental retardation in an increasing number of institutions therefore became a matter of law or policy in many parts of the country.

As the twentieth century progressed, more humane attitudes toward persons with disabilities took hold, but institutionalization remained the primary service paradigm, if for no other reason than to protect these individuals from ignorant members of society. Movement toward a service paradigm of integration gained strength in the 1950s, largely through the influence of the civil rights movement and its contention that the values of social equality and inclusion must finally be extended to all individuals. The efforts of parent and advocacy groups eventually prompted passage of a series of federal, state, and local laws, beginning in the 1970s, that have guaranteed equal rights and access to education and other social services for persons with disabilities. These developments led to a one-third decrease in the institutional population between 1976 and 1986 (Braddock, Hemp, and Fujiura, 1986) and a substantial increase in funding for community-based services, although service capacity continues to lag far behind needs (Davis, 1987).

The current community program paradigm holds that persons with disabilities are best served in their communities rather than in institutions. To achieve the values of social equality and individual dignity, those who follow this paradigm tend to employ the principles of normalization, least restrictive environment, and individualization. Residential services are provided in small facilities rather than training in sheltered workshops, and so on. Unfortunately, community programs throughout the country cannot meet needs due to lack of resources (Scheerenberger, 1987; Smull and Bellamy, 1991).

According to Castellani (1987), normalization lies at the core of the field's shared "political ideology," which has been so successful in promoting deinstitutionalization and other policy changes in support of integration. Normalization as a guiding principle was first enunciated and implemented in Scandinavia in the late 1950s, holding that the "patterns and conditions of everyday life" for persons with disabilities should be as close as possible to sociocultural norms (Nirje, 1969).

Wolfensberger (1972) has been normalization's leading advocate in the United States. Recognizing that normalization had taken on many meanings, Wolfensberger (1983) renamed his version "social role valorization" to underline the importance of transforming persons with disabilities from devalued to valued members of society. To this end he proposed a two-pronged strategy of (a) reducing or preventing the overt signs that observers might use to devalue a person and (b) changing the perceptions and values of society. Debate over the practice implications of normalization and associated principles has often been quite heated.

EMPIRICISTS AND ADVOCATES

Similar to that common in the social sciences, the major division between the subgroups in conflict over normalization is between those who believe that empirical research should guide human affairs and those who instead look to values. This is of course an ideal-typical typology (research is always guided by values, no matter how hidden), yet one that is widely recognized as having some validity. Thus Menolascino and Stark (1990) name researchers and advocates as the prime combatants: "Divisiveness and polarization is taking place as researchers develop theories and make decisions based upon data, whereas advocates tend to utilize philosophical principles that are based on practice needs" (p. 22). We will expand the camp identified by Menolascino and Stark (1990) as "researchers" and by Zigler, Hodapp, and Edison (1990) as "scientists" by using the term *empiricists* to refer to all those personnel in the field who value empirical research as the basis for services. These include not just researchers, but also administrators and a great many service providers, particularly those who use behavioral technologies. The orientations of advocates and empiricists are essentially incommensurate, just as competing Kuhnian paradigms in the hard and social sciences tend to be incommensurate. As Landesman and Butterfield (1987) (representatives of the empirical camp) note, "The controversy is based on differences in faith, experience, and values, and the relative validity of the different positions is untestable" (p. 814).

Some of the differences in the orientations of empiricists and advocates are presented, in ideal-typical fashion, in Table 2-1, which also summarizes the natural supports orientation. The respective principles and practices of empiricists and advocates were extracted from recent articles and responses that explicitly address the problem of conflict between the two camps over normalization (one group of articles: Zigler, Hodapp, and Edison, 1990, and six accompanying commentaries, plus Williams, 1991; a second group: Greenspan and Cerreto, 1989, Landesman and Butterfield, 1987, and Schopler, 1989; a third group: Jacobson, 1989, Mulick and Kedesdy, 1988, and Wolfensberger, 1989).

As shown in Table 2-1, the two camps do share basic values but tend to stress different principles to guide practices. For example, empiricists

TABLE 2-1 Comparison of the Primary Guiding Principles, Service Paradigms, and Practices Associated with Three Distinctive Approaches to Organizing Disabilities Services

	Guiding Principles	Service Paradigm	Practices
Empiricism	Research-based, least restrictive environment, individualization	Direct services by professionals	Perform cumulative *research* to build *theory* as a basis for best *individualized* services by professionals—*integration* should be "to the extent possible"
Advocacy	Values-driven, normalization, integration, individualization	Direct services and advocacy by professionals	Advocate guiding *values* as basis for *transformation* of services/society in order to achieve *normalization* (hence services *community-based*]—*integration* should be total
Natural Supports	Community involvement, self-determination, individualization	Promotion of supports within community	Professionals develop *outreach* and *training* programs to promote *supports* within the community and to help individuals and families achieve *self-determination*—*integration* develops in tandem with supports

may view social equality and community participation as approachable for any particular individual through a continuum of services in which individualized placement is made according to the principle (now legally mandated) of least restrictive environment, which for some individuals could be an institution. On the other hand, the efforts of advocates toward the same ends would more likely stress making service settings "normal" (institutions thus being abolished), with the expectation that this will provide individuals with experiences that boost their self-esteem and their ability to interact and establish relationships in the community.

In a similar vein, individualization is a principle that seems widely shared yet differentially interpreted. For empiricists, it implies that professionals assess the individual using empirically validated instruments to determine an appropriate treatment program in the least restrictive environment. For many advocates, it means that community programs have to be flexible enough to meet individual needs (rather than individuals being inserted into available slots in categorical programs). For natural supports proponents, it means viewing the person as an individual who probably lacks the support networks that most "normal" people naturally develop, so that services should aim to establish relationships that will help meet specific needs identified by individuals and families rather than just by professionals.

Self-determination is being increasingly promoted as a major guiding principle, especially by advocates and natural supports proponents (e.g., Bradley and Knoll, this book, Chapter 1; O'Brien, 1987; Smull and Bellamy, 1991). It has been defined as "the attitude and ability that lead individuals to define goals for themselves and to take the initiative in achieving those goals. Some personal characteristics associated with self-determination are: Assertiveness, creativity, and self-advocacy" (*Federal Register*, Jan. 22, 1991). The impetus for self-determination comes partly from ideological concerns for individual rights but also, importantly, out of practical considerations: persons with disabilities will be much more committed to (and therefore more successful) attaining self-determined service goals than goals decided upon by other people (Deci and Ryan, 1985; Mithaug, 1991). Even persons with severe mental retardation are capable of a surprising degree of self-determination if given appropriate supports (O'Brien, 1987).

THE SUPPORT PARADIGM AS A PRACTICAL RESPONSE

The support paradigm as discussed here is limited to guiding services for persons with disabilities. However, its elaboration flows from developments in the wider context of social welfare services, all of which interact with similar political realities and trends in societal and professional values (Tropman, 1989). As Froland, Pancoast, Chapman, and Kimboko (1981) make clear, the support orientation is relevant for any group dependent on social welfare services. There are literatures on developing natural support systems for the elderly, homeless persons with mental illnesses, and single mothers, for example. In recent years, federal government requests for proposals have begun supporting research and demonstration projects for natural supports in these and other fields.

The support paradigm is essentially a prescription for building supportive relationships within the community in order to make social integration a reality. Natural supports might be provided, for example, by relatives at home, by peers and teachers at school, and by coworkers and supervisors at work (Nisbet and Callahan, 1987). However, natural supports tend to be inadequate in quantity, quality, and consistency. The task of service agencies therefore must shift from providing direct services to establishing substantive support systems tailored to individual needs (Minnesota State Planning Council on Developmental Disabilities, 1987; Smull and Bellamy, 1991). Table 2-2 contrasts some of the guiding principles of the community program paradigm versus the support paradigm.

TABLE 2-2 Principles Guiding Services for Persons with Disabilities: Support Paradigm versus Community Program Paradigm

Support Paradigm Principles	Community Paradigm Principles
People involved seen as partners	Hierarchical provider-client relations
Promote self-determination	Professionals determine what is best
Develop interdependence	Develop client independence
Promote community integration	Develop segregated programs
Promote people-focused outcomes	Apply data-based approaches
Model family- or community-centered approaches	Develop service-centered programs
Support individuals/groups to solve problems	Provide solutions to problems
Offer choice from variety of programs	Prescribe programs
Design individualized approaches	Help individual to fit into program
Develop/activate natural supports	Provide direct services (i.e., artificial supports)
Develop support networks/linkages	Promote individual participation
Promote right to choose	Promote right to participate
Build relationships	Rely on technical experts

A strong case for the support paradigm has been made elsewhere (although sometimes using a different terminology) (Bogdan and Taylor, 1987; Bradley and Knoll, this book, Chapter 1; Minnesota State Planning Council on Developmental Disabilities, 1987; Smull and Bellamy, 1991; Taylor, 1988). We would stress that to be widely accepted and eventually effective, the support paradigm must be seen as a practical solution derived from the natures of the problems it addresses. It will take more than appeals to values and principles, because these are only unifying at a superficial level across, and within, the various camps.

Rather, a primary strength of the support paradigm is that it offers a way of directly promoting integration while addressing severe service shortfalls for which there is no other obvious solution during this period of severe budgetary constraints. As Smull and Bellamy (1991) argue, the present system is actually in a state of "crisis": funds are too scarce, service providers too few, and waiting lists too long to ever be able to serve all those in need through the prevailing community program paradigm.

PARALLELS WITH PRIMARY HEALTH CARE

The crisis situation in disabilities services is analogous to that faced by health care systems throughout the Third World: the supply of personnel, funds, and facilities is incapable of meeting needs according to the desired standards of care, and will remain so into the foreseeable future. The solution is also analogous to that widely adopted in the Third World, out of necessity: promote community involvement, tap community resources, and train community members so that they can take care of most basic tasks, while creating a system of referrals providing access to professional help when needed. This is the essence of the primary health care (PHC) movement (World Health Organization, 1978).

An important issue for PHC has been that of how to most efficiently utilize scarce professional expertise. Commonly, the role of at least some professionals is reoriented away from direct services toward outreach activities and the training of community members to perform basic functions once reserved solely for professionals. "Community health workers" may be volunteers, but experience has shown that much better results are obtained when they are given some form of compensation. They have been described as the "bridge" between the community and the health care system (Ofosu-Amaah, 1983). For services to individuals with disabilities, this bridging function would be performed by family members, coworkers, or other community members given basic training. Again, the possession of self-determination skills by persons with disabilities as well as their significant others is critical for success.

Empiricists (e.g., Landesman and Butterfield, 1987; Zigler, Hodapp, and Edison, 1990) have often stressed the imperative of individualized services based on careful in-depth research, while acknowledging that current research is often of insufficient quality and breadth. But in practical terms, resources are woefully inadequate for providing true individualized research-based attention to even a minority of those in need. The ideal of individualized attention for all can be approached only if professionals train and support persons with disabilities and their significant others so they can better address their own needs and develop stronger relationships with fellow community members.

Empirical research is needed for the development of new systems of services using new methodologies employed by new categories of personnel (such as the support coordinators described by Smull and Bellamy, 1991). There is already a research base on such relevant topics as the development of peer supports among children (e.g., Stainback and Stainback, 1990), of coworker supports (e.g., Shafer, Tait, Keen, and Jesiolowski, 1989), of supports for families (e.g., Singer and Irwin, 1991), of self-determination and self-advocacy skills (e.g., Sievert, Cuvo, and David, 1988), and so on. More research along similar lines is being stimulated by federal government requests for proposals meant to further the aims of the "new paradigm."

Another issue that the support paradigm has the potential to address is that of empathy or caring. Critiques of our current medical system have often asserted that health care is experienced by patients as cold and unfeeling, due to its technological orientation and the hierarchical dominance of professionals (see Kleinman, 1988). Similar charges have been leveled at the disabilities service system. But it is impossible to imagine that overburdened professional service providers, for whom "burnout" is considered an occupational hazard, can satisfy currently unmet needs for empathy of so many persons with disabilities. For that, we must look to the community, as promoted by the support paradigm.

CONCLUSION—EVOLUTION OR REVOLUTION?

Bradley and Knoll (this book, Chapter 1) view the current shift toward the support paradigm (or, in their words, toward "the era of community membership") as the newest stage of an "evolutionary process." However, the changes envisioned in the service system are so extensive that they might better be described as revolutionary, which would be in keeping with Kuhn's (1970) contention that paradigm shifts are indeed revolutions in guiding conceptual frameworks.

In contrast to some support paradigm advocates, we, like Smull and Bellamy (1991), have stressed the practical necessity of the shift to the support paradigm. This approach helps to avoid polemics and offers common ground for the collaboration of advocates, researchers, and professional service providers. Although community-based programs have had notable successes, empiricists and advocates alike have recognized serious shortcomings. If the current paradigm is retained, these shortcomings can only be addressed in terms of more money, more research, more trained professionals—but it should be clear that not enough "more" will be forthcoming from governmental or private sources. These "anomalous data" can be accommodated only by a new paradigm. The support paradigm is the only such paradigm on the horizon that can be used to guide current services into a new era.

The shift need not be particularly threatening. A comprehensive system of outreach, training, and upward referrals would have a need for well-trained researchers and professional service providers that continues to exceed supply. The most significant changes will occur closer to the ground, among those personnel who will need to shift their focus from direct provision to community outreach and natural support promotion.

There will, inevitably, be false starts and bad programs (Smull and Bellamy, 1991), yet the support paradigm does offer real promise of fuller realization of the field's shared values of social equality, individual dignity, and community inclusion/participation. As Bogdan and Taylor (1987) maintain:

> When people with developmental disabilities have to rely exclusively on the services of a particular agency, they are destined not to become part of the community. The more an agency provides, the less others will be involved in a person's life. Only when support is spread throughout the community can people become part of their communities (p. 210).

Acknowledgment: The authors are grateful to Richard Pratt, Thomas Sileo, and Garnett Smith for their comments on earlier drafts of the manuscript.

REFERENCES

Bogdan, R., and Taylor, S.J. (1987). Conclusion: The next wave. In S.J. Taylor, D. Biklen, and J. Knoll (Eds.), *Community integration for people with severe disabilities* (pp. 209–213). New York: Teachers College Press.

Braddock, D., Hemp, R., and Fujiura, G. (1986). *Public expenditures for mental retardation and developmental disabilities in the United States: State profiles* (2nd ed.). Chicago: Institute for the Study of Developmental Disabilities, University of Illinois at Chicago.

Bradley, V.J., and Knoll, J. (1995). Shifting paradigms in services to people with disabilities. In O.C. Karan and S. Greenspan (Eds.), *Community rehabilitation services for people with disabilities.* Newton, MA: Butterworth-Heinemann.

Burrell, G., and Morgan, G. (1979). *Sociological paradigms and organizational analysis.* London: Heinemann Educational Books.

Castellani, P.J. (1987). *The political economy of developmental disabilities.* Baltimore: Paul H. Brookes.

Cozzens, S.E., and Gieryn, T.F. (Eds.) (1990). *Theories of science in society.* Bloomington: Indiana University Press.

Daniels, S. (1990). Disability in America: An evolving concept, a new paradigm. *Policy Network Newsletter* (Doctoral Leadership Training in Vocational/Special Education and Transition Services, The George Washington University), *3*, 1–3.

Davis, S. (1987). *A national status report on waiting lists of people with mental retardation for community services.* Arlington, TX: Association for Retarded Citizens.

Deci, E.L., and Ryan, R.M. (1985). *Intrinsic motivation and self-determination in human behavior.* New York: Plenum.

Froland, C., Pancoast, D.L., Chapman, N.J., and Kimboko, P.J. (1981). *Helping networks and human services.* Beverly Hills, CA: Sage Publications.

Gleason, J.J. (1990). *Special education in context: An ethnographic study of persons with developmental disabilities.* Cambridge: Cambridge University Press.

Greenspan, S., and Cerreto, M. (1989). Normalization, deinstitutionalization, and the limits of research: Comment on Landesman and Butterfield. *American Psychologist, 44,* 448–449.

Horgan, J. (1991). Profile: Reluctant revolutionary. *Scientific American,* May 1991, 40, 49.

Jacobson, J.W. (1989). Behavior modification and normalization in conflict? *Mental Retardation, 27,* 179–180.

Kleinman, A. (1988). *Illness narratives: Suffering, healing, and the human condition.* New York: Basic Books.

Kuhn, T.K. (1970). *The structure of scientific revolutions* (2nd ed.). Chicago: University of Chicago Press.

Landesman, S., and Butterfield, E.C. (1987). Normalization and deinstitutionalization of mentally retarded individuals: Controversy and facts. *American Psychologist, 42,* 809–816.

Masterman, M. (1970). The nature of a paradigm. In I. Lakotos and A. Musgrave (Eds.), *Criticism and the growth of knowledge.* Cambridge: Cambridge University Press.

McFadden, D.L., and Burke, E.P. (1991). Developmental disabilities and the New Paradigm: Directions for the 1990s. *Mental Retardation, 29,* iii–vi.

Menolascino, F.J., and Stark, J.A. (1990). Research versus advocacy in the allocation of resources: Problems, causes, solutions. *American Journal on Mental Retardation, 95,* 21–25.

Meyer, L.H. (1991). Advocacy, research, and typical practices: A call for the reduction of discrepancies between what is and what ought to be, and how to get there. In L.H. Meyer, C.A. Peck, and L. Brown (Eds.), *Critical issues in the lives of people with severe disabilities* (pp. 629–649). Baltimore: Paul H. Brookes.

Minnesota State Planning Council on Developmental Disabilities (1987). *A new way of thinking.* St. Paul: Author.

Mithaug, D.E. (1991). *Self-determined kids.* Lexington, MA: Lexington Books.

Mulick, J.A., and Kedesdy, J.H. (1988). Self-injurious behavior, its treatment, and normalization. *Mental Retardation, 26,* 223–229.

Nirje, B. (1969). The normalization principle and its human management implications. In R. Kugel and W. Wolfensberger (Eds.), *Changing patterns in residential services for the mentally retarded* (pp. 181–194). Washington, DC: President's Committee on Mental Retardation.

Nisbet, J., and Callahan, M. (1987). Achieving success in integrated workplaces: Critical elements in assisting persons with severe disabilities. In S.J. Taylor, D. Biklen, and J. Knoll (Eds.), *Community integration for people with severe disabilities* (pp. 184–201). New York: Teachers College Press.

O'Brien, J. (1987). A guide to life-style planning: Using the activities catalog to integrate services and natural support systems. In G.T. Bellamy and B. Wilcox (Eds.), *A comprehensive guide to the activities catalog: An alternative curriculum for youth and adults with severe disabilities* (pp. 175–189). Baltimore: Paul H. Brookes.

Ofosu-Amaah, V. (1983). *National experience in the use of community health workers: A review of current issues and problems* (WHO Offset Publication No. 71). Geneva: World Health Organization.

Peck, C.A. (1991). Linking values and science in social policy decisions affecting citizens with severe disabilities. In L.H. Meyer, C.A. Peck, and L. Brown (Eds.), *Critical issues in the lives of people with severe disabilities* (pp. 1–15). Baltimore: Paul H. Brookes.

Scheerenberger, R.C. (1983). *A history of mental retardation.* Baltimore: Paul H. Brookes.

Scheerenberger, R.C. (1987). *A history of mental retardation: A quarter century of promise.* Baltimore: Paul H. Brookes.

Schopler, E. (1989). Excesses of the normalization concept. *American Psychologist, 44,* 447–448.

Shafer, M.S., Tait, K., Keen, R., and Jesiolowski, C. (1989). Supported competitive employment: Using coworkers to assist follow-along efforts. *Journal of Rehabilitation, 55,* 66–75.

Sievert, A.L., Cuvo, A.J., and David, P.K. (1988). Training self-advocacy skills to adults with mild handicaps. Journal of Applied Behavior Analysis, 21, 299–309.

Singer, G.H.S., and Irwin, L.K. (1991). Supporting families of persons with severe disabilities: Emerging findings, practices, and questions. In L.H. Meyer, C.A. Peck, and L. Brown (Eds.), *Critical issues in the lives of people with severe disabilities* (pp. 171–312). Baltimore: Paul H. Brookes.

Smull, M.W., and Bellamy, G.T. (1991). Community services for adults with disabilities: Policy challenges in the emerging support paradigm. In L.H. Meyer, C.A. Peck, and L. Brown (Eds.), *Critical issues in the lives of people with severe disabilities* (pp. 527–536). Baltimore: Paul H. Brookes.

Stainback, W., and Stainback, S. (Eds.) (1990). *Support networks for inclusive schools.* Baltimore: Paul H. Brookes.

Taylor, S.J. (1988). Caught in the continuum: A critical analysis of the principle of the least restrictive environment. *Journal of the Association for Persons with Severe Handicaps, 13,* 41–53.

Tropman, J.E. (1989). *American values and social welfare: Cultural contradictions in the welfare state.* Englewood Cliffs, NJ: Prentice-Hall.

Williams, P. (1991). Reaction to Zigler, Hodapp, and Edison (1990). *American Journal on Mental Retardation, 96,* 224–225.

Wolfensberger, W. (1972). *The principle of normalization in human services.* Toronto: National Institute on Mental Retardation.

Wolfensberger, W. (1983). Social role valorization: A proposed new term for the principle of normalization. *Mental Retardation, 21,* 234–239.

Wolfensberger, W. (1989). Self-injurious behavior, behavioristic responses, and social role valorization: A reply to Mulick and Kedesdy. *Mental Retardation, 27,* 181–184.

World Health Organization. (1978). *Primary health care: Report of the international conference on primary health care,* Alma-Ata, USSR, Sept. 6–12. Geneva: Author.

Zigler, E., Hodapp, R.M., and Edison, M.R. (1990). From theory to practice in the care and education of mentally retarded individuals. *American Journal on Mental Retardation, 95,* 1–12.

3

The Influence of Legislation on Services to People with Disabilities

Bryce Fifield and Marvin Fifield

Historians documenting the evolution of the disabilities movement often refer to the laws that affect the lives of people with disabilities (e.g., Berkowitz, Johnson, and Murphy, 1967; Coll, 1973; Glasson, 1900; Keesecker, 1929; Obermann, 1965; Phillips and Rosenberg, 1980; Sarason and Doris, 1969). However, legislation that affects the lives of people with disabilities should be of more than just a passing interest to those who are involved with the disability community. Not only does legislation articulate who is to receive the services, but it also articulates what and how services are to be delivered to people with disabilities. In addition, disability legislation reflects the values, philosophies, and concerns of our society. An understanding of the historical background of legislation that affects the lives of people with disabilities is a necessary step in gaining a thorough understanding of current practices in the rehabilitation field.

Legislation evolves in a political arena that represents a peculiar mix of social values, economic needs, financial expediency, and political compromise. Although it is generally drafted to address emerging national needs, federal legislation often evolves simultaneously with state legislation and case law resulting from litigation. Frequently, it includes references to what were historically viewed to be "best practices" of the period. The values and philosophies of the period are often reflected in the terminology used in the legislation.[1] Legislation must run a gauntlet of opposing views and compete with other issues of national interest through a process of compromise and negotiations (Naisbitt and Aburdine, 1990).

This chapter is divided into two parts. The first part provides a historical overview of the legislation that has shaped the current systems and practices that serve people with disabilities. Concurrent with the overview, brief commentary about the social and historical events that affected legislation is offered. We have also attempted to identify some of the precedents established in early legislation that continue to shape contemporary practices. We first discuss compensation programs for military and work injuries. Later the emergence of rehabilitation and education legislation that provided services rather than compensation is discussed.

The second part of this chapter identifies specific social themes that have been articulated in national legislation shaping current policies and practices in the disabilities field. As might be expected, these social themes have not evolved in a linear or chronological fashion, but have emerged, combined, divided, and dissolved in a number of ways. Understanding the roots of legislation that affects the disabilities community is an important part of understanding the issues the disabilities field currently faces.

HISTORICAL OVERVIEW

The attention governments have given to the welfare of their citizens has varied over the course of history. Prior to the major shifts in Western political power as reflected in documents such as the Magna Carta, the Declaration of Independence, and the U.S. Constitution, rulers have generally assumed little or no responsibility for the welfare of their subjects other than to enforce internal security and collect taxes. Few examples of enlightened concern for the welfare of the governed are scattered amongst a general history that includes mainly neglect and abuse. Most rulers did little more than to permit, and occasionally encourage, religious groups to administer to the needs of the poor, the "crippled," and the sick (Durant and Durant, 1968; May, 1976; Phillips and Rosenberg, 1980; Schulz, 1920).

It wasn't until the fifteenth century that government policies began to reflect greater concern for the welfare of the average citizen than that of

---

[1]We support the current usage of "people first" language. It is accurate and readable, and helps to maintain dignity and individuality. However, such terminology is not historically accurate when referencing or describing previous legislative acts. Non–people first language in this paper is used to maintain historical integrity and continuity.

the ruling class (Durant and Durant, 1968). This trend grew slowly over the next several centuries. Currently, among most Western cultures, citizens look to the state to provide assistance for those unable to meet their own needs, to equalize opportunities, and to help restore benefits lost due to wars, accidents, or natural disasters.

As part of their efforts to recruit and maintain a loyal army, rulers and governments have historically made provisions for warriors who were wounded or disabled in battle (Durant and Durant, 1968). Consequently, early legislation affecting the lives of people with disabilities focused on compensation for wounded or disabled soldiers. Evidence exists that suggests recruitment promises were not always kept, except when wounds were obtained in a manner that demonstrated particular valor or distinction. In such cases, compensation probably depended more on courage and loyalty than the fact that the warrior was disabled. In Europe and most of the Western world, compensation for military service was generally provided in the form of land, titles, or pensions, and was often offered only to senior officers (Glasson, 1900).

Legislative initiatives affecting the lives of people with disabilities in the American colonies had their roots in the public welfare practices of England and northern Europe (Noble, 1980). In North America, the first record of a law that made provisions for disabled soldiers was recorded in Plymouth colony in 1636: "If any man shall be sent forth as a soldier and shall return maimed, he shall be maintained completely by the colony during his life" (White, 1907). A few years later, the statutes of the colony of Virginia outlined a similar law for those "hurt or maimed and disabled from providing for their necessary maintenance and subsistence . . . be relieved and provided for by the several counties, where such men reside or inhabit" (Hening, 1823). The language of the Virginia statute is noteworthy because it expands the Plymouth law by defining the disability of the soldier as a condition that limits his ability to earn a living.

Glasson (1900) reports that similar laws were passed by the colonies of Maryland, New York, Rhode Island, and the provinces of Massachusetts Bay. The Massachusetts Bay Act for Levying Soldiers is noteworthy because it stated that relief should be drawn from the public treasury as ordered by the court (Liachowitz, 1988).

Acting on the recommendations of its special committee on disabled soldiers and seamen, the Continental Congress of the United States passed the first national law addressing disability-related issues just fifty-three days after the Declaration of Independence from England in 1776. The resolution was similar in scope and structure to the Virginia statute. It defined an individual's disability in terms of an inability to continue serving in the army or navy and to maintain a livelihood. It also stated that pensions would be in proportion to the degree of disability, to be determined by their own officials, and would be paid by the applicant's home state, formerly a colony (U.S. Continental Congress, 1800–1801).

The 1776 resolution also provided for a "corps of invalids" as an option for disabled soldiers. The resolution provided for this corps to be "employed in garrisons for guards, in cities, and other places . . . military schools for young gentlemen . . . mathematical schools for the purpose of learning geometry, arithmetic, vulgar and decimal fractions, and the extraction of roots . . . and recruiting services . . ." (U.S. Continental Congress, 1800–1801). The Invalid Corps was formalized in June 1777 and provided full pay rather than a pension from the home state. In 1778 the Continental Congress instituted a provision that deprived disabled soldiers of their pensions if they refused to join the Invalid Corps. The 1778 provision suggests that the Invalid Corps was not proving to be a successful alternative to straight pensions. It also suggests that the Congress was already struggling to control the costs of serving people with disabilities (U.S. Continental Congress, 1800–1801).

These early colonial and national pension laws set precedents for disability practices that are in use today (Liachowitz, 1988). Many of these early precedents continue to be debated and challenged in more contemporary legislation and policies. Among the more notable are the following: (a) disabled veterans would be compensated by public resources; (b) the disability must be related to the veteran's inability to maintain a livelihood, a relationship that requires some sort of test, or medical certification; (c) the amount of pension would be related to previous earnings; (d) care for wounded veterans would be a national obligation; (e) recipients of benefits would have little influence over the provisions that affected their lives.

For the most part, pension provisions established in the late 1700s have continued into the twentieth century. During and after the Civil War, the federal government demanded that pensioners from earlier wars prove their loyalty to the Union (Liachowitz, 1988).

Disabled veterans of the Civil War were treated quite differently, depending on whether they were soldiers for the Union or the Confederacy. Benefits to the disabled veterans of the Confederacy were very limited and the number deserving benefits was great. The benefits provided to veterans in the North were more generous, but were provided in return for service, often without the condition of an injury. It is estimated that more than four million soldiers were wounded during the Civil War. At least half were of such severity that they could not be returned to service. Furthermore, almost half a million died before they could be treated or while they were in hospitals. Thus, between the

North and the South, there were approximately 1.5 million wounded veterans, many with severe disabilities (McPherson, 1988).

During and after the Civil War, the costs of providing needed medical services to those disabled grew to staggering levels. For example, in 1866 more than 20 percent of the total budget for the state of Missouri was used to purchase prosthetic devices for Missouri soldiers with missing limbs (Ward, 1990).

Military pensions for Civil War veterans were not always contingent on injuries (Catton, 1962). A pension grant providing for the wounded veteran was graded on the basis of severity. However, the grant was not related to the soldier's ability to earn a livelihood or his financial status. The dollar amount of military pensions, then as now, is unrelated to the veteran's education, occupation, or socioeconomic class. Disabled veterans have been considered a special class who are rewarded for their service to the country, not on the basis of disability or loss of earning capacity (Glasson, 1900).

Between the Civil War and World War I, there were few new disability pension provisions. However, there was considerable debate about what constitutes eligibility for disability pensions and whether the obligation for funding and administering such pensions should be shouldered by the states or the federal government. In 1888 improved pension provisions for Civil and Indian War veterans were part of the Republican Party National Platform. This was the first time in the United States that a disability issue was addressed as part of a political campaign (Glasson, 1900). Table 3-1 summarizes the early legislation that established compensation for disabilities resulting from military service.

In 1918, as World War I was coming to its close, Congress unanimously enacted a law to provide vocational rehabilitation into civil employment for people with disabilities who had been discharged from the military. This was a new approach by which the disabled veteran could be given job training, rather than a pension. This act was patterned after the vocational education system then evolving in secondary schools (U.S. Congress Joint Committee on Education, 1918).

This early attempt to shift from a pension system to a rehabilitation system had only limited success. Although much of its failure can be attributed to administrative and bureaucratic problems, the act failed to a significant degree because it did not make allowances for shifts in how to provide services to people with disabilities. For example, from a philosophical standpoint, the 1918 act failed to recognize that vocational training and rehabilitation are not the same nor can one approach substitute for the other. This distinction continues to cause controversy in current disability practices.

TABLE 3-1 Early Legislation Affecting Compensation for Disabilities Resulting from Military Service

Year	Action	Impact
1636	New Plymouth laws	Maintenance of soldiers maimed in the course of service.
1644	Colony of Virginia Act X	Maintenance of soldiers maimed or disabled in the course of service. Disability defined in terms of ability to earn a living. Responsibility for relief assigned to counties.
1776	Continental Congress resolution regarding pensions for wounded soldiers and seamen	Pensions in proportion to the degree of disability. Pensions to be paid by applicant's home state. Formed the Invalid Corps.
1778	Continental Congress resolution	Extended military pensions to the widows of officers.
1836	U.S. Congress. An act granting half pay to widows or orphans	Extended military pensions to widows and orphans of all military personnel.
1888	Republican Party platform	Proposed substantial increases in pensions for veterans. The first record of a disability-related issue being included on a political party platform.
1918	U.S. Military Rehabilitation Act	Provided for vocational rehabilitation of veterans disabled in World War I. Unanimously passed by Congress.

Perhaps an even more important philosophical issue overlooked by the vocational rehabilitation provision of the 1918 act was that veterans appear to be valued primarily for what they have done, not for what they are able to do. Unlike civilians with disabilities, their value was not dependent on their potential productivity (Liachowitz, 1988).

Workers' Compensation

As the United States advanced in industrialization, a line of disability-related legislation affecting the private sector emerged, parallelling legislation for disabled veterans. To recruit and provide a source of expanded personnel resources, pensions for disabled workers were provided for particularly hazardous jobs (Glasson, 1900). As with pension legislation, U.S. laws affecting workers' compensation[2] incorporated elements from earlier European laws (Somers and Somers, 1954). For example, compulsory insurance programs were initiated in Germany during the 1800s. These laws also set the precedent of copayments, in which a portion of the cost for these benefits was contributed by the employer. England's first workers' compensation laws were enacted in 1879 (Hanes, 1968).

The first North American laws concerning worker injuries appeared in state statutes around the turn of the century (Rhodes, 1917). Maryland established a cooperative insurance fund in 1902 to compensate municipal workers injured while working in hazardous industries. However, it wasn't until 1906 that Congress passed the first federal workers' compensation law (Somers and Somers, 1954). By 1913, twenty-four states had workers' compensation laws, and by 1919, all but six states had them (Liachowitz, 1988).

Workers' compensation laws in the United States evolved into three major areas: laws governing federal employees (a complex set of laws that differs between federal departments and agencies in terms of eligibility requirements and benefits), state workers' compensation laws for state and local public employees, and state laws that provide a shared responsibility between state and private agencies. This legislation established several precedents for Social Security disability provisions and employer-provided health insurance programs that have become an important part of contemporary employment benefits. Table 3-2 summarizes the legislation that established compensation for disabilities that resulted from work-related injuries.

Vocational Rehabilitation

The relationship between a disability and poverty has been used as one of the primary justifications for disability programs. This relationship was first established in colonial times and became known as the "Duke's Laws" (Staughton, Nead, and McCamant, 1879, reported by

---

[2] The term *workmen's compensation* was changed to *workers' compensation* in the 1970s to reflect the increased number of women employed.

TABLE 3-2   Early Legislation Affecting Compensation for Disabilities Resulting from Work-Related Injuries

Year	Action	Impact
1879	England enacts workers' compensation laws	Provided for compensation for workers injured on jobs.
1902	Maryland Cooperative Insurance Fund	Provided funds to compensate injured and municipal workers in hazardous industries.
1906	U.S. workers' compensation law	Provided compensation for workers injured in hazardous jobs.
1956	Amendments to Social Security Act	Allowed disabled workers to receive pension before reaching retirement.

Liachowitz, 1988). The Duke's Laws first identified charity as a function of government and then grouped together the indigent, poor, and physically deficient as "distracted persons" and prescribed legislative provisions for them (Liachowitz, 1988).

The legislative provisions described to this point assist through compensation or pensions and can be referred to as benefits income maintenance. Such benefits are designed to care for those who are poor due to a disability. Rehabilitation, on the other hand, focuses on providing assistance by restoring the earning power of people with disabilities by teaching skills they can use to earn a living.

At the federal level, the first rehabilitation laws were enacted by Congress in 1918 "to provide for vocational rehabilitation and return to civil employment of disabled persons discharged from the military or naval forces of the United States. . . ." (U.S. Congress Joint Committee on Education, 1918). This law represented the first national statute that linked a disability to eligibility for training in new skills to help gain employment.

The stage for vocational rehabilitation legislation was set in 1914 when Congress, concerned that unskilled workers would be an economic liability on the nation, created the Commission on National Aid to Vocational Education. As a result of the commission, the Vocational Education Act was passed, with provisions for the national government to aid states in developing educational programs in agriculture, trade, commerce, and home economics (U.S. Congressional Commission on National Aid to Vocational Education, 1914). To participate in the vocational education program, states were required to submit a state plan, which was then reviewed and evaluated by a federal board. Those plans favorably reviewed were approved, and funds were awarded to the state by the Department of Labor. This process (state planning, federal approval, and funds awarded on the basis of population) set the precedents by which federal funding has since been distributed to states for most federal programs in health, welfare, and education.

The 1918 law took the concept of vocational education and changed it to vocational rehabilitation, implementing the concept that training veterans in vocational skills was a better policy than giving them a pension (U.S. Congress Joint Committee on Education, 1918). The military vocational rehabilitation program failed for a variety of reasons, most of which were administrative problems.

Two years later, these same elements were brought together in the first civil rehabilitation legislation. This legislation became known as the Smith-Fess Act or the Industrial Rehabilitation Act of 1920 (Public Law 66-234). A considerable amount of congressional debate preceded the Smith-Fess Act, focusing on both the national moral obligations and the economic benefits of rehabilitation. Representative Clyde Kelly asserted that "this great work of human salvage means changing a national liability into a national asset" (U.S. Congressional Record, 1919). Although moral issues were commonly used in justifying vocational rehabilitation programs, such programs were and continue to be viewed primarily in terms of their economic benefits.

Unlike pension programs, vocational rehabilitation programs have been administered primarily through public education. The 1916 Massachusetts statute, which served as a model for the 1918 Vocational Rehabilitation Act, authorized the state Board of Education to return victims of industrial accidents and disease to the workforce (Berkowitz, 1979). Prior to 1920, New York, California, and many other states had their own vocational rehabilitation programs for civilians (Liachowitz, 1988). Like the Vocational Education Act, the Rehabilitation Act allocated funds in proportion to the state's population, a practice in common use today. By 1921, thirty-five states were participating in the federal vocational rehabilitation program. By 1932, forty-four states had joined the State–National Partnership of Vocational Rehabilitation. The bureaucracy for vocational rehabilitation was placed within the Department of Labor and defined strictly as a skills-training program (Berkowitz, 1979).

It is important to recognize the extent to which vocational rehabilitation legislation has been influenced by the economic and social conditions of the day. In particular, the Vocational Rehabilitation Act of 1920 established a number of precedents that have been carried forward as the basis of more contemporary legislative provisions.

Feasibility

Among the early precedents for future rehabilitation legislation was the concept of feasibility. Participation in vocational rehabilitation programs was based on both the need for rehabilitation determined by a disability and the feasibility of rehabilitation into employment. Because the concern of vocational rehabilitation focused on economic benefits, and because individuals with severe disabilities were considered poor risks, even though they might be eligible, they were not considered vocationally feasible. This practice provided for almost certain success of rehabilitation programs by eliminating poor risks based on a presumptive determination made by a rehabilitation counselor. Berkowitz (1979) notes that the secret of successful rehabilitation is being able to focus on good risks. Because people with the most severe disabilities are generally high-risk employees, they were and continue to be eliminated from participation in vocational rehabilitation programs (Berkowitz, 1980).

The issue of participation based on both need and feasibility continues in contemporary vocational rehabilitation programs and is a source of conflict between rehabilitation professionals and consumers. Rehabilitation professionals contend that it makes no sense practically or economically to provide rehabilitation training for those so severely disabled that job placement is not feasible. Consumers counter that for a counselor to determine one's unemployability *before* vocational training is provided is presumptive and that *all* should be given the opportunity for vocational training. The 1992 Vocational Rehabilitation Amendments have modified this procedure by a process that starts with presumed feasibility. It is now the responsibility of vocational rehabilitation counselors to justify on what basis they determine a given consumer is not vocationally feasible (Public Law 102-569).

State-Determined Criteria for Eligibility

Another precedent included in the early rehabilitation legislation was the latitude allowed to individual states to establish their own eligibility criteria. The National Vocational Rehabilitation Program was designed to promote rehabilitation services provided by states. Under the provisions of the act, states were allowed to define their own eligibility criteria for benefits. As a result, there is a wide variation across states in the level of financial support and the benefits provided. The state/federal partnership generates a financial investment at both levels of government, making changes difficult. Each governmental level blames the other for shortcomings and it becomes difficult to defend regulations. Consumers feel they are kept on the sidelines by the rehabilitation bureaucracy at both the federal and state levels. Their only recourse has been to go directly to

Congress and to promote changes in the administration of the program and new provisions by changing the authorizing legislation through amendments. An example of this process can be seen in the 1992 amendments to the Rehabilitation Act (Public Law 102-569) that provide for a state advisory council made up of at least 51 percent consumers to set and approve the order of services for a state and the state eligibility benefit criteria.

Case Method

Another precedent of early rehabilitation legislation is the method by which services are delivered. The rehabilitation program tended to focus on case methods in which each person was considered a distinct set of problems with which rehabilitation workers must deal. The case method approach of the early vocational rehabilitation legislation provided a program designed individually for each consumer. This approach set the precedent for other individual service programs found in later legislation (e.g., individual education plans (IEPs), individual written rehabilitation plans (IWRPs), individualized family service plans (IFSPs), etc.). At the same time, consumers argue that they are often treated as cases to be managed and controlled by the counselor without appropriate consideration given to their wants, their dignity, and their opinions.

The Measurement of Value by Work

Finally, the values that underlie many contemporary rehabilitation programs were articulated in the 1920 Vocational Rehabilitation Act. Among these values supporting the whole notion of vocational rehabilitation is a social judgment that defines one's worth in terms of the work one can perform. Thus, the Vocational Rehabilitation Program has tended to focus on fixing the client by providing vocational skills and then fitting the person into the existing social or employment structure. Job placement and case closure are sometimes seen as more important than the needs, goals, and wishes of the consumer, employment as more important than independence, feasibility as more important than need, and closures as more important than satisfying the needs of the consumer.

From an economic investment standpoint, the Vocational Rehabilitation Program has been extremely successful. Evaluation data suggest that individuals with disabilities who have received training and been placed in employment consistently earn more than those that have not, and data also indicate that they maintain that advantage over time (U.S. House of Representatives Report 102-822, 1992). The Vocational Rehabilitation Act has been very popular in Congress. At each reauthorization the issue of concern to Congress is how to improve the act rather than whether it should be reauthorized.

Such legislative popularity creates its own problems, for each reauthorization provides opportunities for legislators to use the act as a vehicle to address other social problems or special populations of particular interest to a legislator or his or her constituency. As a consequence, numerous special populations and priorities for services have been encouraged. For example, special provisions for the mentally ill, alcohol and drug dependents, those living in poverty, native Americans, and native Hawaiians have been added through the amendments or reauthorization act. The rehabilitation amendments also provide a good opportunity to insert "pork barrel" projects designed for a legislator's home district. Such amendments sometimes have little to do with rehabilitation services.

In 1935 the Rehabilitation Act was incorporated into Title V of the Social Security Act. This doubled the previous authorization level for rehabilitation, and in 1939 the authorization was almost doubled again (Braddock, 1986a). In 1938 the Wagner-O'Day Act, Public Law 75-739, expanded the role of sheltered workshops for the blind (Nazzaro, 1977). This provision set in motion the expansion of sheltered workshops for other disability groups. The use of sheltered workshops targeted for specific disability groups expanded until the 1980s, when other types of employment options for persons with disabilities such as enclaves, crew work, and supported employment started to receive attention.

In 1943, the Borden-LaFollette Act amended and expanded the rehabilitation program with provisions authorizing services to the mentally retarded, blind, and mentally ill. Even more important were the provisions that permitted the use of rehabilitation funds to pay for medical services in a manner similar to the benefits provided to veterans (Nazzaro, 1977). This included the preparation of persons with disabilities to benefit from therapy, medication, or surgery in preparation for vocational training.

Since its inception, rehabilitation legislation has been dynamic, continually expanding to address more comprehensive needs such as research, professional training, nonvocational rehabilitation, supported employment, independent living, civil rights issues, and technology. However, through the various reauthorizations, the basic vocational rehabilitation program (Title I of the Rehabilitation Act) has remained much as it was first established.

One of the unique characteristics of the rehabilitation program is that it is virtually the only broad-spectrum service program for adults with disabilities. Several federal and state programs serve the health and education needs of children with disabilities. Other programs deal with problems incidental to the disability, such as poverty, medical needs, and income maintenance. The Vocational Rehabilitation Program, however, provides one of the few options for service to adults individually designed to address their needs. Since there are few other options, consumers have tried to eliminate, or at least ease, its restrictions for eligibility. Such changes would permit the act to provide more services to those needing long-term care and to serve more severely disabled individuals.

The 1992 reauthorization of the Rehabilitation Act was viewed as the first major opportunity to implement the concepts of the Americans with Disabilities Act (ADA) into service legislation. Using the civil rights framework established by the ADA, the 1992 amendments broadened the definition of feasibility and added the concept of presumed feasibility, requiring the vocational rehabilitation agency to justify a decision of nonfeasibility. Other changes expanded consumer participation, consumer rights, and have expanded various provisions for non-Vocational Rehabilitation Services (Public Law 102-569). Table 3-3 summarizes legislation that has established rehabilitation programs for people with disabilities.

TABLE 3-3   Legislation Establishing Rehabilitation Programs for People with Disabilities

Year	Action	Impact
1916	Massachusetts Rehabilitation Law	Board of Education authorized to return those disabled by industrial accidents or disease to the workforce.
1918	U.S. Military Rehabilitation Act	Provided for vocational rehabilitation of veterans disabled in World War I. Unanimously passed by Congress.
1920	Industrial Rehabilitation Act (Smith-Fess Act)	Funds allocated in proportion to state population. Provided for training of new skills to those disabled by industrial injury. Established an education bureaucracy within the Department of Labor.
1938	Wagner-O'Day Act (Public Law 75-739)	Established sheltered workshops for the blind.
1943	Borden-LaFollette Act	Expanded the rehabilitation program by authorizing services to the mentally retarded, blind, and mentally ill.

TABLE 3-3   *(continued)*

Year	Action	Impact
1973	Rehabilitation Act	Expanded rehabilitation service programs and included Section 504, which provided broad civil rights protection under federal programs for people with disabilities. Independent living provision gave management and control to consumers.
1992	Amendments to the Rehabilitation Act	Uses "people first" language. Separated independent living centers from state rehabilitation agencies. Established consumer-controlled councils that set policies and order of services. Established the precedent of presumed eligibility for services.

Social Security Legislation

Although the preamble to the U.S. Constitution calls for "promoting the general welfare," there was no national system to do so until the Social Security Act was signed in 1935 by Franklin D. Roosevelt. The Social Security Act converted the funds first authorized under the 1932 emergency act into permanent public assistance, financed by a payroll tax of 1 percent on both employer and employee (Berkowitz, 1979).

Like the Vocational Rehabilitation Program, the Social Security program was designed as a federally financed, state-managed program. States received federal funding to provide relief and assistance to indigent dependent children, elderly adults, and the blind. Fiscally, Social Security is patterned like workers' compensation legislation, with contributions by both workers and employers. Other than a small program for the blind (Title VI), the Social Security Act originally offered only general assistance to people with disabilities. The original act provided old age assistance (Title I) and aid to families with dependent children (Title IV). Title X established state and public health authorities and Title V authorized grants to states for maternal and child health and crippled children services (Braddock, 1986a).

In 1950 an amendment to the Social Security Act provided assistance to permanently and totally disabled persons. The underlying assumption of the "permanently and totally disabled" provision equates a disability with poverty and the inability to make a living, thus justifying benefits. Proof that one is permanently and totally disabled determines eligibility, and as an entitlement program, all eligible applicants were accepted into the program (Braddock, 1986a).

In 1956 Congress amended the old age insurance provision to allow a disabled worker to receive a pension before reaching retirement. In 1972 the permanently and totally disabled provision was revised into the Supplemental Social Security Income (SSI) program (Braddock, 1986b).

The Social Security Act with its many amendments has had a major impact on virtually all programs for persons with disabilities. However, as the program has grown and costs have soared, many efforts to contain costs have been initiated. Such efforts often take the form of bureaucratic red tape or provisions designed to ensure that no one ineligible receives benefits. Efforts to guard against such abuse add eligibility requirements and assurances of need, along with periodic reviews. This has had the effect of making the initial approval cumbersome enough that it would discourage those with marginal disabilities.

Originally, income maintenance was provided to states for institutional care of people with disabilities through the 1987 Medicaid and Medicare provision of the Social Security Act. It wasn't until 1981 that amendments to the Social Security Act provided income maintenance and health benefits to families and individuals with disabilities living in non-institutional, community-based settings (Braddock, 1986b). The implementation of the community-based provisions has been slow. A common consumer complaint about the Social Security program is that it continues to promote institutionalization and dependency rather than community integration and independence.

The basic philosophy of the Social Security program is not totally compatible with that of rehabilitation. To participate in Social Security, one must prove that he or she cannot work. If the consumer later becomes employable, he or she becomes ineligible not only for income maintenance offered under Social Security Disability Insurance (SSDI) and SSI, but also for the health benefits offered under Medicaid and Medicare. Thus, to participate at any level, one becomes captive to the program. This serves as a deterrent to pursuing rehabilitation training. To counter this, the 1980 Social Security amendments included provisions in Sections 1619a and 1619b that allowed a recipient with disabilities to retain Medicaid benefits while seeking employment and making an effort to live independently beyond the benefits of Social Security (Public Law 96-265). These two

TABLE 3-4   Social Security Legislation Affecting People with Disabilities

Year	Action	Impact
1935	Social Security Act	Rehabilitation Act incorporated into Social Security Act. Funding authorization for rehabilitation was nearly doubled. Provided general assistance to people with disabilities, aid to families with dependent children, aid to the blind, and grants to states to establish services for crippled children.
1956	Amendments to Social Security Act	Allowed disabled workers to receive pensions before reaching retirement.
1972	Amendments to Social Security Act to establish Social Security Income	Provided income maintenance for those who are permanently and totally disabled.
1980	Amendments to Social Security Act	Provided income maintenance and health benefits to individuals with disabilities living in noninstitutional settings.

provisions have had only limited success in encouraging Social Security recipients to seek employment. Many recipients will not take the chance of losing Social Security benefits or going through the lengthy process of re-instatement if they fail in an employment placement. The Social Security Administration has tried repeatedly to expand the use of Sections 1619a and 1619b by providing training to rehabilitation providers and consumers (National Association of Rehabilitation Facilities, 1988). Table 3-4 provides a summary of Social Security legislation that affects people with disabilities.

Educational Legislation for Persons with Disabilities

Because public education was primarily considered a state and local responsibility, the early education laws for people with disabilities came from the individual state legislatures. Prior to 1900, the only federal education legislation was targeted toward specific disabilities. For example, federal legislation established St. Elizabeth's Hospital for the Insane in 1855 (Public Law 32-4) and the Columbia Institute for the Deaf in 1857 (Public Law 34-46). The American Printing House for the Blind was established in 1879 (Public Law 45-146)(Nazzaro, 1977).

The first significant federal support for public education for people with disabilities was provided through the National Defense Education Act in response to the Russian space program, which launched Sputnik in 1957. It may seem ironic that federal support for education, particularly education for children with disabilities, was first linked to national defense. However, during the Cold War, staying ahead of the communist countries was a national priority, even if it meant spending federal money on education.

An amended provision of the National Defense Education Act (Public Law 85-864) provided funds for mental retardation research and under Public Law 85-926 authorized the first federally supported programs to train teachers of children who were mentally retarded. Although the disability "mental retardation" was mentioned by name, it was used generically (Aiello, 1976). "Teachers of the mentally retarded" referred to special education teachers who served students with a variety of learning problems. By 1960, sixteen institutions of higher education were sponsoring special education traineeships, and a cadre of teachers and teacher-trainers were being prepared (Braddock, 1986a). Table 3-5 summarizes education legislation affecting people with disabilities.

The National Defense Education Act of 1958 (Public Law 85-864) illustrates how many federal provisions addressing the needs of people with

TABLE 3-5 Legislation Affecting the Education of People with Disabilities

Year	Action	Impact
1958	National Defense Education Act (Public Law 85-864)	Funded research in mental retardation and supported programs to train teachers of children with mental retardation.
1963	Maternal and Child Health and Mental Retardation Planning Amendments (Public Law 88-156)	Required states to conduct studies on the extent and incidence of mental retardation and initiate planning to provide services.

Table 3-5   *(continued)*

Year	Action	Impact
1963	Mental Retardation and Community Mental Health Center Construction Act (Public Law 88-164)	Authorized construction of research and training facilities to address the needs of people with disabilities. Established the Division on Education of the Handicapped in the U.S. Office of Education.
1975	Education for All Handicapped Children Act (Public Law 94-142)	Provided federal funds to teach children with disabilities in public schools. Outlined the rights of children with disabilities and their parents to due process in the development of the individual educational plan.
1986	Part H Amendment to Public Law 94-142	Provided educational intervention services to infants and toddlers with disabilities and those at risk of developing disabilities.

disabilities became law. Such initiatives often lack the broad-based popularity or support in Congress needed to stand on their own. Sponsors of disability legislation often attach their provisions as amendments to more popular legislation. This strategy helps the provisions move through congressional committees with fewer delays. Under such a strategy, the task of the sponsor is to prevent the provisions from being stripped from the bill.

CONTEMPORARY LEGISLATIVE THEMES

Without question, the major breakthrough in terms of federal programs for persons with disabilities occurred under the administration of President John F. Kennedy. Nine months after President Kennedy took office, he established the President's Panel on Mental

Retardation, consisting of twenty-one distinguished physicians, scientists, educators, lawyers, and consumers. The panel organized itself into six task forces addressing prevention, education and habilitation, law and public resources, biological research, behavior and social research, and coordination. Following a year of work, the panel published its report (President's Panel on Mental Retardation, 1962).

Although the work of the panel focused on mental retardation, it outlined legislative needs and programs that applied to almost all disabilities. Braddock (1986b) notes that President Kennedy's panel ushered in the modern era of federal concern for people with disabilities. During the past thirty years, almost every piece of disability legislation can be traced back to selected recommendations made by the President's Panel. What is perhaps even more important is that virtually every recommendation of the President's Panel has found its way into law. The ninety-five recommendations of the President's Panel have formed the basis of today's federal assistance programs for people with disabilities (Fifield and Fifield, 1993).

One of the many important precedents established by the President's Panel was that of consumer participation in policy planning. Consumers who participated on President Kennedy's panel brought a different set of questions than those posed by professionals and distinguished scientists. Consumers challenged commonly held notions by noting that many of the problems they experienced were caused not by their disabilities but by the environment provided by society. This environmental concern was further nourished by the emergence of ecological and environmental issues that were gaining increased attention in the 1960s. Civil rights, consumerism, normalization, and environmental issues all emerged out of the early 1960s as important conceptual reference points for future legislative provisions.

Consumer participation on the President's Panel was minimal by today's standards. However, their concerns were heard and recorded. The increasing participation of people with disabilities in the development of policies and priorities marked a change in the makeup of the players making decisions about national disability legislation. The legislation that emerged from the context of increased consumer participation addresses five evolving social concerns: protection and care, development and opportunities, rights, environmental issues, and consumer responsiveness.

Protection and Care–Referenced Legislation

The "new era" initiated by President Kennedy's panel focused significant attention on correcting living conditions and upgrading health services for people with disabilities. Examples of this legislation include the Maternal and Child Health and Mental Retardation Planning Amendments of 1963 (Public Law 88-156) and the Mental Retardation Facilities and Community Mental Health Center Construction Act (Public Law 88-164). Public Law 88-164 authorized the construction of research facilities, university-affiliated facilities, and specially designed state facilities for diagnosis, treatment, education, and training of people with disabilities. Title III of the act was an education bill. As with other federal aid to education, to be passed by the Congress it had to be concealed in more popular legislation, which in this case was health legislation. Title III expanded the teacher training provisions authorized under the National Defense Education Act and added a research authority. This act also added a Division on Education of the Handicapped to the U.S. Office of Education, as part of the cabinet-level Department of Health, Education, and Welfare. New standards for health care, sanitation, and safety were also promulgated.

Protection and care–referenced legislation was initially introduced with the Social Security Act of 1935. In 1950 Title XIV established a federal categorical public assistance program for persons with disabilities, Aid to the Permanently and Totally Disabled. The 1956 amendments authorized benefits for adults disabled in childhood, referred to as the Aid to Dependent Children's Benefits. It was again extended in 1972 through the Supplemental Security Income program, which replaced the Aid to the Disabled program, and provided a national minimum income for persons who are elderly, blind, or have a disability.

Developmental-Referenced Legislation

One of the basic assumptions underlying protection and care legislation is the application of the medical model for meeting the needs of people with disabilities. The medical paradigm views a disability as a condition, calling for a treatment based on a diagnosis. The medical paradigm establishes a patient/doctor relationship, with other providers considered "allied health" personnel. The objectives of medical treatment are to cure, eliminate, or ameliorate the condition. Conditions that cannot be cured with medical treatments are considered chronic, requiring ongoing or long-term care.

Disabilities have long been considered the responsibility of the health field. Historically, this was appropriate because of the special health problems that accompanied a disability. Until the advent of modern medicine, accidents or wounds were feared more for the resulting infection than for the disability they may cause. As such, disabilities have been labeled in categories like diseases. These categories typically focus on the cause of

the disability. Virtually all legislation, regulations, eligibility requirements, and professional correspondence used such categories until the
1970s. Even today, much of the current health and care language continues
this precedent.

The rehabilitation field, however, has found it more practical to focus
on the functional limitations resulting from the disability and to concentrate their efforts on rehabilitation and correcting the limitation through
training rather than to concentrate on the causes of disabilities.

Western society tends to think of the standard human model as "able-
bodied," that is, having all human functional abilities. An inability to
perform a typical life function is considered an impairment or functional
disability (Office of Technology Assessment, 1982). Following this logic, a
disability can be described as a loss of normalcy. The severity of a disability
is the discrepancy between a person's functional ability and "normalcy"
or "able-bodiedness." We generally hold that such a discrepancy or impairment can be breached by therapy, education, and intervention. Even those
disabilities that occur before or during the child's birth and early developmental stages (i.e., developmental disabilities) can be improved by intensive intervention, learning opportunities, and living in an environment as
near normal as possible (Office of Technology Assessment, 1982).

To a significant extent, this approach is as much a statement of belief
as it is a scientific principle. Inherent in it is a value statement about what
it is and means to be a human being and have human potential. This has
become known as the Developmental Principle (Kozlowski, Hitzig, and
Helsel, 1983). In the late 1960s, legislation was drafted that addressed this
principle with provisions designed to enhance normalization and the rights
of persons with disabilities.

Between 1965 and 1975, developmental-referenced legislation separated itself from protection and care legislation by redefining and broad-
ening the concepts of intervention, treatment, and therapy. Developmental-referenced legislation focused on maintaining and restoring
physical, social, vocational, and cognitive skills. Planned, sequential,
and proactive treatment was stressed rather than cure or care. Goals
were identified, and techniques to measure progress in achieving such
goals were developed.

Although developmental-referenced provisions are found in many
pieces of legislation, it is the Developmental Disabilities Act of 1970
(Public Law 91-517) that has been most clearly identified with this trend.
The purpose of the act was to better meet the needs of individuals with
developmental disabilities by addressing the gaps in services that occurred
between services authorized by other legislation. The Developmental Disabilities Act was advocacy legislation that addressed many of the issues

consumers and advocacy organizations had been pressing and were first recognized by the President's Panel. The act established a planning council in each state, with consumers constituting a majority of the council's members. These councils were responsible for monitoring, planning, and advocating for improved disabilities services.

University-affiliated programs were authorized to provide leadership to the developmental disabilities field, and projects of national significance were funded to provide creative and innovative solutions to targeted problems. The consumer and advocacy provisions of the Developmental Disabilities Act set it apart from previous disability legislation. These features were particularly notable because they established a formal mechanism for bringing consumers and advocates for consumers into the planning and program monitoring process. As a consequence, various reauthorizations of the act have made it a trendsetter, like a legislative trial balloon. Many of the new service elements, delivery models, as well as the evolving philosophy of services to persons with disabilities were first introduced in the Developmental Disabilities Act. They have since been added as major provisions in other pieces of legislation. Examples of such provisions include a functional definition of a disability, protection and advocacy, community-based services, case management, supported employment, early intervention, and assistive technology.

Developmental-referenced provisions were added to the 1973 amendments to the Rehabilitation Act (Public Law 93-112). However, the most significant disability legislation of the 1970s was the Education for All Handicapped Children Act (EHA) of 1975 (Public Law 94-142). This act started with a value statement that all children with handicaps were capable of learning and benefiting from the opportunities that education offered. Thus, all children, regardless of their disability or its severity, are entitled to a free and appropriate education. EHA not only stated it, but also provided federal dollars to facilitate the education of children with disabilities (albeit less money than authorized). The law was also an entitlement program for which all handicapped children appropriately diagnosed were eligible. In 1986 Part H of Public Law 94-142, the Early Inter- vention Provisions, extended developmental services to infants and toddlers with disabilities and those at risk.

Rights-Referenced Legislation

Among the more significant social conflicts that emerged during the 1960s was the civil rights movement. During this period, the rights and needs of minority groups became the subject of open forums.

Minorities of all types emerged from this general social turmoil, demanding recognition. The Civil Rights Act of 1964 (Public Law 88-352, the tenth amendment) asserted fundamental human rights and guaranteed numerous protections. The passage of this act and the activities that both preceeded and followed it included efforts to ensure that people with disabilities also had rights that needed protection in legislation.

The first rights-referenced disability legislation was the Architectural Barriers Act of 1968 (Public Law 90-480). This act required all federal buildings to be accessible to people with disabilities. Standards for accessibility were later refined and incorporated into Section 504 of the Rehabilitation Act of 1973, Public Law 93-112. Section 504 became the landmark rights legislation of the 1970s and the foundation for later rights provisions. In essence, Section 504 prohibits discrimination on the basis of a handicap to any program receiving or benefiting from federal financial aid. Section 504 is of particular interest because of the implementation regulations and definitions that it generated. Section 504 provided the first federal statutory definition of a disability, a definition that has been used extensively in subsequent legislation.

Other laws also incorporated rights-referenced legislation in their provisions. For example, Public Law 94-142, as an entitlement program, set in law the right of children with handicaps to a free and appropriate public education. The 1975 amendments to the Developmental Disabilities Act added the Bill of Rights for Persons with Disabilities and established a protection and advocacy agency in each state. State protection and advocacy agencies were assigned the responsibility of ensuring that the rights of persons with disabilities were not violated by state, public, or private service agencies. In 1988, Congress passed the Civil Rights Restoration Act, reaffirming its intent to secure rights for persons with disabilities and overturning several court cases that had narrowed the definition, scope, and consequences of previous legislation.

The most significant disabilities legislation in the last quarter century was the landmark Americans with Disabilities Act (ADA) of 1990 (Public Law 101-336). This legislation expanded previous legislation, which for the most part was restricted to nondiscrimination by government agencies and agencies receiving federal support. The ADA expanded these provisions into the private sector and to all public services. It would be difficult to exaggerate the significance of the ADA, for it is a statement of belief and policy that will continue to be defined and interpreted in the years to come. Table 3-6 summarizes legislation addressing the rights of people with disabilities.

TABLE 3-6 Legislation Addressing the Rights of People
with Disabilities

Year	Action	Impact
1968	Architectural Barriers Act	Mandated access to federal buildings.
1970	Developmental Disabilities Act	Established state planning councils with a majority of their membership to be made up of consumers.
1973	Rehabilitation Act	Expanded rehabilitation service programs and included Section 504, which provided broad civil rights protection under federal programs for people with disabilities.
1974	Amendments to the Developmental Disabilities Act	Established a protection and advocacy agency in every state.
1975	Education for All Handicapped Children Act (Public Law 94-142)	Provided federal funds to teach children with disabilities in public schools. Outlined the rights of children with disabilities and their parents to due process in the development of the individual educational plan.
1987	Amendments to Developmental Disabilities Act	Required states to conduct studies of the effectiveness of programs serving people with disabilities and the satisfaction of consumers of such services.
1988	Civil Rights Restoration Act	Reaffirmed congressional intent to secure rights for people with disabilities.
1990	Americans with Disabilities Act	Assured the rights of people with disabilities to access the services of the private sector.

TABLE 3-6 *(continued)*

Year	Action	Impact
1992	Amendments to the Rehabilitation Act	Uses "people first" language. Separated independent living centers from state rehabilitation agencies. Established consumer-controlled councils that set policies and order of services. Established the precedent of presumed eligibility for services.

Environmental-Referenced Legislation

The Architectural Barriers Act of 1968 (Public Law 90-480) was not only rights-referenced, but it also addressed a particularly troublesome environmental barrier—access to federal buildings. Since the early 1960s, consumers had been arguing that the problem to be fixed was not always the individual but often the environment. Environmental-referenced provisions focused on eliminating environmental barriers to buildings, information, services, and opportunities. Like developmental and rights provisions, environmental legislation reexamined definitions and values.

The first environmental-referenced legislation called for hospital and institutional reform and improvement. As the movement for normalization, mainstreaming, and inclusion advanced, it became apparent that community buildings, sidewalks, communication systems, transportation, and technology had barriers built into them that prevented or restricted their utilization by people with disabilities. Important community services were often provided in locations and at times that were convenient to providers and service agencies but not to consumers. The Independent Living Provisions of the 1973 Vocational Rehabilitation Act shifted the locus of the problem and the locus of control by empowering management and control of the program to consumers (Public Law 93-112). The independent living philosophy is that people with disabilities are not patients who should be grateful for whatever the provider offers but consumers, taking responsibility for their own lives. Consistent with the independent living philosophy, the environment needed to be examined to identify those features that prohibited or impeded access to opportunities, choices, generic services, and so on.

The least restrictive environment provisions of the Education for All Handicapped Children Act also is an environmental-referenced provision. The amendments to Public Law 94-142 during the end of the 1980s, which increased attention to mainstreaming and least restrictive placement, focused on improving the fit between the person with a disability and the regular education environment.

In 1982 the Office of Technology Assessment published a report exploring the role of technology for people with disabilities (Office of Technology Assessment, 1982). This study pointed out that technology, especially new technological advances in space exploration, the military, and industry, can be the vehicle by which many environmental barriers can be overcome. The term *rehabilitation technology* was first used to describe the devices and services used to facilitate workplace accommodation. In 1986 the Older Americans Act used the term *assistive technology*, which was later defined in 1987 amendments to the Developmental Disabilities Act as the devices and services used to achieve independence, productivity, and integration.

The Technology-Related Assistance Act of 1988 (Public Law 100-407) expanded the definition and provided funding to develop and disseminate information about assistive technology in an effort to increase the availability and use of assistive technology by persons with disabilities. Since 1988, assistive technology has been an expanding provision included in the Individuals with Disabilities Education Act of 1991 and the 1992 amendments to the Rehabilitation Act. Advancements in assistive technology have made it feasible to implement many of the provisions of the Americans with Disabilities Act.

Consumer-Referenced Legislation

Throughout history, society has viewed people with disabilities as different and has almost always described them in negative terms. Even functional descriptions have taken on negative connotations over time. The terms *handicapped* and *client* were used interchangeably throughout the 1970s and 1980s. But these terms also implied a dependent relationship in which the provider was the decision maker. The independent living philosophy challenged this dependency, replacing it with self-determination.

The term *consumer*, even though it is still somewhat technically incorrect, has come to reflect the type of relationship that should exist. The first consumer-referenced provisions were those that strengthened the decision making, options, and independence of the consumer.

Consumer-referenced legislation outlined provisions for increased consumer representation on policy and advisory councils. The Developmental Disabilities Act of 1970 mandated 51 percent of the state council to be consumer members. The 1977 Rehabilitation Act amendments required the membership of independent living boards to have a majority representation of consumers. The Education for All Handicapped Children Act (Public Law 94-142) strengthened the role of parents through the individual education plan process, and the Vocational Rehabilitation Program required "clients" to sign off on their individual written rehabilitation plan. Each successive reauthorization of these major pieces of legislation has aggressively strengthened the level and depth of consumer participation in the disabilities service system.

In 1987, the reauthorization of the Developmental Disabilities Act further increased the role of people "consuming" disability services. The 1987 reauthorization required state planning councils to conduct statewide studies of the effectiveness of service programs and the degree of satisfaction among primary consumers with such services.

The Technology-Related Assistance Act of 1988 not only used "people first" language, but also used the term *consumer* throughout the act's provisions. The expression "consumer-responsive statewide program of technology-related assistance" was used, calling attention to the fact that the consumer was the reference point and services were to be responsive to the consumer's need.

The Americans with Disabilities Act was not only focused on disability rights and environment, but it also strengthened consumer responsiveness by using language that addressed dignity, choice, and participation. In addition, people-first language was used in the 1991 reauthorization of Public Law 94-142, the Individuals with Disabilities Education Act (IDEA), as it was in the 1992 Rehabilitation Act amendments. The various provisions of these reauthorizations further strengthened consumer participation in planning, monitoring, setting priorities, and making decisions in the development of individual service plans.

CONCLUSION

Legislation has had a profound influence on the disability field. It has not only altered what services are available to people with disabilities and how such services are provided, but it plays a key role in defining how people with disabilities are included in broader social roles.

The laws enacted by our governments that impact the lives of people with disabilities can be both proactive and reactive. The language and provisions of legislation are influenced by political, economic, moral, theoretical, practical, and other factors.

These same factors also impact the implementation and interpretation of legislation. Policies and procedures often deviate from the social imperative that led to the legislation's enactment. As a consequence, the intent of Congress is restated, qualified, and often becomes more prescriptive in subsequent amendments and reauthorizations. These changes are reflected not only in the revised provisions, but also in the language and terminology used. Figure 3-1 shows some of the significant changes that have occurred in the rehabilitation field as reflected in legislation over the past thirty years.

A frequent misunderstanding among people working in the disabilities field is that laws are static. Many hold that once a piece of legislation has been passed, certain problems will go away as a result. As this review of the legislation of the past thirty years has shown, such is not the case. Legislation develops. Themes emerge from the enactment and enforcement of laws passed by our governments. From these themes, new problems emerge that require new solutions. Often the new solutions find their way into the policies and principles that form the foundation for a new generation of legislation.

The historical perspective of legislation that affects the lives of people with disabilities reflects our country's early, timid steps toward addressing individual differences. The legislation of the past quarter century suggests that our efforts are perhaps becoming a little more assertive. Yet as a nation and as a society, we can do a far better job at recognizing the dignity, independence, and unique needs of all people, including those who have disabilities.

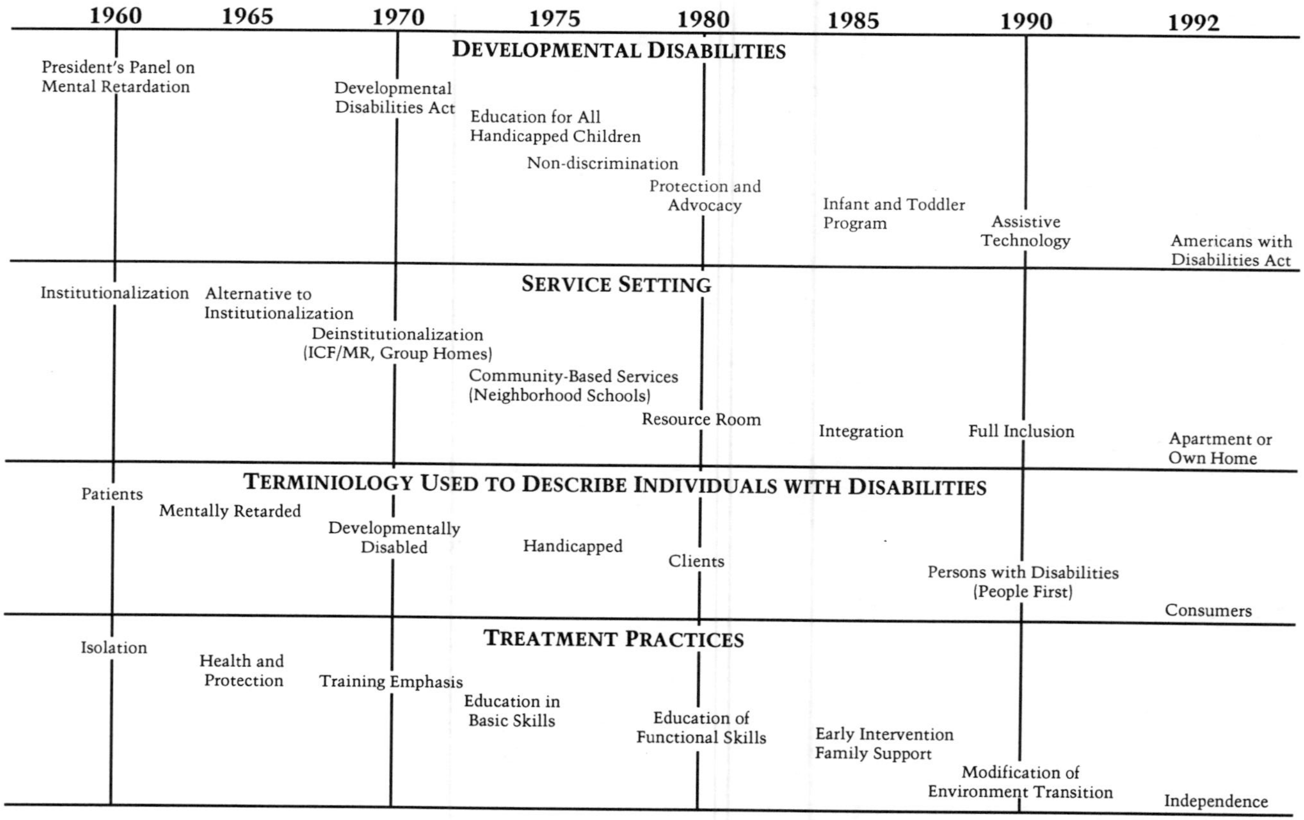

FIGURE 3.1 Paradigm Shifts over the Past Thirty Years

REFERENCES

Aiello, B. (1976). Especially for special educators: A sense of our own history. *Exceptional Children, 42*(5), 244–252.

Berkowitz, E.D. (1979). *Disability policies in government programs.* New York: Praeger.

Berkowitz, E.D. (1980). *Rehabilitation: The federal government's response to disability, 1935–1954.* New York: Arno Press.

Berkowitz, M. (1963). *Rehabilitating the disabled worker: A platform for action.* Report of the National Institute on Rehabilitation and Workmen's Compensation, University of Michigan, June 1962. Washington, DC: U.S. Department of HEW.

Berkowitz, M., Johnson, W.G., and Murphy, E.H. (1967). *Public policy toward disability.* New York: Praeger.

Braddock, D. (1986a). Federal assistance for mental retardation and developmental disabilities I: A review through 1961. *Mental Retardation, 24*(3), 175–182.

Braddock, D. (1986b). Federal assistance for mental retardation and developmental disabilities II: The modern era. *Mental Retardation, 24*(4), 209–218.

Catton, B. (1962). *The army of the Potomac: Mr. Lincoln's army.* Garden City, NY: Doubleday.

Coll, B.D. (1973). *Perspectives in public welfare: A history.* Washington, DC: U.S. Department of HEW, SRS.

Durant, W., and Durant, A. (1968). *The lessons of history.* New York: Simon and Schuster.

Fifield, B., and Fifield, M. (1993). *The evolution of university-affiliated programs for the developmentally disabled: Changing expectations and practices.* Report submitted to the Administration on Developmental Disabilities. Logan: Utah State University, Center on Persons with Disabilities.

Glasson, W.H. (1900). *History of military pension legislation in the United States.* Columbia University Studies in History, Economics and Public Law, *XII*(3), 1–130.

Hanes, D.G. (1968). *The first British workmen's compensation act. 1897.* New Haven: Yale University Press.

Hening, W.W. (Ed.) (1823). *Statutes at-large Virginia: 1619–1792* (13 volumes). New York: Bartow.

Keesecker, W.W. (1929). *Digest of legislation for education of crippled children.* U.S. Department of Interior, Bureau of Education, Bulletin No. 5. Washington, DC: U.S. Government Printing Office.

Kozlowski, R.E., Hitzig, W., and Helsel, E. (1983). *Future directions in adult services.* Position Paper No. 3. Columbus: Ohio Developmental Disabilities Planning Council.

Liachowitz, C.H. (1988). *Disability as a social construct.* Philadelphia: University of Pennsylvania Press.

May, H.F. (1976). *The enlightenment in America.* New York: Oxford University Press.

McPherson, J.N. (1988). *Battle cry of freedom.* New York: Ballantine.

Naisbitt, J., and Aburdine, N. (1990). *Megatrends 2000.* New York: Avon Books.

National Association of Rehabilitation Facility Monograph Series (1988). *Incentives to work for SSI and SSDI recipients.* Washington, DC: Author.

@REF = Nazzaro, J.N. (1977). *Exceptional timetables: Historical events affecting the handicapped and gifted.* Reston, VA: Council for Exceptional Children.

Noble, J.H. (1980). New directions for public policy affecting the mentally disabled. In J.J. Bevilacqua (Ed.), *Changing government policies for the mentally disabled.* Cambridge, MA: Ballinger.

Obermann, C.E. (1965). *A history of vocational rehabilitation in America.* Minneapolis: Denison.

Office of Technology Assessment (1982). *Technology and handicapped people.* Washington, DC: U.S. Government Printing Office.

Phillips, W., and Rosenberg, J. (Eds.) (1980). *The origins of modern treatment and education of physically handicapped children.* New York: Arno Press.

President's Panel on Mental Retardation (1962). *A proposed program for national action to combat mental retardation.* Washington, DC: U.S. Government Printing Office.

Rhodes, J.E. (1917). *Workmen's compensation.* New York: Macmillan.

Sarason, S.B., and Doris, J. (1969). *Psychological problems in mental deficiency.* New York: Harper & Row (1st ed., 1949).

Schulz, G.F. (1920). The cripple in primitive society. *American Journal of Care for Cripples, VIII,* 335–346.

Somers, H.M., and Somers, A.R. (1954). *Workmen's compensation: Prevention, insurance, and rehabilitation of occupational disability.* New York: Wiley.

U.S. Congress Joint Committee on Education (1918). *Hearings concerning the bill proposing military vocational rehabilitation: HR 12212.* April 30–May 1. Washington, DC: U.S. Government Printing Office.

U.S. Congress, Public Law 32-4, Federal Legislation Establishing St. Elizabeth's Hospital for the Insane (1855).

U.S. Congress, Public Law 34-46, Columbia Institute for the Deaf (1857).

U.S. Congress, Public Law 45-146, American Printing House for the Blind (1879).

U.S. Congress, Public Law 64-347, Vocational Education Act of 1917.

U.S. Congress, Public Law 65-178, Military Rehabilitation Act of 1918.

U.S. Congress, Public Law 66-234, Civilian Vocational Rehabilitation Act of 1920—Smith-Fess Act.

U.S. Congress, Public Law 66-236, Vocational Rehabilitation Act of 1920.

U.S. Congress, Public Law 74-271, Social Security Act of 1935.

U.S. Congress, Public Law 75-739, Wagner-O'Day Act of 1938.

U.S. Congress, Public Law 76-19, An Act to Provide for Reorganizing Agencies of the Government, and for Other Purposes (1939).

U.S. Congress, Public Law 82-590, An Act to Amend Title II of the Social Security Act (1952).

U.S. Congress, Public Law 85-864, National Defense Education Act of 1958.

U.S. Congress, Public Law 85-926, Expansion of Teacher Training for the Mentally Retarded (1958).

U.S. Congress, Public Law 88-156, Maternal and Child Health and Mental Retardation Planning Amendments of 1963.

U.S. Congress, Public Law 88-164, Mental Retardation Facilities and Community Mental Health Centers Construction Act of 1963.

U.S. Congress, Public Law 88-352, Civil Rights Act of 1964.

U.S. Congress, Public Law 89-750, Education of the Handicapped Act of 1966.

U.S. Congress, Public Law 90-480, Architectural Barriers Act of 1968.

U.S. Congress, Public Law 91-517, Developmental Disabilities Service Facilities Construction Act of 1970.

U.S. Congress, Public Law 93-112, Rehabilitation Act of 1973.

U.S. Congress, Public Law 93-516, Rehabilitation Act Amendments of 1974.

U.S. Congress, Public Law 94-103, Developmental Disabilities Assistance and Bill of Rights Act of 1975.

U.S. Congress, Public Law 94-142, Education for All Handicapped Children Act of 1975.

U.S. Congress, Public Law 96-265, Social Security Amendments of 1980.

U.S. Congress, Public Law 97-35, Omnibus Budget Reconciliation Act of 1981.

U.S. Congress, Public Law 99-457, Education of the Handicapped Act Amendments of 1986—Part H.

U.S. Congress, Public Law 100-407, Technology-Related Assistance for Individuals with Disabilities Act of 1988.

U.S. Congress, Public Law 101-336, Americans with Disabilities Act of 1990.

U.S. Congress, Public Law 101-476, Education of the Handicapped Act Amendments of 1990—Individuals with Disabilities Education Act.

U.S. Congress, Public Law 102-569, Rehabilitation Act Amendments of 1992.

U.S. Congress, An Act to Amend an Act Entitled "An Act to Provide for Vocational Rehabilitation and Return to Civil Employment of Disabled Persons Discharged from the Military" (1919).

U.S. Congressional Commission on National Aid to Vocational Education (1914). Report of Hearings on House Document 1604 Pursuant to Joint Resolution 16 (63-2), published January 1, 1914.

U.S. Congressional Record (1919). Vol. 58, October 14, p. 6914.

U.S. Continental Congress (1800–1801). *Journal of Congress: Containing the proceedings from September 5, 1774, to November 3, 1778* (13 volumes). Philadelphia: Folwell's Press.

U.S. House of Representatives Report 102-822 (1992).

Ward, G.C. (1990). *The Civil War: An illustrated history.* New York: Random House.

White, T.R. (1907). *Commentaries on the Constitution of Pennsylvania.* Philadelphia: Johnson Press.

4

□ □ □
□ □ □
□ □ □

Ethical Challenges in Supporting Persons with Disabilities

Stephen Greenspan and Peter Love

INTRODUCTION

The community revolution in disability services is being carried out by professionals and advocates who believe strongly that much of what used to be, or in some cases still is, standard practice is immoral. Because a sense of moral outrage is central to this revolution, one must consider ethics—that is, the study of morality—if one is to begin to understand that revolution. This chapter on ethics also addresses concern over the increased "ethical risk" (Wetle and Besdine, 1982) of certain labeled populations, a risk based on the negative stereotypes inherent in the terms used to describe them (e.g., "retread," "tard") and on their disadvantaged social status. Wolfensberger (1991), for example, has pointed out that people with disabilities are becoming increasingly marginalized as a result of two simultaneous social trends: the shift to a service-based economy and the emergence of a disability industry that is dependent on its subject populations' dependency.

As indicated in Chapters 1 and 2, the community revolution in disability services—referred to simply as the "community revolution"—involves a paradigm shift away from fitting persons into programs and toward fitting programs to persons, away from segregation and toward integration. Implicit in this evolving service model is a set of moral judgments about the rightness—both in terms of efficacy and human rights—of making human services more respectful of the preferences, dignity, and personhood of the individuals being served. This paradigm shift is at least in part driven by a sense that the new way of providing services is morally superior to the old way.

As discussed by several commentators (Bradley and Knoll, Chapter 1, this book; Schwartz, 1992), the community revolution in disability services is driven by a new awareness that people with severe disabilities are, in fact, full members of the human race, have full value as human beings, and are entitled to the same moral and civil rights, respect, and dignity as people who lack the designation of "disabled." While it may seem overly polemical to imply that services provided before the community revolution (and in many programs still today) fail to demonstrate full acknowledgment of the value of persons with disabilities, this chapter will demonstrate the essential truth of this generalization.

In virtually all systems of ethical analysis (save for the largely discredited "ethical egoism"), it is accepted as a given that moral agents have equal value, and that their needs (regardless of merit or accomplishments) should be given equal weight. The critical problem is in the definition of *moral agents*. As pointed out by Regan (1983) in his insightful analysis of the problem of animal rights, even the greatest of moral philosophers (such as Kant) have excluded from the definition of *moral agents* those beings considered incapable of exercising moral reasoning or of experiencing suffering from moral injustice. Hicks (1971) has extended this argument to suggest that people with mental retardation should not be considered persons in the full sense, as indicated in this passage: "Why not have the courage to accept . . . that there doubtless are many creatures who, although being of the human race, do not qualify as persons" (Hicks, 1971, p. 346).

Depending on the era and society, groups considered less than fully human have included children, members of various minority groups, women, people with serious cognitive impairments, and animals. The failure to include a class of beings as moral agents has fundamental importance for how they are treated, as it is considered permissible to make exceptions to the applicability of moral principles (such as the Golden Rule) to beings considered not to be moral agents. It is not accidental, therefore, that every liberation movement in history has had the central aim of convincing oppressors of their shared commonality with the oppressed.

Central to any ethical analysis is the value that the actor places on the other actors and on the various outcomes. The infamous Tuskegee study (Jones, 1981)—in which the U.S. Public Health Service allowed syphilis to remain unchecked for several decades in black men, without informing them that they had syphilis, that they were in a study, or that they were untreated, in order to study the natural history of the disease—was carried out on a population (African-Americans) whose lives were especially devalued in that region of the country (the rural deep South) and time (the first half of the twentieth century). Even given the lack of emphasis on informed research consent at that time (a situation that changed largely as a result of that study), it is dubious if such a study could have been carried out on people considered to be "normal" (i.e., whites). A more recent example, and one more relevant to the focus of this chapter, is the Willowbrook study carried out in the late 1950s and early 1960s, in which children with mental retardation were involuntarily infected with hepatitis B, in an experiment aimed at examining the natural history of the disease (Rothman and Rothman, 1984). One of the justifications for this (from the perspective of 1994, appalling) research program was the incredible argument that subjects of the study were better off than fellow residents because they received better medical care.

In a similar vein, practices (institutionalization in early childhood, sterilization, and so on) that many today would consider inhumane were routinely carried out on people with disabilities for two reasons: (1) because the proposed end (protection of the individual and of society) was considered to justify the means (just as in the Tuskegee study, where the end—furtherance of what today would in fact be considered weak science—was used to justify the means of deceitfully denying treatment to people who were sick); and (2) because the people on whom these practices were carried out were significantly devalued by the physicians, other professionals, and laypeople who were involved.

A more extreme (perhaps the most extreme) example of the link between devaluation of persons with disabilities and justification of inhumane practices is, of course, the treatment of persons with disabilities in Nazi Germany. The practice of exterminating persons with disabilities (which preceded the broader Holocaust of Jews, gypsies, and others) was clearly based on a view of such individuals as lacking full humanity, as lacking a capacity to have a worthwhile quality of life, and as a category of beings whose continued existence was considered an unreasonable imposition on the broader society (Wolfensberger, 1981).

As Boggs (1986) indicates, most of the literature on ethics and severe disability emphasizes biomedical issues, particularly those that involve life and death, such as the withholding of medical treatment to newborns (the Baby Doe cases) or elderly persons, sterilization, and organ transplantation from anencephalic infants (Coulter, 1988). The role of aversive stimulation in behavioral programming with self-abusive individuals has also attracted considerable interest and debate (Repp and Singh, 1990).

Much less attention has been paid, however, to ethical aspects of everyday life and services for persons with disabilities. Yet the development of ethical guidelines for everyday transactions involving people with disabilities is likely to be more important for most such individuals than the current emphasis on medical issues.

Given that the "support revolution" largely involves a change in everyday relationships between consumers and the people who work with them, in the balance of this chapter we will emphasize the role of ethical theory in guiding the everyday treatment of persons with disabilities. Because of its central role in providing an ethical framework for changing the way in which persons with disabilities are allowed to live their everyday lives, we first discuss the "normalization principle."

THE ROLE OF NORMALIZATION THEORY

There are two major approaches to ethical theory: "consequentialist" (also known as teleological or utilitarian) and "nonconsequentialist" (also known as deontological or Kantian). Consequentialist theorists believe that the only criterion necessary for evaluating the rightness of some action is whether it produces a sufficiently good outcome for society or for the affected population. In contrast, nonconsequentialist theorists believe that likely outcomes, while relevant to evaluating a particular course of action, do not in themselves provide a sufficient basis for making such a judgment. Rather, it is necessary to determine through logical analysis whether the action conforms to some universally desirable principle, such as Kant's famous dictum that people should always be viewed as ends rather than as means to some other end.

Both consequentialist and nonconsequentialist arguments have been made to support the community revolution in disability services, just as they were formerly made to support models of service that are now in disrepute. A consequentialist argument against residential institutions and sheltered workshops (two bulwarks of the prerevolutionary way of doing things) is that more normalized and less restrictive settings (found, for example, in supported living or supported employment) provide essential opportunities for people to acquire community living skills. A nonconsequentialist argument against such approaches, on the other hand, would emphasize the importance of protecting such basic human rights of people with disabilities as the right to choose one's own lifestyle, the right to be happy, and so on.

Arguments against such innovations, on the other hand, tend to be largely consequentialist in nature, since, in order to justify the denial of basic human rights, a nonconsequentialist argument would require one to make the unpopular assertion that persons with disabilities lack full humanity. Consequentialist arguments tend to emphasize that certain practices are necessary to protect individuals with disabilities from the dangerous, even life-threatening, consequences of placing people with limited ability in less protected settings. For example, supporters of the use of aversive techniques to decrease the frequency of self-injurious behavior argue (consequentially) that they are highly effective methods and are needed to protect people from death or disfigurement. Opponents of such interventions, on the other hand, do point out (also consequentially) that humane nonaversive interventions can be just as effective, but their main (nonconsequentialist) argument is that the use of aversives is a form of torture that has no place in a civilized society, regardless of its efficacy.

The community revolution is often viewed as a triumph of a particular ethical doctrine known as the "normalization principle." This principle was first formulated in Scandinavia by Bank-Mikkelsen (1969) and Nirje (1976) and is today known in the United States mainly through the writings of Wolfensberger (1980a). The essence of the normalization principle is that persons with disabilities should be treated in a manner that allows them to participate both symbolically and actually in roles and lifestyles that are "normal" for persons of their age and culture.

An implication of such a principle is that many practices once standard and considered perfectly acceptable in the disability field now are considered to violate the dignity, self-worth, and rights of people with disabilities. These include such practices (ranging from more to less serious) as hosing people down in communal showers, having people appear in public in a state of undress, referring to adults as children or otherwise portraying them as having the characteristics of children, having people live and work in the same setting, and taking people on outings in large segregated groups. Unfortunately, many of these attitudes and practices remain in force in the lives of many people with disabilities. Despite the two decades since the dissemination of normalization theory, many current practices continue to violate the principles of the theory.

Adherents of the normalization principle have been influential in bringing about a number of major policy changes. Among the most far-reaching of these is the policy of deinstitutionalization. While deinstitutionalization is not identical to the normalization principle, and some have argued that some community settings can be less in congruence with the principle than some institutions (Schwartz, 1992), there is fairly widespread agreement that attainment of anything approaching a normal lifestyle is difficult if not impossible within most institutional contexts.

Given that institutions are rapidly becoming a thing of the past in many states, the challenge posed by the normalization principle is to ensure that the community settings in which people live, work, and recreate operate in a manner that truly allows people with disabilities to participate in normal social roles and lifestyles. Many difficulties remain in promoting the understanding that normalization is not just a matter of geography and physical location but a fundamental shift in underlying attitudes and beliefs. The paradigm shift underlying the move from placing people into settings (i.e., sheltered workshops and group homes) to bringing supports to people in more natural settings (through, for example, supported employment and supported living) is a natural outgrowth of the application of the normalization principle. Thus, the community revolution is, to a large extent, a revolution that is based on the normalization principle.

Although it is generally assumed that the normalization principle constitutes a unitary ethical framework, the original European formulation (associated mainly with Nirje) and the most widely known American formulation (associated mainly with Wolfensberger) differ in at least one fundamental respect. The Nirje version represents a nonconsequentialist ethical theory in which living a normal lifestyle is seen as a basic human right of people with disabilities; the Wolfensberger formulation represents a consequentialist ethical theory in which living a normal lifestyle is a means to a broader social end, which is greater acceptance and valuation of people with disabilities.

Nirje (1985; Perrin and Nirje, 1985) has made clear the view that normalization theory is a universal deontological ethical system, in which the rights of all members of a democratic society are applied to people with disabilities who, in the past, were typically denied such rights. Central to the right to live a normal lifestyle, in Nirje's view, is the right to exercise lifestyle choices and preferences. Included in this right is, according to Nirje's view, the right to choose to engage in behaviors and lifestyles that are deviant or atypical (at least to the extent that deviant or atypical behaviors are tolerated for anyone in that society). Thus, if nonhandicapped people in a particular society are allowed to keep their immediate environments messy, wear outrageous clothing, espouse outrageous political views, and have homosexual relationships, there is no legitimate reason to deny the exercise of such choices to people with disabilities.

Wolfensberger (1980b), on the other hand, has made quite clear that his main concern in formulating his version of normalization theory is to bring about a change in the way that people with disabilities are portrayed and perceived. And he has stated that allowing unfettered freedom to persons with disabilities to act in excessively provocative or deviant ways (for example, through political organizing) would be an unacceptable threat to such a desired end.

A central issue for Wolfensberger is reducing what he refers to as "image deviance." This is the tendency to present people with disabilities, either directly (through excessive visibility) or indirectly (by juxtaposing their programs to symbols like cemeteries or junkyards), in a way that suggests that they are devalued or even surplus. A major motivating factor for Wolfensberger in thus portraying people with disabilities in a normal and nonoffensive manner is to prevent them from suffering the same fate in this country as they did in the native Germany of his formative years. In recently calling for a change in the name of normalization to "social role valorization," Wolfensberger (1983) stated that he hopes to clear up confusion about, and opposition to, the philosophy, which he attributes to the lack of a name that conveys a clear meaning. It may be argued, however, that much of the confusion and opposition stems from the maintenance of a definition—"the use of normal means to achieve normal ends"—that lacks specificity. An even greater source of such opposition may stem, however, from what many human service professionals see as the overly rigid manner in which the system is applied.

This rigidity is reflected in the tendency to evaluate agencies and programs (through PASS and PASSING) on the basis of external appearances alone, with no weight given (or allowed to be given) to the circumstances leading up to those appearances (Wolfensberger and Glenn, 1975; Wolfensberger and Thomas, 1983). Thus, allowing someone with cerebral palsy to sit in a wheelchair would be seen as a sign of image deviance, even if the recommended alternative (sitting on a beanbag, for example) would be physically painful or harmful for that individual.

Particularly galling to many persons who might otherwise be very sympathetic to the principle of normalization is the explicit instruction in the PASS and PASSING scoring manuals to avoid taking into account consumer choice when scoring a particular practice. (There is a section on consumer choice, but scoring in other sections is not affected by whether a behavior is chosen by a consumer or imposed on the consumer.) Thus, the presence of a doll collection in a consumer's room would be seen as a sign of age devaluation, even if the doll collection was the client's own particular hobby (as is the case with many educated professional adult women). In line with the tendency to ignore individual client choice is the tendency to impose Wolfensberger's own (to some extent culturally biased) value judgments about what activities or symbols are signs of "normal" or "deviant" images. Thus, taking consumers bowling is used as an example, in social role valorization (SRV) training sessions, of a tendency to devalue consumers, even though it is one of the most widely engaged-in forms of recreation in this country and even though it may be very enjoyable to the people going bowling.

Such a value judgment by SRV trainers undoubtedly reflects Wolfensberger's view that persons with disabilities should be allowed or encouraged to engage in only those behaviors that conform to his particular view of what is appropriate or highly valued (and bowling is presumably suspect because Wolfensberger associates it with working-class people). In line with the discussion of "dual standards" later in this chapter, the admonition that people with disabilities never be allowed to be presented in what Wolfensberger considers a negative light (regardless of circumstances or preferences) means that they must be made to live up to standards (for example, always dressing in one's best clothes) that few people in this society adhere to or find tolerable.

The focus by Wolfensberger on image deviance and external conformity to what he considers "normal" is to us an indication that the Wolfensberger approach has more in common with the pre–community revolution way of viewing and treating people with disabilities than may be commonly appreciated. Both provide essentially utilitarian justifications for treating individuals as a homogeneous class, regardless of individual preferences, with such treatment being justified by ends that are portrayed as being in the interest of either the consumer or the larger society. In the case of Wolfensberger, the types of treatments he advocates are undoubtedly more humane and likely to be more congruent with individual preferences than was the case formerly. But we, along with many other critics (e.g., Dybwad, 1969), find it difficult to accept an ethical formulation in which individual consumer happiness, satisfaction, and rights are subordinated to the presumed interest of the class of persons with disabilities.

Our purpose in pointing out that Wolfensberger's is not the only formulation of normalization theory is to indicate that some of the bitter opposition to normalization by many disability professionals and researchers (e.g., Landesman and Butterfield, 1987) may be a form of "throwing the baby out with the bath water." If it were more widely understood that normalization (in the original Nirje version) can be viewed from a rights perspective, in which personal choice (which typically, but not always, would result in image normality) is paramount, then we believe much of the opposition to this highly useful and influential doctrine would cease.

Our own bias (as was undoubtedly evident in the preceding pages) favors a Nirje/Kantian or rights-based interpretation of normalization theory (Greenspan, 1992). However, our objection to the Wolfensberger strain of normalization theory is less to its principles than to the dogmatic manner in which those principles are often applied. Such dogmatism is not the exclusive purview of SRV advocates. Certainly, it is possible to apply the Nirje emphasis on choice in an overly rigid and harmful manner, as when a person with limited capacity for reflection is asked to make important choices without being given help that might be needed in understanding the nature and consequences of those choices. When working with people with disabilities (especially serious cognitive disabilities), one must always walk a fine line between paternalism (making decisions for people) and failing to give people the help that they need and depend on to function effectively. The application of ethical principles to real life is often difficult because of the frequency with which different ethical principles (in this case, "respect for autonomy" and "protection" or "diligence") may conflict. An ethical and reflective professional must become adept at navigating such territory.

THE PROBLEM OF PATERNALISM

Everyday relationships between "professionals" (using the term loosely to include all paid workers, including paraprofessionals) and persons with disabilities have, historically, been characterized by a good deal of paternalism. The ethical underpinnings of the community revolution, and such ethical formulations as the normalization principle, are to a large extent efforts to get professionals to reduce, if not eliminate, their paternalistic tendencies. Perske (1972) has introduced the concept of "dignity of risk" to assert the rights of persons with disabilities to experience the consequences of their choices.

Paternalism, according to one dictionary (Merriam-Webster, 1985, p. 862), refers to "a system under which an authority undertakes to supply needs or regulate conduct of those under its control in matters affecting them as individuals. . . ." In terms of one's professional relationship to individuals with whom one works, the term describes an uneven balance of power in which virtually all decision making and authority reside in the hands of the professional. In contrast to paternalism, the professional role vis-à-vis persons with disabilities can be defined, according to Bayles (1989), as the "agency" model (in which the consumer possesses all of the power); the "friendship" model (similar to the agency model, but characterized by greater warmth and commitment); and two models, "contract" and "fiduciary," in which power is shared equally, with the professional exercising authority in certain areas of expertise (e.g., how to write a legal brief or perform a surgical procedure) but with the consumer possessing ultimate authority in how the relationship is defined (e.g., whether to file a lawsuit or undergo a procedure).

Underlying the paternalistic model, according to Bayles (1989), is a view of the consumer as someone lacking the competence to make his or her own decisions. Most professions have made efforts, through revisions in their codes of conduct, to counteract their historical tendencies toward paternalism. Medicine, perhaps the most paternalistic profession of all, has now firmly established the "autonomy" principle (Beauchamp and Childress, 1983): the obligation to respect the authority of persons to make medical decisions on their own behalf, on the basis of information provided in a neutral way by physicians. In the disability field, on the other hand, paternalism remains deeply rooted and is very difficult to eliminate (Wikler, 1979).

One of the central difficulties of paternalism in disability services lies in the problem of distinguishing between two variants: strong and weak. Strong paternalism involves making decisions for someone whose access to autonomy is not questioned but who makes decisions that another agent is in disagreement with. Weak paternalism involves making decisions for someone who is perceived as having difficulty accessing autonomous decision-making premises (e.g., a person prevented from killing himself or herself while depressed or under the influence of psychoactive substances). Weak paternalism is generally perceived as ethically permissible (or, at any rate, more ethically permissible), while strong paternalism is generally not considered permissible.

In disability services, the perception has been that a majority of persons with disabilities (particularly those with cognitive limitations) have sufficiently limited access to autonomy as to justify the substituted decision making of weak paternalism. The reality, however, is that the vast majority of people with disabilities (including cognitive limitations) do have access to autonomy (sometimes with assistance, but more often not). This fact suggests that much of the weak paternalism that is perceived as ethically permissible is, in reality, a form of strong paternalism that should be considered much less acceptable than it is. Both kinds of paternalism are based on a tendency to view all persons with disabilities, particularly when cognitive limitations are involved, as lacking the competence to make sensible or safe decisions. Thus, *paternalism* is an appropriate term to characterize a style of behavior that seems to be rooted in a view of people with disabilities as childlike, and a view of professionals as carrying out some of the responsibilities of parents.

Although both variants of normalization theory contain strong objections to the infantilization tendencies so prevalent in everyday interactions with people with disabilities, the Wolfensberger (SRV) variant may be considered more willing to tolerate a degree of paternalism than the Nirje (classical normalization) model. This is because the notion that it is the responsibility of staff and agencies to ensure that their clients act or appear in ways that reduce image deviance—in spite of individual preferences or tendencies to the contrary—accepts a paternalistic view of the role of professionals vis-à-vis persons with disabilities.

The community revolution may be characterized, to some extent, as an effort to shift the professional role from paternalism closer to the fiduciary/ contract model (equal power) or agency/friendship model (consumer power) just discussed. Thus group homes, while based in the community, are seen as reflecting an earlier service paradigm (Bradley and Knoll, Chapter 1, this book) and, while a major advance against large institutions, still are grounded in a paternalistic definition of staff-consumer relationships. Supported living, in which the person owns or leases his or her home, and in which staff function as support persons rather than quasi-bosses, is—at least in theory—a model in which power is shifted to the consumer. In fact, as two examples gathered from an evaluation of community residences in Connecticut (Dunaway et al., 1991) show, paternalism—while reduced—is anything but unknown in supported living settings.

One such example involved a man ("Mr. Jones") with a very mild disability who lived in his own apartment with a roommate. He was a gracious host to one of our interviewers and invited her to share a meal with him and his roommate. He was very interested in the questions being asked and gave lengthy, well-thought-out, and very appropriate answers. The support person, who happened to be there during the meal, continually interrupted Mr. Jones, pointing out that he was ignoring his food, and that he should eat it before it got cold.

The other example involved a man ("Mr. Smith") who has a moderate cognitive impairment and who resided in his own condominium. Mr. Smith, who has his own job and is really quite independent, has a problem with shoplifting. One day he brought home a small item that he had stolen from a drugstore. The support person discovered this and not only ordered Mr. Smith to return the item, but also accompanied him to ensure that he did so—as though Mr. Smith were a small child.

Both examples, however well-intended the support persons, can be characterized as highly paternalistic. The behaviors that the staff wished to correct, however much they were seen by those staff as problematic or deviant, are well within the range of behaviors that "normal" people engage in. Thus, paternalistic behavior may be considered to be symptomatic of a kind of double standard, in which persons with disabilities are made to conform to standards of behavior that are actually higher than those tolerated in the community at large. This tendency toward a dual standard was termed by the late Marc Gold (1973) as the "deviance-competence hypothesis." By this he meant that we are more likely to tolerate deviance from norms or from perfection in persons considered "competent," because such deviation (aside from being seen as a right) is considered merely a form of individual variation or eccentricity; in persons defined as "incompetent," however, even small variations from norms or from perfection are interpreted as symptoms of the individual's "problem," and thus as deficiencies needing to be eliminated through behavioral programming.

Critics of this rights position are likely to argue (as supporters of restrictive practices tend to do) that one must look at the consequences of allowing persons with disabilities too much freedom. Poor hygiene is a frequent problem for persons with serious disabilities and often poses impediments to their employment and acceptance by persons in the broader community. The cost of allowing unrestricted freedom to persons with disabilities, in line with this argument, would be to allow them to suffer the highly negative consequences stemming from the fact that they are, indeed, incompetent in many important areas. The rights position would be seen by such critics as hopelessly romantic and out of touch with reality, and equally likely to lead to problems for consumers as for agencies.

There is, obviously, some truth to such criticism, but one can argue the obverse as well and show that there is a habitual tendency to underestimate the ability of persons with all levels of disability to rise to the occasion offered by allowing greater freedoms (Dunaway et al., 1991). Furthermore, advocates for a civil libertarian position are not necessarily calling for a complete end to direction and teaching, but rather for increased sensitivity to preference, choice, and lifestyle variation, and greater reflection by caregivers about the appropriate limits of their interference in the lives of the persons with whom they work. Central to such a reevaluation is the need to separate (a) what is truly a requirement for order and safety from what is merely a matter of preference and convenience for agencies and staff, and (b) what are reasonable and necessary risks for consumers from what are risks that might be considered to be unreasonable and unnecessary.

No discussion of paternalism can be complete without some mention of the appropriateness and limits of "behavior modification." Currently, there is much debate over the ethics of using aversive punishments and highly restrictive behavioral interventions to alleviate seriously self-injurious or aggressive behaviors (Repp and Singh, 1990). However, there has been relatively little discussion of the paternalistic (i.e., unequal power distribution) quality of behavior modification itself.

When "behavior therapy" (typically using classical conditioning methods) is used with many nondisabled people to alleviate habit disorders, such as smoking, there is a clear adherence to the contractual/fiduciary model of professionalism, in which consumer participation and right to termination of treatment are clearly respected. In behavior modification, which is typically used with children or with adults with disabilities (and which is based mainly on operant methods), determination of treatment goals is made by professionals, and the target of the intervention has little or no power to authorize or terminate treatment (and may not even be informed that he or she is the subject of behavior modification).

The paternalistic tendency, that is referred to above as the "deviance-competence hypothesis," is reflected not only in a tendency to remediate mildly deviant (but within normal limits) behaviors such as those displayed by Smith and Jones, but also in a tendency to "overprogram," that is, to target behaviors for improvement that may be, in fact, above average for the general population. This was reflected in an example we observed in a study in the state of Washington (Dunaway et al., 1992), when a facility had developed a program to increase prosocial behaviors in a gentleman who was the most well-liked individual in the facility, and whose social competence probably exceeded that of many of the professionals who worked with him.

Because behavior modification works, and because there is a tendency to view in favorable terms (financially and otherwise) agencies that have "active treatment" plans, typically defined as behavioral interventions, for all of their clients, there is a tendency to engage in gross overprogramming, with insufficient attention paid to whether such overprogramming constitutes an infringement on the rights of consumers (Bannerman, 1990). Yet, such intrusive and paternalistic uses of behavior modification in everyday life are never brought to the attention of human rights committees, as such committees are seen as existing mainly to deal with more "serious" matters. Overprogramming is seldom seen as a problem, because it is difficult for professionals to acknowledge that one can have too much of a good thing.

Unquestioned use of behavioral techniques to decrease the frequency of "problem behaviors" or characteristics is grounded in the undeniable fact that such techniques are usually effective. Behavior modification has been seen as generally compatible with the goals of the community revolution, because (a) it typically results in a more harmonious and positive relationship, replacing ineffective and inhumane practices such as verbal abuse and restraint; and (b) in emphasizing the functional nature of maladaptive behavior, behavior modifiers offer alternatives to the excessive reliance on psychotropic medications. The utility of behavioral programming is typically cited as support for the morality of its use (Axelrod, 1990). Such ethical arguments may have some validity when applied to behaviors that are injurious or life-threatening (e.g., head banging) but become problematic when applied to behaviors that involve an individual's lifestyle (e.g., hygiene, choice of friends or sexual partners, use of money) or perceived deviance. Furthermore, it has been pointed out that interventions that focus only on behaviors or symptoms are often less effective than interventions that adopt a more ecological analysis of an individual's underlying "communicative intent" (Donnellan, et al., 1984).

Behavior modification embraces a wide variety of methods, ranging on a continuum from fairly nonrestrictive and nonaversive to very restrictive and aversive. Hierarchies for locating methods along this continuum have been developed (Morris and Brown, 1983) in response to the need for developing mechanisms and guidelines to protect the rights of persons with disabilities from interventions that are potentially harmful. An example of an intervention at the low (noncontroversial) end of the continuum would be "differential reinforcement," whereby a caregiver pairs ignoring of a relatively benign undesired behavior (say, whining) with prompt reward of a desired incompatible behavior (say, appropriate social verbalization). Another such intervention would be "response cost," that is, denying some privilege (e.g., going on an outing) to deal with some behavior deficiency (e.g., not doing one's chores). Preferably, but often not, these two should be rationally related to each other. The noncontroversial nature of this type of intervention stems from the lack of any overt coercion or physical punishment, although it may be argued—because of the power differential between staff and persons with disabilities inherent in most facilities—that there is always covert coercion.

An example of an intervention in the intermediate (more controversial) range would be "time-out" or "overcorrection," in which some form of physical coercion (being placed in a time-out room or being made to do certain movements) is used to deal with certain forms of undesirable behaviors. An example of an intervention at the high (controversial) end of the continuum would be the use of electric shock (e.g., the SIBIS device), pinching, ammonia spray, and so on, to bring about decreases in the frequency of self-injurious behaviors.

Two ways in which the community revolution has influenced the practice of behavior modification are (1) the widespread implementation of prior-approval mechanisms, to guard against the unnecessary and uncontrolled use of aversive methods; (2) a strong bias against using coercive methods in even the intermediate range; and (3) a strong emphasis on seeking and trying alternative methods whenever possible. Thus, there has been much written about the communicative function of maladaptive behavior. This means that one should try to determine what need the person engaging in the maladaptive behavior is trying to express and one should seek to meet that need (or communicate with him or her about it) before assuming that punishment is needed. There appears to have been a marked decrease in the use of time-out and other mild forms of punishment in exemplary programs. However, in nonexemplary programs, and where staff are poorly trained or supervised, there is still a tendency to rely excessively on time-out and other forms of punishment.

The current primary controversy in the behavior modification field is over whether more extreme forms of aversive intervention, such as electric shock, have a legitimate role in dealing with the behaviors of people with severe disabilities. As in other controversies involving values, the basis of the debate is between those who take the utilitarian position that aversives have been shown to be effective for some individuals (Axelrod, 1990) and those who take the deontological position that aversives are inherently dehumanizing and represent an abusive violation of human rights (Donnellan and LaVigna, 1990). To cover their bets, advocates for this point of view also typically attempt to demonstrate the utilitarian position that nonaversive alternatives can and do work if only they are tried (McGee et al., 1987).

Until recently, there has been little questioning of the moral rightness of behavior modification in general, with such questioning directed mainly at those interventions at the high or intermediate ends of the restrictiveness hierarchy. The gradual evolution of the service delivery system into such settings as "supported living" has, however, caused some commentators to wonder whether even relatively benign forms of behavior modification, such as response-cost, are compatible with the value base underlying that revolution. This is because behavior modification, by definition, involves a paternalistic model in which the person whose behavior is being modified is placed in a dependent, childlike position and typically has no say in the choice of behaviors targeted for modification or in the choice of consequences used to bring about that modification.

Furthermore, precisely because they "work," there is a tendency to overuse techniques such as response-cost to coerce lifestyle decisions and behaviors that, but for the disability status of the "client," would be considered no one else's business. For example, a punishment such as grounding from recreational outings as a "natural consequence" of inappropriate behavior (e.g., passing gas) on an agency's van might be appropriate, although it comes close to violating a basic right (which is typically exempted from response cost). The next step, however, would typically be to use grounding, or the threat of grounding, as the habitual punishment for a broad range of behaviors—such as keeping one's room neat—that have no "logical" connection to the consequence and that, one might argue, are not appropriate targets for modification in adults. Thus, the attack on behavior modification is, in part, a philosophical attack on the appropriateness of one set of persons (staff) telling another set of individuals (consumers) what to do solely because of their disability status. Such a state of affairs becomes even more problematic when the intervention is carried out in a setting—the home owned or leased by the consumer—in which the staff person is technically a visitor but in reality often has higher status than the resident.

CONCLUSION

In all professions there is an implicit and often explicit status differential between professionals and consumers. The potential abuse of the greater power of the professional has given rise to codes of ethical conduct designed to redress some of this imbalance. Because this status differential in the field of disability services has historically been seen in the light of benevolent paternalism, there has been less concern over potential abuses of power than has been the case in other areas of professional practice. The community revolution in disability services, with its emphasis on individual rights, choice making, and self-expression, has brought to light many areas of potential abuse of this power differential.

One obstacle to bringing about the development of increased attention to ethical obligations is the considerable confusion still remaining over where to situate disability services in the human services field. Because disability services are typically subsumed under specific disciplines (e.g., medicine, education, vocational rehabilitation, social work), it is assumed that the codes of conduct for those fields will govern the behavior of workers in the disability field. However, as indicated by Greenspan and Negron (1994) with respect to practices in educational settings: (1) professional codes differ widely in their provisions and relevance to disability issues, (2) dissemination and enforcement of ethics codes vary widely from one discipline to another and have no applicability to people identified with another (or no) discipline, and (3) many workers (both those considered professionals and those considered paraprofessionals) fail to identify with a specific discipline. This suggests the possible need to (1) define disability services as its own distinct field with its own distinct code of conduct and (2) develop enforcement mechanisms (located within oversight organizations as well as within service agencies) that are taken seriously by individuals and agencies alike.

REFERENCES

Axelrod, S. (1990). Myths that (mis)guide our profession. In A.C. Repp and N.N. Singh (Eds.), *Perspectives on the use of nonaversive and aversive interventions for persons with developmental disabilities* (pp. 59–72). Sycamore, IL: Sycamore Publishing Co.

Bank-Mikkelsen, N.E. (1969). A metropolitan area in Denmark: Copenhagen. In R. Kugel and W. Wolfensberger (Eds.), *Changing patterns in residential services for the mentally retarded.* Washington, DC: President's Committee on Mental Retardation.

Bannerman, D.J. (1990). Balancing the right to habilitation with the right to personal liberties: The right to eat too many doughnuts and take a nap. *Journal of Applied Behavioral Analysis, 23,* 79–89.

Bayles, M.D. (1989). *Professional ethics* (2nd ed.). Belmont, CA: Wadsworth Publishing Company.

Beauchamp, T.L., and Childress, J.F. (1983). *Principles of biomedical ethics.* New York: Oxford University Press.

Boggs, E.M. (1986). Ethics in the middle of life: An introductory overview. In P.R. Dokecki and R.M. Zaner (Eds.), *Ethics of dealing with persons with severe disabilities.* Baltimore: Paul H. Brookes.

Coulter, D.L. (1988). Beyond Baby Doe: Does infant transplantation justify euthanasia? *Journal of the Association for Persons with Severe Handicaps, 13,* 71–75.

Donnellan, A.M., Mirench, P.L., Mesaros, R.A., and Fassbender, L.L. (1984). Analyzing the communicative functions of aberrant behavior. *Journal of the Association for Persons with Severe Handicaps, 9,* 201–212.

Donnellan, A.M., and LaVigna, G.W. (1990). Myths about punishment. In A.C. Repp and N.N. Singh (Eds.), *Perspectives on the use of nonaversive and aversive interventions for persons with developmental disabilities* (pp. 33–57). Sycamore, IL: Sycamore Publishing Co.

Dunaway, J., Granfield, J., Norton, K., and Greenspan, S. (1991). *Costs and benefits of residential services for persons with mental retardation in Connecticut.* Storrs, CT: Pappanikou Center of the University of Connecticut.

Dunaway, J., Norton, K., Bear, J., Greenspan, S., and Granfield, J. (1992). *Residential services for persons with mental retardation in the state of Washington.* Olympia, WA: Legislative Budget Committee.

Dybwad, G. (1969). Action implications, U.S.A. today. In R. Kugel and W. Wolfensberger (Eds.) *Changing patterns in residential services for the mentally retarded.* Washington, DC: President's Committee on Mental Retardation.

Gold, M.W. (1973). Research on the vocational habilitation of the retarded: The present, the future. In N.R. Ellis (Ed.) *International Review of Research in Mental Retardation,* Volume 6 (pp. 97–141). New York: Academic Press.

Greenspan, S. (1992). Normalization si, SRV no. *The Pappanikou Center Brief, 4,* 8–9.

Greenspan, S., and Negron, E. (1994). Ethical obligations of special services personnel. *Special Services in the Schools, 8,* 185–209.

Hicks, J.C. (1971). Respect for persons and respect for living things. *Philosophy, 46,* 346–348.

Jones, J.H. (1981, 1993 expanded edition). *Bad blood: The Tuskegee syphilis experiment.* New York: The Free Press.

Landesman, S., and Butterfield, E.C. (1987). Normalization and deinstitutionalization of mentally retarded individuals: Controversy and facts. *American Psychologist, 42,* 809–816.

McGee, J.J., Menolascino, F.J., Hobbs, D.C., and Menousek, P.E. (1987). *Gentle teaching: A non-aversive approach to helping persons with mental retardation.* New York: Human Sciences Press.

Merriam-Webster. (1985). *Webster's Ninth New Collegiate Dictionary.* Springfield, MA: Author.

Morris, R.J., and Brown, D.K. (1983). Legal and ethical issues in behavior modification with mentally retarded persons. In J.C. Matson (Ed.), *Treatment issues and innovations in mental retardation* (pp. 61–95). New York: Plenum.

Nirje, B. (1976). The normalization principle. In R. Kugel and A. Shearer (Eds.), *Changing patterns in residential services for the mentally retarded* (rev. ed.). Washington, DC: President's Committee on Mental Retardation.

Nirje, B. (1985). The basis and logic of the normalization principle. *Australia and New Zealand Journal of Developmental Disabilities, 11,* 65–68.

Perrin, B., and Nirje, B. (1985). Setting the record straight: A critique of some frequent misconceptions of the normalization principle. *Australia and New Zealand Journal of Developmental Disabilities, 11,* 69–74.

Perske, R. (1972). The dignity of risk and the mentally retarded. *Mental Retardation, 10,* 24–27.

Regan, T. (1983). *The case for animal rights.* Berkeley, CA: University of California Press.

Repp, A.C., and Singh, N.N. (1990). *Perspectives on the use of nonaversive and aversive interventions for persons with developmental disabilities.* Sycamore, IL: Sycamore Publishing Co.

Rothman, D.J., and Rothman, S.M. (1984). *The Willowbrook wars.* New York: Harper & Row.

Schwartz, D.B. (1992). *Crossing the river: Creating a conceptual revolution in community and disability.* Brookline, MA: Brookline Books.

Wetle, T., and Besdine, R.W. (1982). Ethical issues. In J.W. Roe and R.W. Besdine (Eds.), *Health and disease in old age.* Boston: Little, Brown.

Wikler, D.I. (1979). Paternalism and the mildly retarded. *Philosophy and Public Affairs, 8,* 377–392. Also in R. Satorius (Ed.) (1983), *Paternalism* (pp. 83–94). Minneapolis: University of Minnesota Press.

Wolfensberger, W. (1980a). A brief overview of the principle of normalization. In R.J. Flynn and K.E. Nitsch (Eds.), *Normalization, social integration and community services.* Baltimore: University Park Press.

Wolfensberger, W. (1980b). A call to wake up to the beginning of a new wave of "euthanasia" of severely impaired people. *Education and Training of the Mentally Retarded, 15,* 171–173.

Wolfensberger, W. (1981). The extermination of handicapped people in World War II Germany. *Mental Retardation, 19,* 1–7.

Wolfensberger, W. (1983). Social role valorization: A proposed new term for the principle of normalization. *Mental Retardation, 21,* 234–239.

Wolfensberger, W. (1991). Reflections on a lifetime in human services. *Mental Retardation, 29,* 1–15.

Wolfensberger, W., and Glenn, L. (1975). *Pass 3* (2nd ed.). Vol. I: *Handbook.* Vol. II: *Field Manual.* Toronto: National Institute on Mental Retardation.

Wolfensberger, W., and Thomas, S. (1983). *PASSING* (2nd ed.). Toronto: National Institute on Mental Retardation.

5

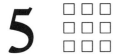

Elements for a Code of Everyday Ethics in Disability Services

Stephen Greenspan and Peter F. Love

INTRODUCTION

Although the normalization principle has obvious relevance for the development of policies—and the evaluation of services and programs—that benefit people with disabilities, it does not, in either of its formulations (see Chapter 4), provide us with a code of conduct that might guide the behavior of individual professionals or paraprofessionals. The need for such a code in training, supervising, and disciplining persons who work in this field has become increasingly pressing.

The community revolution, with its emphasis on individual planning and natural supports, has introduced a new level of complexity and unpredictability into the daily decision-making process in the field. Workers in disability programs are increasingly moved away from institutional norms and guidelines and toward reliance on their own values. Since there is a divergence of ideas of what represents a "good" for persons with disabilities, there is a need for a universal code of conduct to which agencies, professionals, and other workers may subscribe.

Ethical codes do exist for various professions involved in disability services such as nursing, medicine, psychology, and social work (Gorlin, 1990). Aside from the fact that few of the illustrations contained in those codes involve persons with disabilities, enforcement of a professional organization's code applies only to persons who belong to that organization. Membership in one's own relevant professional organization is not typically required for persons who work for disability agencies, and even if one did belong to such an organization, there is the real possibility that a person whose conduct is of concern to you may not be a member of the same profession or professional organization. Finally, the majority of people who work in the disability field—direct care staff (under whatever job title might apply in a particular setting)—typically lack training in a generic discipline and may not, therefore, strictly qualify as "professionals."

As the first author and a colleague argued in a recent paper (Greenspan and Negron, 1994) aimed at educators but equally applicable to adult services workers, the solution to this problem may be to recognize that there are universal obligations that apply to all (regardless of status or educational background) who work in human services in general, or disability services in particular. While these obligations are spelled out in the codes of conduct of various professional organizations, they are derived from universal notions of morality and would still be operative regardless of one's professional status or organizational membership.

As will be discussed in the concluding section of this chapter, the development, dissemination, and enforcement of such codes should become the responsibility of each service-providing agency (private and public), as well as agencies funding such services, and not be viewed solely as the responsibility of specific professional organizations. We will present a framework that provides a basis for a code of conduct having widespread applicability for human services in general and disability services in particular. This framework, first developed in Greenspan and Negron (1994), contains ten principles, derived from the general literature on professional ethics (Bayles, 1989) and reflected in a wide variety of fields, including bioethics (Beauchamp and Childress, 1983), mental health (American Psychological Association, 1992; Herlihy and Corey, 1992), regular and special education (Strike and Soltis, 1985; Howe and Miramontes, 1992), and many other disciplines.

These ten principles (listed in Table 5-1) constitute a comprehensive framework for guiding the obligations that individuals have to consumers (in this case, people with disabilities). Although this list has wide applicability to many fields and was not developed specifically with the needs and characteristics of persons with disabilities in mind, such a framework is highly congruent with the theory of normalization (particularly as expressed in the writings of Nirje). In fact, one might even argue that it is a fundamental requirement of the normalization principle that the same ethical obligations that define the conduct of all "professionals" (which, to restate, is a term we use to cover a broad range of human services employees, regardless of level of training) should also apply equally to people with disabilities. In the following pages, we shall illustrate this

TABLE 5-1   Ten Professional Obligations Toward Clients

1. Discretion: No blabbing
2. Candor: No lying
3. Competence: No quackery
4. Fairness: No discrimination
5. Loyalty: No dual relationships
6. Protection: No cover-ups
7. Autonomy: No power-tripping
8. Diligence: No goofing off
9. Honesty: No stealing
10. Respect: No attacking

point, by providing—after a brief explanation of each of the ten principles—one or more examples of how the principle is sometimes violated in the course of everyday interactions with people who have disabilities.

OBLIGATION 1: DISCRETION

This principle involves the requirement that all professionals exercise self-control in their verbalizations or other forms of communication. Most of the emphasis in writings about this requirement has been on the importance of respecting "confidentiality," that is, of not violating the trust placed in them by consumers by disclosing sensitive information that they have learned in the course of working with those consumers. However, discretion is a broader concept that involves a certain carefulness in communicating, with both consumers and others. For example, a discreet professional thinks twice before revealing overly personal information about himself to consumers, or before volunteering information (whether critical or not) about other professionals, and so on. While the discretion requirement is sometimes used as a smokescreen to avoid complying with the obligation to show "candor" (see Obligation 2), ethical professionals must learn to find an appropriate balance between these two ethical requirements.

One unavoidable outcome of the community revolution, which stems from support professionals (particularly in residential settings) becoming involved in many aspects of the everyday lives of people with disabilities, is the learning of intimate details about the people with whom they work.

These details, involving sexual and other behaviors that would typically be considered private and normal, are seen as fair game for discussion at planning meetings and are often seen as symptoms needing alleviation. Furthermore, in many agencies little effort is made to ensure that such information is shared only with people who need to know it. In schools, careless sharing of sensitive information often takes place in the teacher's lounge, where many people may be present who lack any need or right to know information such as IQ scores, family problems, health problems (including HIV infection), and psychiatric reports.

This lack of discretion often seems to serve the demands of a secondary agenda for people working in the disability field (i.e., distancing from the "clients"). Detailed discussions of weight gain, menstruation, toileting behaviors, and so on often occur at planning meetings in front of people who are the focus of the meetings, regardless of the topics' relevance to the person's real needs or quality of life. People without disabilities would consider such discussions impolite at best and offensive at worst. This often has the net effect of downgrading the status of the person with a disability to an object of discussion.

OBLIGATION 2: CANDOR

All persons, whether they are professionals or not, are under a universal moral and ethical obligation to tell the truth. When dealing with persons with disabilities, or their parents/guardians, there is often a tendency to hold back some portion of the truth. This sometimes happens, for example, at planning meetings when professionals adopt a united front and keep to themselves divisions of opinion or information that might support objections that could be raised by the consumer or his or her representative.

This relatively easy acceptance of behavior (e.g., lying by professionals) that would be considered both ethically and socially unacceptable in relation to people without disabilities is supported by the twin histories of the use of deception in behavioral research and attitudes toward child rearing. These attitudes have been transferred to the field of disability services. Both are typically subsumed under the justificatory rubric of "for their own good."

Another common justification for lying to consumers surfaces when professionals seek to manipulate their behavior. For example, with one moderately cognitively impaired man in his fifties, residential staff tried various ploys to coerce him into taking a daily bath in the evening (something imposed by the residential manager rather than any health requirement, and fiercely resisted by the client). One regular tactic involved turning on the water in the bathtub and saying to the consumer, "Come on, I want to show you something in the other room." The consumer would start to walk down the hall and would get very upset when he heard the water running in the bathtub.

Praise that is administered in an exaggerated way is also a form of lying that should be avoided both as a matter of principle and also because it often backfires (Greenspan, 1985). Caregivers often assume, mistakenly, that when one praises an accomplishment that is flawed, the only way to do so is by making a false-positive characterization of the person (for example, saying a bad artwork is terrific or an incompetent artist is a good artist). Rather, one can honestly (and more effectively) give praise in such a situation by praising the effort ("You're really working hard at learning to paint") or some particular aspect of the work that you like ("There's a lot of yellow there. I like yellow").

As with violations of other ethical principles, professionals often find themselves tempted to lie in order to bring some benefit to the client. Examples include falsely filling out an insurance form on behalf of the consumer, giving false information in a criminal investigation of the consumer, or making a diagnostic classification that does not really fit the individual but that makes him or her eligible for some program or entitlement.

Principled professionals make every effort to avoid lying, regardless of the temptations or benefits that are believed to accrue. In the disability field, as in other walks of life, honesty is the best policy.

OBLIGATION 3: COMPETENCE

Virtually all codes of conduct emphasize the importance of professionals practicing within the limits of their competence. This obligation holds even when the professional possesses a license or certificate that allows (or does not prohibit) a particular action or procedure. Thus, the professional is expected to be reflective about his or her own qualifications, and to carry out only those activities that he or she possesses the training or skills to carry out. If the professional feels that he or she lacks appropriate training or experience, the person either should seek to get appropriate training or supervision or should refuse to do the procedure, even if ordered to do so by a superior.

One agency was providing supported living services to a young woman with intellectual and emotional disabilities. When the woman became pregnant, the agency's director was asked if he could incorporate into his agency's residential program a component involving parenting education and support. Although this administrator, his agency, and staff lacked expertise or background in parenting interventions, he agreed to the request. The services were inappropriate and inept, and serious problems ensued for the mother and her child.

Another case: One nursing trainee was acting as case manager for a young woman with a severe disability. In this capacity, she met one day with the young woman's parents to help them deal with their feelings about her possible move to a group home. During this meeting, the trainee was informed that the young woman's parents were experiencing marital difficulties, and she was asked if she might provide some marriage counseling. Although the trainee lacked training or expertise in marriage counseling, she agreed to provide the service, without arranging supervision. The counseling was incompetently provided and probably did more harm than good. Even if a better outcome had followed, however, it would clearly have been more appropriate for the trainee to decline the request and make a referral to another agency or professional. Since the trainee's primary role was as case manager for the young woman, the service also violated the loyalty principle—prohibiting dual relationships (see Obligation 5)—and should have been declined on that ground as well.

Violation of the competence obligation is common around the use or recommendation of psychotropic medications. An article of faith (approaching a political correctness litmus test) among many in the forefront of the community revolution is that psychotropic medications are overprescribed and are often unnecessary, if not harmful to consumers. Human rights committees have been set up to monitor the use of so-called behavior-modifying drugs and other controversial practices. These committees (most of whose members typically lack training or qualifications in psychopharmacology) will sometimes second-guess the prescription of particular drugs or dosage levels for particular consumers and will bring persistent pressure to bear on prescribing physicians to lower dosage levels. While such pressures are not necessarily bad, committee members sometimes show little humility in approaching a task for which they typically lack expertise. We are familiar with more than one case in which the result of such meddling has proven both psychologically and physically detrimental to the affected clients. While it is appropriate, and even beneficial, to require physicians to explain their use of particular medication strategies, it is inappropriate for persons lacking medical training to presume to practice medicine without a license.

Sometimes, this also occurs when direct care staff who have an interest in alternative herbal-based therapies attempt to persuade clients or family members to substitute folk remedies for physician-prescribed treatments. Certainly, one of the factors contributing to the tendency of disability professionals to step outside their realms of competence has been the relative lack of malpractice litigation in this area of human services. While it is not our position to suggest that such litigation is necessarily desirable, it has served in other fields (e.g., medicine) to make professionals more cautious about overstepping the bounds of their competence.

The issue of competence also sometimes arises in the application of operant conditioning techniques (under the general rubric of "behavior modification") to reduce the frequency of undesirable behaviors or increase the frequency of desirable behaviors on the part of consumers. In Chapter 4 we raised issues of possible inequity in applying such techniques to change lifestyle choices that are not necessarily problematic for the consumer or others. Even when targeting behaviors that are problematic, however, it should not be assumed that anyone, regardless of training or experience, can design and implement such interventions. There are many cases in which professionals with virtually no understanding of the principles or techniques of behavior modification used the term to describe interventions that bore little resemblance to what a qualified professional would have designed. Incompetently designed behavioral interventions are likely, at best, to fail and, at worst, to inflict harm on consumers.

The same is also sometimes true when an agency or professional whose main experience with behavioral interventions has been with one category of disability (e.g., delinquency) attempts to apply these techniques to another category of disability (e.g., autism) in which the professional or agency has had no experience or training. Interventions that may be justifiable when used with individuals whose behavior has been instrumentally learned may be a form of unjustifiable cruelty when used with individuals whose behavior is an expression of underlying brain pathology. Regardless of the claims of some theorists for the universality of behavioral principles, professionals must always ask themselves if they possess the qualifications to treat a particular variety of disability or a particular set of symptoms.

OBLIGATION 4: FAIRNESS

Most professional codes of conduct contain a provision that professionals avoid discriminating against or for consumers on the basis of their status, wealth, influence, or racial/ethnic background. This principle is often violated, for example, when a parent with a "connection" to an agency trustee or director is able to get his or her son or daughter served ahead of wait-listed individuals. A less pernicious, but still problematic, example of this phenomenon is reflected in the tendency of agencies to make their resources and services available to those who are able to launch the most persistent, sophisticated, and sometimes litigious campaigns.

Such a tendency obviously works to the detriment of people who are poor or disadvantaged. We're aware, for example, of a caseworker for a state adult services agency who was told by his supervisor that he was "too ethical" in helping unsophisticated (often minority) applicants to redo their applications for services to make a stronger case for eligibility.

The obligation to be fair also can be applied to the tendency (as we have noted repeatedly) to apply a double standard in restricting lifestyle choices and idiosyncrasies of people with disabilities. Thus, a person with a disability who becomes a parent is likely to be scrutinized and reported to child protective authorities at the first sign of inadequacy (Budd and Greenspan, 1984). The first author has reported on one such case (Greenspan, 1992), in which two perfectly competent parents were prevented from taking their newborn son home from the hospital for days because of their physical limitations—they both used wheelchairs and had limited upper-body strength. The same hospital that subjected these individuals to various forms of harassment (including an occupational therapy evaluation) would probably not, however, assume it had a right to question the right of an able-bodied but crack-addicted single teenage mother to take her baby home.

OBLIGATION 5: LOYALTY

This principle cautions professionals to avoid dual relationships, otherwise known as conflicts of interest. A dual relationship exists when one uses a consumer to meet a need of one's own, through a relationship that is separate from one's professional or work-related relationship. A relatively innocent, although still problematic, example of this would be hiring a consumer to perform some personal chore such as cleaning one's apartment or babysitting. A somewhat less innocent example would be selling, or allowing one's spouse to sell, items such as Tupperware to a consumer through a business activity that the professional or his or her spouse engages in that is separate from his or her primary role vis-à-vis the consumer. Perhaps the most reprehensible form of dual relationship of all (one prohibited in most ethical codes and, under certain circumstances, by criminal statutes as well) would be to enter into a sexual relationship—consensual or otherwise—with a consumer.

Dual relationships are often well intended, and for that reason are engaged in quite commonly (Herlihy and Corey, 1992). They are to be avoided, however, because they have a high likelihood of exploiting the consumer and because they place the professional in a situation in which his or her interests are likely to conflict with the consumer's. Such a situation occurred when a housekeeping aide—who was a regional Amway distributor in her spare time—persuaded a male consumer to join Amway under her sponsorship, thus giving her a percentage of any of his future earnings. While the professional in this case probably believed quite sincerely that she was doing the consumer a big favor, and while he quite enthusiastically believed that this was a great opportunity for him, it proved quite harmful to him by diverting attention and resources from pressing problems and becoming the latest in a long string of failure experiences. Even if the outcome of this dual relationship had been more successful for the consumer, however, it was grossly inappropriate for the professional to have used her position of trust with the consumer to essentially sell him on an activity in which she stood to gain something.

Even in their most innocent form (hiring a consumer to clean one's house or babysit), such relationships always have the potential of unwitting exploitation. For example, a consumer may not feel free to say no or ask for more money. The word *loyalty* is used to describe this principle because a dual relationship always involves some dilution of a professional's primary loyalty, namely, to the consumer's interests. Furthermore, even when nothing improper is really occurring, dual relationships are always viewed with suspicion by others.

One form of dual relationship that is quite common involves a situation in which a member of an agency's board of trustees (which, among other things, evaluates the performance of and sets compensation levels for the agency's director) is hired by the agency to perform some task (e.g., draw up architectural plans) within the board member's outside professional role. Such an arrangement is always suspect, because one can question whether the decision to award the contract or to approve the director's salary would have been made if either individual did not stand to gain (in the other relationship) from making such a decision.

Another common form of such a relationship occurs when someone performing a task for a consumer in one capacity (e.g., as a psychologist doing an assessment of the consumer) makes a referral to himself or herself for another activity (e.g., mental health counseling) in the professional's outside practice. Even if the professional is uniquely qualified to perform the task to which he or she is making the referral, such a referral is typically ethically inappropriate.

Clearly, special vigilance must be exercised to avoid letting "best intentions" lead to problematic relationships.

OBLIGATION 6: PROTECTION

This obligation involves the expectation that professionals will report to appropriate authorities colleagues who behave unethically, illegally, or who endanger the welfare and rights of consumers. One's obligation to the welfare of consumers should always be paramount and should take precedence over solidarity or friendship with coworkers or fear of consequences (ranging from social or physical ostracism to termination of employment) as a result of being a "whistle-blower."

This obligation is, obviously, frequently ignored, no less so in the disability field than in other fields, such as medicine, where practitioners are notoriously reluctant to pass judgment on their colleagues. Even in obvious cases of physical or sexual abuse, it is not uncommon for professionals to look the other way rather than run the risk of being seen as a "stool pigeon" by peers.

Professionals have a clear ethical (and, in some cases, legal) obligation to protect the rights and well-being of clients, by reporting to employers, state funding/regulatory agencies, or police any instances of abusive, neglectful, or unsafe treatment of clients.

OBLIGATION 7: AUTONOMY

Virtually all professional codes of conduct emphasize the consumer's right to freedom from coercion or undue influence by professionals. As noted in our discussion of paternalism in Chapter 4, professionals must respect a consumer's right to decide what is in his or her best interest, even when the professional has good reason to think that decision is flawed. In most professions, the professional's role is a delimited one, having freedom typically (but not always) to decide what method is most appropriate to achieve a goal that is typically determined by the consumer, in consultation with the professional. The consumer retains the right to terminate or withdraw from the relationship with the professional, as does the professional from the relationship with the consumer (except in cases where it would conflict with the diligence principle, by constituting a form of negligence).

This ideal notion of the autonomy principle is a difficult (even if quite relevant) one to apply to disability services. This is because people with disabilities are considered to have (and often do have) limitations of social and practical intelligence (Greenspan, 1979, 1981) that cause them to make poor decisions. For this reason, weak (i.e., benevolent) paternalism is more likely to characterize professional relations with people who have disabilities than with people who do not. To counteract this tendency, respect for autonomy of lifestyle choice is the central emphasis in classical (Nirjean) normalization theory, as discussed in Chapter 4.

Ironically, as is often the case in the disability field, abuse of the obligation to respect autonomy sometimes occurs through actions intended to comply with it. This is commonly the case when parents or guardians act as surrogate decision makers for their presumably incompetent child or ward. In one state (Dunaway et al., 1992), for example, parents have been given veto power over any decision to deinstitutionalize their adult son or daughter, even when the consumer strongly requests deinstitutionalization, and even when (as is often the case with people who are institutionalized) the parent has had virtually no contact with the son or daughter for decades. Furthermore, parents and other family members are often deferred to by professionals as if they had the authority of legal guardians even though the consumer (as is the case for most people with disabilities) may never have been declared legally incompetent.

The community revolution represents an attempt to change the nature of services to give the consumer more control over his or her life and lifespace. Thus, in the typical supported living arrangement, the professional drops in at prearranged times to provide whatever supports are needed (e.g., money management, activities of daily living), while respecting the fact that he or she is a guest in the consumer's home. This is presumed to contrast with the situation in group homes, in which various limits are set by staff on consumer freedoms, such as access to kitchen or food, and punitive consequences, such as loss of privileges, are meted out for violations of these limits. Taking the concept of autonomy one step further, there is even consideration being given to a voucher approach in which consumers would be able to fire a residential support agency when dissatisfied with services received and to transfer resources to another agency of their choosing.

Changing the ecology of the living setting alone, however, does not guarantee that the nature of the consumer-staff relationship will change in all respects. Thus, we are aware of one person in his own apartment who refers to his residential support person as "my boss," a characterization that is never corrected. We are also aware of a residential support person who gave instructions to a resident about when and where he could have sexual relations in his own apartment. While many professionals working in a support capacity do have an understanding of (and may even welcome) the need to adopt a more collaborative approach to consumers, others have apparently not gotten the message. And, of course, the continuation of a dependency on staff may be something craved and actively sought by consumers themselves.

At the core of the principle of autonomy is the principle of informed consent. For most people, the "information" part of informed consent is acquired through an education process and the ability to relate past experiences to a present situation. A challenge posed by the community revolution is to respect the autonomy of consumers while helping them to understand and evaluate the various options open to them. Sometimes, however, growth for people with disabilities, as for everyone else, can only come through experiencing the consequences of bad choices. An aspect much noted in normalization theory is the "dignity of risk," that is, allowing people with disabilities not only the right to make choices but also to experience the full range of consequences of those choices. Logical as this notion may be, however, it is difficult for human services professionals (who tend, to their credit, to be caring individuals) to allow people who are believed to lack age-typical decision-making skills to suffer consequences of their choices when those consequences (e.g., jail or serious harm) are sufficiently serious. In addition, the education process used to obtain informed consent is often seen by many professionals as burdensome.

OBLIGATION 8: DILIGENCE

This term refers to the obligation to make a reasonable effort to discharge one's responsibilities toward a consumer. As indicated by Bayles (1989), this may be the most violated of all of the universal obligations of professionals. An example of a lack of diligence would be a failure to send in forms requested to assist a consumer in getting financial entitlements. Another example would be failure to keep a promise to a consumer. A group home worker, for example, who promises to send presents to a consumer's family before a holiday is not exercising diligence if she fails to keep this promise until well past the agreed-upon mailing date.

When professionals undertake to do a job for a consumer, they are expected to do it to the best of their ability, and with an acceptable degree of effort. Ideally, one would expect all who work in the disability field to take pride in their work, and to have more than a "clock-watcher" mentality. This means that, on occasion, more than usual effort might be required to deal with some crisis or special problem. Such diligence is especially needed in such community revolution–inspired roles as job coach or independent-living support person.

Diligence involves not only making an effort to do a good job, but also doing things on time. In one case, a physical therapist was hired to evaluate the feeding practices in an agency serving persons with severe physical disabilities. The reason for the referral stemmed from a complaint from an advocacy organization to the effect that the staff feeding consumers lunch were too few in number, were improperly trained and supervised, and engaged in potentially unsafe practices such as feeding consumers too fast.

The professional doing the evaluation had a reputation for being an excellent evaluator but also a serious procrastinator, whose reports were typically submitted long after they had been promised. In this case, the report—recommending changes in feeding practices—was handed in three months late. Unfortunately, during this three-month period, one consumer contracted aspiration pneumonia and died, an outcome that might have been avoided if the recommended changes had been made earlier.

The obligation of diligence typically extends (as do all of these obligations) not only to individual workers but also to agencies and their administrators as well. Often, there is a reversal of priorities, as agency needs take precedence over consumer needs. An example of this occurred when an administrator of a sheltered workshop instructed a counselor not to recommend supported work (that would have been provided by another agency) for a consumer clearly ready for such a transition, in order to retain the funding attached to that individual. An opposite example of the same ethical violation occurred when an agency accepted funding, for similar reasons, for supported living placement of an individual clearly not ready for this level of independence.

OBLIGATION 9: HONESTY

This obligation refers to the absolute requirement that one resist the temptation to misappropriate ("steal") money or goods belonging to consumers, as well as to one's employer. Such behavior is prohibited by virtually all codes of professional conduct but also by general notions of morality (say, the Ten Commandments), as well as by criminal statutes.

Because people with disabilities are often limited in their ability to budget and keep track of their money, balance their checkbook, and shop independently, they often depend on support people to assist them with these activities. In supported living settings, such assistance may be given in an informal manner, without the controls and bookkeeping procedures that are likely to be in place in group homes. It is, therefore, much easier for support staff—who are often underpaid—to exploit clients financially if they are so inclined.

The obligation to resist any violation of a consumer's trust, by being scrupulously honest in handling the consumer's money or goods, is derived from the notion of a "fiduciary" (Sokolowski, 1991). Professionals are expected, in carrying out their role, to keep the consumer's interests always in the forefront, and to behave in a trustworthy manner.

OBLIGATION 10: RESPECT

This obligation requires professionals to deal with persons with disabilities in a manner that affirms their morale and feelings of self-worth. The history of relations with people with disabilities is one that emphasized defects and unworthiness. The community revolution, as mentioned in the opening section of Chapter 4, is based on a view of persons with disabilities as having the same value as everyone else. The obligation to treat consumers with respect is, therefore, central to the community revolution.

The requirement to treat consumers with respect is, as with the other nine obligations outlined in this chapter, a generic requirement driving all interactions between professionals and consumers (Koppelman, 1984). This requirement has special importance in the disability field. As suggested by Wolfensberger's (1983) attempt to rename normalization "social role valorization," actions that symbolize full valuation of persons with disabilities are at the heart of what normalization—and the community revolution—are all about.

One way in which advocates of the community revolution have attempted to indicate a newfound respect for the people they work with is through the development and use of terms considered nonoffensive to people with disabilities, and which connote that the persons being referred to have full membership in the human race. Thus, in the disability field, more than in most other fields, the terms one uses are seen as indicators of one's value orientation. An aspect of this process that is aggravating to some is the tendency for terms adopted as part of this revaluation process (and seen as great reforms when adopted) to become themselves repudiated a few years later as the moral equivalent of racism. Thus, the term *retardates* was adopted in the scientific literature in the 1960s as a humane alternative to the previous use of terms such as *idiot, imbecile,* and *moron,* but anyone using the term *retardates* today would be seen as both out-of-fashion and having very bad values. The basic point underlying the shift in terminology is the belief that terms that emphasize defects or deficiency are essentially dehumanizing, and reflect (or encourage) a devaluation of the persons referred to.

Thus, the new trend in terminology is generally referred to as "People First language" (Parker, 1982; Williams and Shoultz, 1982), that is, language that emphasizes the humanity of the people being referred to. People First is the name of a national self-advocacy organization for persons who were formerly institutionalized, and has as its unofficial logo a bell jar bearing the slogan "Label jars, not people." A requirement of People First language is that disability terms be used as nouns representing charac-teristics of people, rather than as nouns (or adjectives) representing catego-ries of people. Thus, it is standard practice to refer to "persons with (or who have) mental retardation" or "persons with autism," and so on; it is con-sidered unacceptable to refer to "mentally retarded persons," "the men-tally retarded," "schizophrenics," "the handicapped," and so on.

While the shift toward People First language has been largely accepted, in part because disability journal editors and book publishers now insist on it, there are some who resist this trend. For example, Haywood (1986) was the sole holdout in an edited volume, and his chapter contained a note indicating that he insisted on using the term *mentally retarded people* rather than the editors' preferred term *people with mental retardation.* Interestingly, Wolf Wolfensberger and the late Burton Blatt, two of the patron saints of the community revolution, have never given in to the pressure to use People First language, and their many books and articles continue to use terms such as *mentally retarded children.* This resistance has never been fully explained (Wolfensberger is reported to be working on a publication on the subject), but one can assume that it reflects both an unstated annoyance over the awkwardness of the new terminology as well as a stated refusal to be dictated to by self-appointed guardians of "political correctness" over a matter that they consider to be of peripheral impor-tance.

Of course, Wolfensberger himself brought the issue of terminology to the forefront in his emphasis on "image deviance" as a central theme of normalization theory. PASS and PASSING are both tools developed by Wolfensberger and colleagues (Wolfensberger and Glenn, 1975; Wolfens-berger and Thomas, 1973) to determine the extent to which service agen-cies conform in their practices to the requirements of the normalization principle. In these instruments, agencies are marked down if they describe themselves or their facilities in ways that might indicate some devaluation or condescension toward the persons served. Thus, it is considered poor form for an agency serving mainly adults with disabilities to include the word *children* in its title or building signs.

Similarly, Wolfensberger has pointed out that many programs for per-sons with disabilities use facility names (such as "Ranch") or action terms (*serviced* as opposed to *served*) that imply that those who reside or are served in these programs are not fully human. In addition to arguing for changes in the use of agency and building names, Wolfensberger and other leaders of the community revolution have pointed out the pervasiveness with which staff tend to refer to adults with disabilities as childlike (e.g., by commonly referring to them as "kids" or as "boys" and "girls"), a practice related to the tendency to decorate rooms with dolls and otherwise indicate that the service recipients are not competent or fully adult persons. (See Chapter 4 for a more in-depth discussion of this issue.)

On a micro level, there are many ways in which professionals can convey disrespect to persons with disabilities besides the terminology they use to characterize them. One way is to do a great deal of criticizing and focusing on deficiencies; effective and ethical professionals always make an effort to create a climate of affirmation and approval, one marked by warmth and positive reinforcement. While negative feedback and limit-setting are necessary on occasion, professionals should save these responses for when they are really needed, and should provide far more praise than punishment (Greenspan, 1985).

Abusive behaviors, whether verbal/psychological, physical, or sexual, are also obviously prohibited under the obligation to be respectful. It is unethical (and, depending on the behavior, illegal) to abuse clients. The use of aversive techniques under the rubric of behavior modification is considered by some rights-oriented authorities to constitute abuse (McGee et al., 1987), although others—emphasizing the utilitarian advantages of such techniques—argue that aversives have their place (Axelrod, 1990). Nevertheless, it is now recognized that there are clear limits on the methods that can legitimately be used to modify the behavior of persons with disabilities. Principled professionals are obligated to rely primarily on reinforcement techniques, using punishment sparingly and only when its need is clearly documented.

CONCLUSION

It is an essential feature of revolutions in any field to challenge those assumptions that guide the daily unreflective behavior of workers in that field. For workers in the disability field, a number of assumptions about people with disabilities have often guided their daily behavior. These assumptions are grounded in a global deficit model and lead to the belief that people with disabilities are invariably incompetent, dependent, morally ignorant, without impulse control, and in need of protection.

One of the more notable benefits of the community revolution has been to provide a growing number of living counterexamples to this set of assumptions. These counterexamples allow us to make new assumptions based on the achievements of people with disabilities who have demonstrated independence, competence, moral sensitivity, and intelligence. This new history lays the necessary experiential foundation to challenge the dominant paradigm.

In the disability field, ethical issues have been approached by agencies primarily from an individual rights perspective. Oversight function is typically provided through a committee structure that focuses on the violation of individual's rights rather than systemic issues. Information sharing about ethical issues is achieved primarily through what in many agencies is called "values training." Again, this values training tends to focus on language and attitudinal issues of staff people rather than on any systemic concerns.

Two critical elements have, to date, been missing from the traditional approach taken by agencies toward ethical issues: (1) accountability and (2) training. There are two features of the current service delivery system that make agency accountability for breaches of ethical conduct problematic. The first of these is the process of resource allocation. Typically, funding for disability services is in the control of large state or federal bureaucracies. It is in the nature of large bureaucracies to emphasize accountability on a micro level (e.g., compliance with specific regulations) and to pay less attention to the macro-level (e.g., decency of treatment) issues that may often have a greater impact on the daily lives of the people being served. It is hoped that state-level quality assurance mechanisms will begin to focus more on such decency of treatment issues, including the perspectives of people being served, than has been the case in the past.

Another barrier to accountability is the tendency of agencies to adopt politically correct operational principles but to have inadequate mechanisms for internal or external critique. For example, few agencies have specific safeguards for whistle-blowers. Fear of ostracism from peers and even dismissal is a powerful disincentive for direct care staff to call attention to ethical violations.

The best way to encourage ethical accountability may be to provide incentives to smaller units of service delivery (e.g., residential and vocational support agencies, and individual settings within those agencies) to create "ethical communities" in which all participants—staff and consumers—are encouraged to become ethically accountable.

Creating mechanisms for ethical accountability would also help to eliminate the second major impediment to ethical conduct: the lack of specific training and discourse involving everyday ethical matters. Staff training in most agencies typically focuses on concrete aspects of client care. This has the unintended consequence of separating people with disabilities further from the mainstream of society by focusing on their disability. For example, the second author has had experience with a training program that addresses issues of "client violence." Totally lacking from this training was any perspective on either the ecological context in which violence occurs (e.g., the tendency for such episodes to occur more often with particular staff-consumer dyads) or a sense of the commonality of reasons for violent behavior between people with disabilities and those without (e.g., when one's self-esteem or sense of autonomy is challenged, we all tend to "lose it"). Thus, what is often missing from training is a sense of the fundamental obligations of fairness, decency, and respect that should pervade our relationships with all human beings, regardless of their disability status.

In most professions, ethical codes of conduct are enforceable by a variety of mechanisms ranging from censure by one's peers to being barred from practice. The disability field has yet to adopt a unified professional identity that would allow for similar powerful mechanisms of enforcement. However, an integral part of this search for identity must be a commitment to a set of guiding ethical principles and the enforcement mechanisms that will give them life and meaning.

REFERENCES

American Psychological Association (1992). *Ethical principles of psychologists and code of conduct.* Washington, DC: Author.

Axelrod, S. (1990). Myths that (mis)guide our profession. In A.C. Repp and N.N. Singh (Eds.), *Perspectives on the use of nonaversive and aversive interventions for persons with developmental disabilities* (pp. 59–72). Sycamore, IL: Sycamore Publishing Co.

Bayles, M.D. (1989). *Professional ethics* (2nd ed.). Belmont, CA: Wadsworth.

Beauchamp, T.L., and Childress, J.F. (1983). *Principles of biomedical ethics.* New York: Oxford University Press.

Budd, K.S., and Greenspan, S. (1984). Mentally retarded mothers. In E.A. Blechman (Ed.), *Behavior modification with women.* New York: Guilford Press.

Dunaway, J., Norton, K., Bear, J., Greenspan, S., and Granfield, J. (1992). *Residential services for persons with mental retardation in the state of Washington.* Olympia, WA: Legislative Budget Committee.

Gorlin, R.A. (1990). *Codes of professional responsibility* (2nd ed.). Washington, DC: Bureau of National Affairs.

Greenspan, S. (1979). Social intelligence in the retarded. In N. Ellis (Ed.), *Handbook of mental deficiency: Psychological theory and research* (2nd ed.). Hillsdale, NJ: Erlbaum.

Greenspan, S. (1981). Defining choldhood social competence: A proposed working model. In B.K. Keogh (Ed.), *Advances in special education,* Volume 3 (pp. 1–39). Greenwich, CT: JAI Press.

Greenspan, S. (1985). An integrative model of caregiver discipline. *Child Care Quarterly, 14,* 30–47.

Greenspan, S. (1992). Parenting—the ultimate dignity of risk. *The Pappanikou Center Brief, 4,* 11–12.

Greenspan, S., and Negron, E. (1994). Ethical obligations of special services personnel. *Special Services in the Schools, 8,* 185–209.

Greenspan, S., Shoultz, B., and Weir, M.M. (1981). Social judgment and work success of mentally retarded adults. *Applied Research in Mental Retardation, 2,* 335–346.

Haywood, H.C. (1986). Commentary. In P.R. Dokecki and R.M. Zaner (Eds.), *Ethics of dealing with persons with severe disabilities.* Baltimore: Paul H. Brookes.

Herlihy, B., and Corey, G. (1992). *Dual relationships in counseling.* Alexandria, VA: American Counseling Association.

Howe, K.R., and Miramontes, O.B. (1992). *The ethics of special education.* New York: Teachers College Press.

Koppelman, L. (1984). Respect and the retarded: Issues of valuing and labeling. In L. Koppelman and S.C. Moskop (Eds.), *Ethics and mental retardation* (pp. 65–86). Dordrecht: D. Reidel Publishing Co.

McGee, J.J., Menolascino, F.J., Hobbs, D.C., and Menousek, P.E. (1987). *Gentle teaching: A non-aversive approach to helping persons with mental retardation.* New York: Human Sciences Press.

Parker, J.P. (1982). *We are people first: Our handicaps are secondary.* Portland, OR: Ednick.

Sokolowski, R. (1991). The fiduciary relationship and the nature of professions. In E.D. Pellegrino, R.M. Veatch, and J.P. Langan (Eds.), *Ethics, trust, and the professions: Philosophical and cultural aspects.* Washington, DC: Georgetown University Press.

Strike, K.A., and Soltis, J.F. (1985). *The ethics of teaching.* New York: Teachers College Press.

Williams, P., and Shoultz, B. (1982). *We can speak for ourselves.* London: Souvenir Press. Reprinted by University of Indiana Press.

Wolfensberger, W. (1983). Social role valorization: A proposed new term for the principle of normalization. *Mental Retardation, 21,* 234–239.

Wolfensberger, W., and Glenn, L. (1975). *Pass 3* (2nd ed.). Vol. I: *Handbook.* Vol. II: *Field Manual.* Toronto: National Institute on Mental Retardation.

Wolfensberger, W., and Thomas, S. (1983). *PASSING* (2nd ed.). Toronto: National Institute on Mental Retardation.

PART
II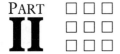

Implementation Issues

Whereas the first part explored conceptual, legislative, and ethical underpinnings of the paradigm of support, this part examines some of the implementation issues that organizations and systems should consider as they make the shift. The five chapters here address management issues, collaborative teamwork, the roles of parents and families, multicultural considerations, and the development of natural supports.

To provide appropriate forms of support to people with disabilities in the natural environments in which they live, work, and play, those who are providing support ultimately need to be supported themselves. The emergence of the support services approach will, therefore, require new methods of management and administration. These new methods emphasize flexibility rather than formalism and consumer well-being rather than conformity to internal or external regulation. In Chapter 6, James Gardner discusses the eclipse of conventional management structure and formalism and describes new management models. Included in his discussion are the anticipated changes that will shape the transition and influence the manner in which organizations are managed within the new support paradigm.

This shift away from management models based on efficiency to those that promote effectiveness is essential to implement current best practices in creating support services for people with disabilities. In Chapter 7, Beverly Rainforth, Michael Giangreco, Pamela Smith, and Jennifer York advocate for a team approach that assures a consumer focus, support from professionals to achieve consumer goals through the integration of services with one another, and the provision of services in the community settings where consumers prefer to live, work, attend school, and use their leisure time. Their chapter examines a collaborative team approach that extends beyond the traditional interdisciplinary model to be more consistent with current best practices and services for people with disabilities.

Viewing family members as equal partners to professionals and other service providers within an effective collaborative team is consistent with the views expressed by Bonnie Shoultz and Patricia McGill Smith in Chapter 8, on the shifting roles of parents and families. They review the history of parent activism and the impact that such activism has had on public policy and human service systems. The "parents' movement" grew out of parental resistance to commonly accepted professional practices such as parent-blaming and patronizing attitudes and beliefs on the part of professionals. Activist parents want relationships characterized by equal partnerships with professionals and professionals who are aware of and willing to admit the limits of their knowledge. Many federal and state laws and priorities are demanding the focused attention of families and consumers in overseeing the implementation of legislation and in influencing regulatory and funding processes. In the future it is expected that parents and other family members will become increasingly sophisticated in their understanding of the service systems they must turn to for assistance.

The growth of parent organizations also implies that professionals will be faced with the growing demand for culturally competent services and the need to develop creative strategies for meeting this demand. Typically, service delivery and professional training has encouraged the adoption of a dominant culture perspective. As a result, professionals may be inadvertently oppressive to people with disabilities with varied cultures, world views, and different perspectives. Generally speaking, services to consumers representing racial or ethnic minorities remain inadequate. In Chapter 9, on multicultural influences, Farah Ibrahim believes that the reason for this inadequacy is attributable to professional training models developed for mainstream Americans. She argues that it is now time to create service and training approaches that respect the cultural needs of consumers and their families. She proposes a multidimensional strategy and presents a model for assessment and intervention that includes a professional training approach to enhance cultural sensitivity.

The field continues to shift to the support framework with its emphasis on individual choices and flexibility. Typically, these services are provided through paid supports and/or professionals. It is expected, however, that individuals and/or their families will also have access to various natural supports, which include family, friends, neighbors, and others who subscribe to and promote many of the same values, beliefs, and traditions as the consumer and his or her family. The development of such natural supports is an essential component of the growth of the support framework represented by the new paradigm. The assessment of natural supports in community services is the focus of Chapter 10, by Robert Schalock. His chapter includes a discussion of the basic principles of natural support, a description of a model for assessing natural supports, and a discussion of the implications of using natural supports. Schalock believes that natural supports are attractive because they are consistent with the field's emphasis on community integration and quality of life. He describes a three-step model that includes an inventory of the natural supports available to the person, a determination of the discrepancy between needed and available supports targeting needed additional supports, and ways to assess the needed supports.

6 □□□ □□□ □□□

Maintaining Quality and Managing Change: Administration in Transition

James F. Gardner

INTRODUCTION

Administration in the field of rehabilitation, disability, and health services organization has traditionally focused on the attainment of organizational goals by working through people and the utilization of other resources in formal organizational settings. However, as organizational goals, physical settings, and administrative structures change, the purpose, content, and process of management and administration will undergo a transformation. The changes in individual disciplines will both cause and reflect changes in the management of rehabilitation programs.

Valerie Bradley and James Knoll (1995, Chapter 1 in this book) have pointed to the shift from institutionalization and segregation to a model of deinstitutionalization and the developmental model in the 1970s. It is important to note, however, that the major characteristics of the community integration paradigm—the developmental model and behaviorism—originated in the institution and were adapted by community programs as state-of-the-art practice.

This same adaptation process took place in management practice. Management models and practices were taken from the large institution, applied to smaller residential settings in the community, then to group homes, and finally to supervised apartment living programs (Smull, 1989).

These models and practices incorporated defined hierarchies of authority; centralized decision making; maintained an emphasis on written policy, procedure, rules, and documentation; and transferred bureaucratic personnel management and staff supervision practices. This mechanistic orientation is associated with a high degree of formalism in terms of internal policy and procedure and external regulation (Gardner and Chapman, 1991).

These mechanistic management models and practices remained functional because the goals, models, and structures for community habilitation and rehabilitation programs did not undergo any radical change. Residential and work preparation programs took place in smaller, community-based settings, but there was no significant change in the function of the programs that would require a change in the form of organization or management.

The recent emergence of the support service model does require a new form of organization and management. Family support services, supported employment, and supported integrated living evolved in the 1980s as new program models. But the new program models will be constrained by outdated organizational models and management practices that are characterized by high degrees of formalism. The mechanistic management models that evolved in large residential and rehabilitation facilities and that were adapted in community service programs will not facilitate the development of support service programs, the extension of informal support networks, and consumer decision making.

THE ECLIPSE OF STRUCTURE AND FORMALISM

Traditional quality assurance systems have incorporated an imposing array of regulation, policy, and procedures. These comprehensive regulatory systems are offered as a method for protecting "vulnerable populations." People with significant disabilities are often vulnerable and need adequate protection from abuse and neglect. As such, the new community integration paradigm must contain the necessary systems and individual protections.

However, the potential for abuse and neglect is only one reason for the pervasive regulations and rules that govern both institutional and community programs. The existing systems of regulations are also artifacts of a previous management and administrative system that operated large institutions and public bureaucracies. The continued utilization of mechanistic management models and practices is well illustrated by examining the extent of formalism in community-based services and supports.

The degree of formalization in an organization is determined by a number of variables. The extent of rules, procedure, and regulation is related to contextual variables such as large size, complex technology (and the possibility of significant risk), critical and uncertain outside environments (Daft, 1988). Nuclear power plants, blood banks, and university hospitals have more rules than street vendors and owner-operated businesses.

During the past fifteen years the term *high reliability organization* has been applied to organizations in which errors of decision or accidents can have catastrophic consequences. Air traffic control systems, petrochemical plants, and nuclear power plants incorporate internal control systems that stress reliability more than efficiency or flexibility (Perrow, 1984). Large residential institutions and community service programs have often attempted to increase reliability and predictability through an emphasis on formalism. Formalism is often a key attribute of mechanistic organizations. The term *mechanistic* is applied to organizations that are characterized by regulations, rules, policy and procedure, centralization, and a clear hierarchy of authority (Burns and Stalker, 1961).

Tight control typically exists in stable environments with routine technology, large size, and an emphasis on efficiency. Mechanistic management controls include functional structure, bureaucratic control, formal information and reporting systems, and generally infrequent innovation. The decision-making process is characterized by rational analysis, and there is an articulated goal of cooperation between units.

Henry Mintzberg's (1989) analysis of an overly mechanistic organization emphasizes regulations and rules as attributes of the "machine organization." The goal of the machine organization is to eliminate surprises and uncertainty. The operating work is routine and the work processes are highly standardized. Tasks are generally simple and repetitive.

The structure of machine organizations includes large-size operating units, relatively centralized power for decision making, strong administrative structures, and sharp distinction between line and staff. Mintzberg's characteristics of the machine organization include the following (pp. 134, 136–137):

- Staff analysts who do the standardizing emerge as a key part of the structure.
- Rules and regulation permeate the entire system.
- Power clearly rests at the top.
- Hierarchy and chain of authority are paramount concepts.
- Attempts are made to eliminate all possible uncertainty so the organization can run smoothly and without interruption.
- The machine organization is a structure with an obsession—namely, control.

- The emphasis on control leads to closed systems that become immune to external influence.

The bureaucratic machine model also exists in a modified form as a professional bureaucracy. Professional bureaucracies differ from machine models in the decentralization of power among the various professionals in the organization. In addition, professional norms and rules of behavior can substitute for the rules and regulations of the organization itself. The impact on individuals with disabilities and support staff, however, is much the same for both bureaucratic models. The standardization of behavior resulting from professional norms produces the same type of conformity and control achieved by the rules of the machine bureaucracy (Heffron, 1989).

The bureaucratic machine and professional models do enable organizations to develop standardized responses to critical situations. Hospitals, services for people with disabilities, and fire departments operate as machine and professional bureaucratic organizations.

The limitation of machine organizations, however, is found in their very success. As performance systems, they are designed for repetition and productivity. Performance systems are not designed for adaptation, problem solving, or innovation (Segal, 1974; Skrtic, 1987).

Organizations serving people with disabilities have organized as machine (and professional) organizations in an attempt to minimize risk. The machine organization is most notable in large residential centers or sheltered vocational settings. However, as community-based services have evolved as alternatives to institutional programs, they have retained many of the characteristics of machine organizations.

THE ALTERNATIVE OF ORGANIC MANAGEMENT MODELS

The alternative to machine and professional bureaucracies is organizational design based on organic controls. Organic control models would fit the changing and nonroutine environments offered by informal support programs and in integrated service programs where task and technology will change with individual needs. Organic control models are associated with small size and effectiveness rather than efficiency (Daft, 1988).

Organic control models exist in uncertain environments where the task and technology are not repetitive and routine. Organic models have decentralized structures and control behaviors by management of values, norms, and tradition rather than rules alone. There is a stress on face-to-face communication and frequent innovation that may be driven from the bottom rather than the top. Decision making may allow for more trial and error and the organization tolerates more conflict between units (Robbins, 1990).

The organic management form would stress employee decision making and interaction rather than formalized policy and procedure (Koontz and Weihrich, 1990). As such it would decentralize decision-making responsibility, increase consumer autonomy, and decrease the relative role of the professional.

Mechanistic and organic systems are models of organizational structure. In practice, few organizations incorporate all the characteristics of either an organic or mechanistic system. However, the shift in paradigms as noted elsewhere in this book does suggest a movement from the mechanistic to the organic control system. In addition, the transformation in services and supports is consistent with the emerging trends in management. Rosabeth Moss Kanter (1989, p. 84) notes that managers are "watching hierarchy fade away and the clear distinctions of title, task, department, and even corporation, blur."

Kanter identifies five characteristics of the new managerial environment:

1. The pathways for exercising influence and making change have increased.
2. The use of influence is shifting from the vertical to the horizontal plane, from hierarchy to peer networks.
3. The separation of supervisor and worker is decreasing, particularly in terms of access to information, influence, and control over work.
4. External coalitions and networks are sources of internal power.
5. Career mobility is increasing, but the routes are more ambiguous.

The shift in paradigms in services to people with disabilities and the increasing emphasis on commitment to communities and families, an emphasis on human relationships, person-centered programming, and choice and control will require acknowledgment and adaptation of some of the characteristics of the new management models. The management literature identifies some of the variables that must be considered in the transition from a model of mechanistic control to one of organic control.

TRANSITION IN MANAGEMENT MODELS

Smaller, community-based support and service agencies connected to informal systems of natural support will exist in changing environments, and the resulting internal management system to cope with the environmental uncertainty will be looser, more free-flowing, and adaptive. The organic management form would stress employee decision making and interaction rather than formalized policy and procedure (Koontz and Weihrich, 1990).

Community-based programs connected to the informal support service network will decentralize decision-making responsibility. Increased consumer autonomy and support networks will decrease the relative role of the professional and increase the responsibilities of staff in dispersed program settings, informal support providers, and families. Professionals are already taking on new roles as orchestrators, coordinators, and facilitators of dialogue within support systems. Staffing patterns currently include parents and volunteers exercising leadership responsibilities (Kagan et al., 1987).

This decentralization and delegation of authority will occur only if there is a corresponding increase in management control and information feedback systems. Managers can delegate only when there is a sufficient information control system that allows them to monitor the delegated responsibilities. The management control system in the open system community-based option must be flexible, practical, and applicable to each individual manager. The management communication system in place today relies on occasional observation, written logs, records, and documentation. It is more subjective than objective, and exceptions to expectation form the basis for action.

The management information systems of the future, especially in the decentralized service system, will be based on face-to-face contact and computerized information systems. Decision processes and management structures will be transformed as organizations move from using data to using information (data that have been analyzed) (Cetron, Rocha, and Luckins, 1988). Managers will have access to habilitation program information to determine the effectiveness of programs. Staff and individuals with disabilities will communicate, schedule, and report through integrated information systems. The future management control system will stress the measurement and correction of individual and group staff performance to ensure that organizational objectives (and the plans to attain them) are accomplished (Cain and Taber, 1987).

Current trends and anticipated changes can be analyzed by examining some of the contextual dimensions and structural variables that will shape the transitions. Contextual dimensions describe the organizational setting that influences the choice of internal control processes. Key contextual dimensions (Daft, 1988) that will influence the manner in which organizations are managed include:

- *Environment*   From an organizational perspective, the shift in paradigms will result in people with disabilities living, working, and socializing in natural environments. Natural environments are less certain and less controlled than organizationally directed environments. However, from the perspective of the individual with a disability, the degree of control in natural settings will be greatly increased.

- *Technology*   The technology employed in providing supports and services to people with disabilities in integrated, natural communities will vary by individual and environment. From the organizational perspective, individual choice, multiple environments, and an increasing emphasis on supports will greatly expand the range and diversity of technology employed in the field of rehabilitation.
- *Size*   The size of organizational units in the field of rehabilitation has decreased and will continue to decrease as supports and services are integrated into natural settings. Instead of organizing services for many individuals in congregate settings, individualized supports and services will be provided to people in decentralized and geographically dispersed settings. This will result in a less concentrated focus on paid organizational staff.
- *Goals*   Organizationally, goals will be redirected from organizational efficiency to effectiveness in providing supports and services to individuals to enable them to accomplish their own goals in community life.

Structural variables and internal outcomes refer to the manner in which the organization is managed given the particular mix of contextual dimensions.

- *Structure*   The shift in paradigms is resulting in service and support systems with less formalization, specialization, and standardization. Less formalization is evident in the amount of written documentation, policy, and procedure that is tolerated in support services and service programs in integrated community settings. Specialization, defined as the degree to which organizational tasks are subdivided into separate jobs, and standardization, defined as the extent to which similar work activities are performed in a uniform manner, are both decreasing as the focus of service and supports shifts from institutional to integrated community settings.
- *Communication and feedback*   There will be a shift from formal information systems to face-to-face communication. The implementation of formal information systems in integrated community settings and natural support systems will be restricted. Communication, monitoring, and feedback will be accomplished by advocates and case managers.
- *Control*   The methods of organizational control will shift from bureaucratic forms of hierarchy, rules, regulation, policy, and procedure to clan controls of shared values, commitment, and shared traditions. This will present the public sector with a major dilemma. How can it exercise its responsibility to ensure health and safety, prevent abuse and neglect, and maximize the taxpayers' investment without resorting to mechanistic forms of organizational control?
- *Innovation*   The degree of innovation in the provision of support services and in offering services in integrated community settings will increase

dramatically. By definition, mechanistic control systems are designed to control and limit innovation.

- *Decision making*   There will be a dramatic shift in the locus and methodology of decision making. Individuals with disabilities will be making more and more decisions about their own lives. In addition, trial and error as a decision-making process, rather than rational analysis by a professional team, will become more pronounced.
- *Decentralization*   The decentralization of decision making and hierarchy or authority will continue to erode as the decision-making responsibility is assumed by people with disabilities and their natural support systems.

NEW METHODS OF ORGANIZING

Developing an organic service model requires attention to five variables:

1. A customer-driven service system
2. Broadened responsibility for decision making
3. Experiential learning for staff and people with disabilities
4. Standards as performance indicators for staff and organization
5. Leadership and management by mission, vision, and norms

A Customer-Driven Service System

The development of organic management systems begins with a customer-driven system. But the provider must first identify the customer. At various times the customer can be the state agency that provides operating funds, the licensing and certifying agency that permits operation, parent and advocacy groups that can exert pressure and influence, or people with disabilities. This identification is critical because organizing to serve the funding source is far different than organizing to meet the goals of people with disabilities.

Service providers must develop services that directly and immediately address individual goals and preferences rather than professionally designated problems or needs. Services should be goal driven and not anchored in an individual's limitations, deficits, or problems. In reality, most people derive their goals after considering their interests and their abilities. Most people with limited aptitude for mathematics would not entertain a career as a mathematician. An interest in the ocean and biology might cause them to pursue work in oceanography.

In addition, providers need to pay attention to the behaviors of individuals. The nonverbal communication in behavior can indicate boredom, apathy, and lack of interest in particular services (Donnellan et al., 1988). Individuals should choose to participate in services that are goal oriented. Placement in a training program to address a need identified by staff is not a consumer-driven service. Individuals placed in such training programs may exhibit seemingly dysfunctional behaviors in an attempt to communicate dissatisfaction (Weiss, 1990).

The customer-friendly service system is one whose basic design ensures customer satisfaction. The physical facility, the policies, procedures, and communication should be based on customer preferences (Albrecht and Zemke, 1985).

The focus on the customer inverts the organizational hierarchy. The responsibility of the executive director and senior staff is to ensure that middle managers and service associates have the necessary skills, information, and supports to deliver the services that customers expect. The organizational hierarchy, then, exists to meet the needs of the employees who are serving the customer. The hierarchy becomes an enabler and a support; employees serving people with disabilities are the customers of the hierarchy. Treating colleagues and "subordinates" as customers flattens the hierarchy (Holtry, 1991). The satisfaction of coworkers and "subordinates" with the support received from the hierarchy becomes an important quality indicator in the organization.

Broadened Responsibility for Decision Making

The method for nonroutine problem resolution in the machine organization is direct supervision. Specialization, standardization, hierarchy, and narrow functionalism inhibit informal communication (Mintzberg, 1989). The tradition of interdisciplinary process, while promoting interaction between disciplines, pertains to formal interaction within the context of a plan.

In a customer-driven organization, the impetus for change will come from what has been considered the bottom of the organization. Employees will lack the direct supervisory control over key processes. Staff will need to develop a greater tolerance for ambiguity as they begin to conceptualize new consumer-driven outcomes for service (Albrecht and Zemke, 1985). The cooperation and information exchange in the interdisciplinary process has to be extended beyond the annual team meeting and incorporated as an operating norm.

Decentralized problem solving around consumer needs will require access to information and a broader view of the organization and its expectations of the customer. Organic management models will mandate that staff make decisions and managers will serve as mentors and teachers for staff. Leaders emerge as they learn to influence and persuade without direct authority (Bennis, 1989).

Above all, the middle managers must redefine their roles from supervisor to mentor and coach. This requires on-the-job, day-to-day communicating to the staff the expectations and visions of the organization and providing daily feedback on collective performance. This emphasis on the middle manager shifts the focus of attention from how well the new employee is performing to how well the coach is teaching. How the new employee performs often depends on the capability of the coach. The weakest link in the current service delivery system is the lack of a regular feedback process for the people providing services to the customer (Albrecht and Zemke, 1985; Rice and Rosen, 1991).

The typical support and service programs provide few opportunities for systematic feedback. One-to-one pre-service and in-service training are limited. Feedback from supervisors is generally related to performance of duties and not the specifics of teaching and mentoring new staff.

The Focus on Experiential Learning

The focus on a customer-driven service system and broadened responsibility for decision making will cause some initial discomfort for professionals. They will be called on to perform tasks for which they have neither training nor an organized empirical base from which to make decisions about professional practice. More important, the unambiguous ends toward which professional practice is directed, and the stable institutional context for undertaking the process to accomplish those ends, will be confused. Complexity, uncertainty, and value conflicts will cloud the ends of professional practice.

The technical rationality associated with academic preparation and the norms of professional practice must allow for professional reflection in action (Schon, 1983). This requires an adaptation of the professional knowledge to individual circumstances and situations associated with the person with the disability. Professionals will describe their work less in terms of discipline process and empiricism and more in terms of "experience, trial and error, intuition, and muddling through" (Schon, 1983, p. 43). New situations become times of surprise and confusion when alternative solutions are found by reflecting on knowledge and experiences from the past.

This model of reflection in action is contrary to the dominant model of professionalization and the operation of the professional bureaucracy. Instead of producing objective knowledge, professionalization unrandomizes the complexities and ambiguities of practice and produces standard programs that represent the traditions and conventions of a particular professional subculture (Kuhn, 1970; Schein, 1972; Skrtic, 1987). This leads directly to the pigeonholing phenomenon, wherein the professional defines the perceived consumer need in terms of the defined standard programs.

The role of the reflective practitioner has application for staff development. The focus on teaching and mentoring emphasizes learning through experience. The knowledge gained through experience in problem solving produces new insights and leadership skills (Kouzes and Posner, 1987). The teaching and mentoring then becomes a process for developing leadership within the organization. In addition to serving as teacher and mentor, the middle manager is also a source of future leadership talent within the organization. Warren Bennis (1989, p. 182) has noted the need for "an organization's commitment to providing its potential leaders with opportunities to learn through experience in an environment that permits growth and change."

The organic model rests on the premise that organizations can learn, adapt, and change. Information and decision making are decentralized. The responsibility for the future of the organization rests not at the top of the hierarchy but within the organization. The answers to problems are found throughout the organization. People with disabilities, employees, and the organization are part of a problem-solving and learning experience.

However, experiential learning on the part of employees and individuals with disabilities means that senior management must push decision making down to people with disabilities and employees who directly provide supports and/or services. In service settings, including those in human services, empowerment requires the replacement of highly standardized and mechanistic decision process with looser structures that enable consumers and employees to individualize their own skills and approaches (Rowitz, 1991). Robert Waterman (Albrecht and Zemke, 1985, p. 73) has observed that "When managers guide instead of control, the sky's the limit on what people can accomplish."

The Role of Standards

Standards for services define the expected outcomes of service for people with disabilities and the level of performance for employees and the organization to achieve those outcomes. Standards are the measures of quality. The standards communicate to employees expectations for their level of performance. Outcome standards focus attention on outcomes of service and supports for people with disabilities. People with disabilities should both choose and be satisfied with the outcomes of supports and service. Outcomes achieved by and for the organization cannot substitute for consumer outcomes as the measure of quality. Measures of organizational effectiveness and efficiency such as numbers of people assessed and number of people placed in competitive employment do not address outcomes of quality for the individual.

Standards must reflect quality from the customer's point of view: no other point of view is as important. Management of human services, like management in the rest of the U.S. service industry, must begin with an identification of the customer's experience with that service. The organization develops strategies to monitor the customer's experience with the provision of services. Standards that do not reflect the customer's view of quality will focus on internal agency measures of productivity and/or process. These typically include the number of people served, cost reduction, short-term profit, or the number of people placed.

Process standards function as organizational norms. They define the manner in which individuals, programs, and organizations perform to produce outcomes of quality for the individual. Process standards communicate to staff the policies and procedures for performing assessments, conducting team meetings, or presenting behavior intervention programs to a human rights committee. They become the informal guides to individual and organizational behavior.

Outcomes for the individual rather than organization process provide the best criteria for determinations of quality. In addition, the emphasis on process enlarges the role of the professional in the habilitation and rehabilitation process. As in health care, process measures will "give primacy to the practitioners who are the high priests in charge of its technical mysteries and who also generate and control the information needed to assess it" (Donabedian, 1982, p. 118).

Finally, organizations can use standards to enhance rather than assure quality. A focus on quality assurance leads to a preoccupation with compliance with the full range of variables that impact service quality. Standards then become the basis for inspection and enforcement. Success depends on demonstrating compliance with more than the minimum set or number of standards.

As methods of enhancement, standards focus attention on the limited number of variables that account for the significant outcomes for individuals served by the organization. For example, the Pareto Principle indicates that in a cluster of related variables, the most important variables are only a small proportion of the total (Rowe et al., 1989). In the vernacular, "20 percent of the employees do 80 percent of the work," or "10 percent of the customers are responsible for 90 percent of the firm's income." In terms of quality, 20 percent of the variables account for 80 percent of the organization's quality outcomes.

A quality enhancement orientation stresses the importance of the first 20 percent of the variables. Quality assurance, in contrast, focuses on compliance with the full range of variables. As a result, attention is focused on those variables that have minimal impact on individuals and the organization. As indicated in Table 6-1, a focus on variables 1 through 4 accounts for 95 percent of the outcome. A continued focus on variables 5 through 10 will address only 5 percent of the outcome. Standards should focus attention on the variables that make a difference in outcomes for the individual.

The variables that account for individual outcomes are expressed in a set of performance standards. There must be a match between the perception of customer expectation and the actual specifications for the delivery of services and supports. Zeithaml, Parasuraman, and Berry (1990) have identified the following four factors that influence quality specifications for services.

1. *Management is committed to service quality.* This commitment is present when the management treats service quality as a key strategic goal. Indicators of commitment might include the following:

- Organizational units have resources to improve service quality.
- There are formal internal programs for enhancing the quality of services.

TABLE 6-1   The Pareto Principle and Quality Concepts

Variable	% of Quality Outcome	Cumulative %
1	60	60
2	20	80
3	10	90
4	3	93
5	2	95
6	2	97
7	1	98
8	0.8	98.8
9	0.7	99.5
10	0.5	100

- Staff who enhance the quality of services for individuals are more likely to be rewarded than staff who achieve other goals.
- Senior managers and the board of directors are committed to delivering quality services.

2. *Management has the perception that quality is feasible.*   There is a belief that customer expectations can be met. Innovation and creativity are the keys to fulfilling expectations. The organization is ready to alter the way it does business to meet expectations of customers. Feasibility indicators include the following:

- The organization has the capability of meeting customer expectations.
- Existing operating systems maximize the attainment of customer expectations.
- Given a choice, the customer would choose your service because he or she believes that expectations will be met.
- The organization is willing to alter policy and procedure to better meet the needs of customers.

3. *There is consistency in the provision of services.*   Customer expectations result in consistent services across program environments. Indicators of consistency include the following:

- Customer expectations direct all services.
- All employees are knowledgeable about individual consumer expectations.
- The organization implements formal programs to promote coordination and consistency with other service programs and with specialized and generic services and supports.

4. *Service quality goals result from identification of consumer standards and expectations rather than organization standards.*   In some instances, organizations design, measure, and monitor internal process standards that consumers may not care about and overlook those standards of quality that consumers consider important. The quality standards have several characteristics:

- The standards are specific and indicate to employees the expected measures of process and outcome.
- Employees understand and accept the standards.
- The standards focus on key variables that account for the most important outcomes for consumers.

- Standards are measured and reviewed, and regular feedback is provided to consumers and employees.
- Employee performance improve when standards are challenging but realistic; unrealistically high standards frustrate staff.

The Role of Mission

The mission statement connects the services of the organization with the outcomes for the individual. A *mission statement* is a concise definition of the organization's purpose. Mission statements are based on values, reflect expectations for people with disabilities, and project a vision for the current and future state of the organization (Pfeiffer, Goodstein, and Nolan, 1986). Mission statements address three service variables: who is the customer, what are the services/supports, and how are they provided.

Values are the building blocks of service organizations. Values are statements of fundamental beliefs that guide daily decision making. Organizations, like individuals, are guided by basic values. Organizational values may be consistent or they can clash. Sometimes the organizational values are well defined and acknowledged; other times the values are not discussed and operate in the informal organizational system (French and Bell, 1984). In extreme cases the values that exist in the informal system clash with the articulated values of the formal system.

Organizational values change. The alterations in values result from the growth patterns of organizations, changes outside the organization in legislation, financing, and the demands and expectations of society. The shifting values of organizations require a periodic reexamination of the guiding principles of organizations. The senior management of an organization can conduct a values audit to identify the formal values, the values of the informal organizational system, and the congruity between the two.

One study (Dalkey et al., 1972) revealed that students at the University of California at Los Angeles identified the following ranked values that contributed to their quality of life (Rubinstein, 1975):

1. Love
2. Self-respect
3. Peace of mind
4. Sex
5. Challenge
6. Social acceptance
7. Accomplishment

8. Individuality
9. Involvement
10. Well-being (economic, physical)
11. Change
12. Power (control)
13. Privacy

Another group study conducted by the American Academy of Arts and Sciences ranked the values expected to be most important in the year 2000. The values were as follows:

1. Privacy
2. Equality
3. Personal integrity
4. Freedom
5. Law and order
6. Pleasantness of environment
7. Social adjustment
8. Efficiency and effectiveness of organizations
9. Rationality
10. Education
11. Ability and talent

The development of mission statements often begins with the values audit, in which the members of the organization identify the guiding values and principles. This listing is appended to the mission statement and reviewed annually.

In addition to values and guiding principles, organizations define their assumptions about the people for whom they are delivering services and supports. These expectations are extensions of both individual and organizational values. These assumptions dictate how staff and organizations view the future for people with disabilities. High expectations for individuals result in the provision of opportunities for development. Opportunity, in turn, enables individuals to achieve future outcomes. Low expectations lead to vicious circles in which limited opportunity causes low achievement and the low achievement confirms the original belief in low expectation.

The final step in developing the mission statement is to define the future direction of the organization. The organization examines the external environment, its own values and assumptions about people with disabilities, and its current and projected resources to define the future direction that best matches the expectations and goals of the people with disabilities who will receive services and supports.

The mission statement links organizational goals and objectives, resources, and priorities with outcomes for people with disabilities. A functional mission statement brings clarity and commitment to organizational purpose. The mission statement enables the organization to focus attention on the outcomes for individuals rather than internal measures of productivity, efficiency, or effectiveness. Without a strong mission statement that links organizational goals with expectations of consumers, the agency frequently focuses on the internal measures and becomes more and more efficient at accomplishing the wrong outcomes.

The Role of Leadership

Quality is a leadership responsibility that requires the presence of mission and standards. The mission enables the leader to articulate a purpose, and the standards define an expected level of personal and organizational performance. Neither mission nor standards directly result in quality of services. Rather, leaders motivate employees to achieve performance standards and accomplish missions.

There is a vast literature on leadership theory and research (Stogdill, 1974), but the link between leadership and quality of services is more recent. Peters and Austin (1985) described the leaders who moved other individuals to innovate and improve quality. J. M. Juran (1985, 1986) defined quality as the responsibility of the top-level management. W. Edward Deming's (1982) 14 Points represent a plan for top-level management to increase quality.

Leadership is perhaps even more important in the service sector. Zeithaml, Parasuraman, and Berry (1990) note that "The key is genuine service leadership at all levels of an organization—leadership that offers the direction and inspiration to sustain committed servers. Managing is not enough" (p. 4). They identified the four major characteristics of service leaders:

1. *Service vision* Service quality is the key factor in the organization's future.
2. *High standards* They aspire to legendary standards since good services may not be good enough to differentiate their organization from the competition.
3. *In-the-field leadership style* They are out in the field coaching, praising, and listening.
4. *Integrity* They do the right thing even when it may be costly or inconvenient.

In their study of quality and the service economy, Karl Albrecht and Ron Zemke (1985, p. 168) also define quality of service as a "top management issue." Service management is described as a top-down, whole-organization approach that starts with the nature of the customer's experience and creates strategies and tactics that maximize the quality of that experience. In the service economy, quality is determined by customer perception. The customer's perception of the service experience alone is the key to quality.

Albrecht and Zemke (1985) recognize that leading and managing in the service arena is different than managing the production of a commodity. Leading and managing in the service sector requires a greater tolerance for ambiguity and an ability to cope with less than complete control in key processes. It requires an appreciation of people-related skills and a capacity to deal with constant change.

Effective leadership will also require a recognition that sources of motivation are changing. Old bureaucratic incentives are being replaced by motivation based on entrepreneurial opportunity (Kanter, 1989), and several of these have applicability in the field of rehabilitation. People are motivated when they can connect their work with the mission of the organization. The sense of importance motivates. In addition, greater control over the pace and content of work adds motivation. Finally, the opportunity to learn new skills and to apply new insights based on reflection on experience, and on the enhanced recognition and reputation for successful accomplishment and leadership, will motivate rehabilitation managers.

CONCLUSION

The emergence of a new paradigm for the provision of supports and integrated community service will require new methods of management and administration. But management and administration may not be enough. In the rapid evolution of new program forms and technologies, managers and administrators will have to stay in front of the change curve. They can do so only by leading the change.

Leadership in the field of rehabilitation will face the same issues and concerns confronting service industries today. Leading and managing the coordinated support system in integrated community settings will require new values, skills, and insights. Leadership is the key element for linking new management models, new forms of mentoring and supervision, and quality outcomes for people with disabilities.

The role of leadership in human services will be particularly important in the transition to community membership and functional support. The traditions of management in human services are derived from the machine organization. Leaders will have to develop new organic forms of organization that both protect individuals from abuse and exploitation and promote the quality of life.

REFERENCES

Albrecht, K., and Zemke, R. (1985). *Service America: Doing business in the new economy.* New York: Warner Books.

Bennis, W. (1989). *On becoming a leader.* Reading, MA: Addison-Wesley.

Bradley, V.J., and Knoll, J. (1995). Shifting paradigms in services to people with disabilities. In O.C. Karan and S. Greenspan (Eds.), *Community rehabilitation services for people with disabilities.* Boston: Butterworth–Heinemann.

Burns, T., and Stalker, G.M. (1961). *The management innovation.* London: Tavistock.

Cain, E., and Taber, F. (1987). *Educating disabled people for the 21st century.* Boston: Little, Brown.

Cetron, M., Rocha, W., and Luckins, R. (1988). Into the 21st century: Long-term trends affecting the United States. *The Futurist,* July–August, 29–39.

Daft, R.L. (1988). *Organization theory and design.* New York: West Publishing.

Dalkey, N., Rourke, D., Lewis, R., and Snyder, D. (1972). *Studies in the quality of life: Delphi and decision making.* Lexington, MA: D.C. Heath.

Deming, W.E. (1982). *Quality, productivity, and competitive position.* Cambridge: MIT Center of Advanced Engineering Study.

Donabedian, A. (1982). *Explorations in quality assessment and monitoring.* Volume 11: *The criteria and standards of quality.* Ann Arbor, MI: Health Administration Press.

Donnellan, A.M., LaVigna, G.W., Negri-Shoultz, N., and Fassbender, L.L. (1988). *Progress without punishment: Effective approaches for learners with behavior problems.* New York: Teachers College Press.

French, W.L., and Bell, C.H. (1984). *Organization development: Behavioral science interventions for organization development.* Englewood Cliffs, NJ: Prentice-Hall.

Gardner, J.F., and Chapman, M.S. (1991). Staffing issues in the early 21st century: Labor supply, program models, and technology. In L. Rowitz (Ed.), *Mental retardation in the year 2000.* New York: Springer-Verlag.

Heffron, F. (1989). *Organization theory and public organizations: The political connection.* Englewood Cliffs, NJ: Prentice-Hall.

Holtry, J. (1991). Total quality control: A breakthrough approach to teamwork. In Y.K. Shetty and V.M. Buehler (Eds.), *The quest for competitiveness: Lessons from America's productivity and quality leaders.* New York: Quorum Books.

Juran, J.M. (1985). Catching up: How the West is doing. *Quality Progress*, November 1985, 18–22.

Juran, J.M. (1986). The quality trilogy. *Quality Progress*, August, 19–24.

Kagan, S., Powell, D., Weissbourd, B., and Zigler, E. (1987). Past accomplishments: Future challenges. In S. Kagan, D. Powell, B. Weissbourd, and E. Zigler (Eds.), *America's family support programs: Perspectives and prospects* (pp. 365–380). New Haven: Yale University Press.

Kanter, R.M. (1989). The new managerial work. *Harvard Business Review*, November–December, 85–92.

Koontz, H., and Weihrich, H. (1990). *Essentials of management* (5th ed.). New York: McGraw-Hill.

Kouzes, J.M., and Posner, B.Z. (1987). *The leadership challenge.* San Francisco: Jossey-Bass.

Kuhn, T. K. (1970). *The structure of scientific revolutions* (2nd ed.) Chicago: University of Chicago Press.

Mintzberg, H. (1989). The machine organization. In H. Mintzberg (Ed.), *Mintzberg on management: Inside our strange world of organizations.* New York: Free Press.

Perrow, C. (1984). *Normal accidents: Living with high risk technologies.* New York: Basic Books.

Peters, T., and Austin, N. (1985). *A passion for excellence.* New York: Random House.

Pfeiffer, J.W., Goodstein, L.D., and Nolan, T.M. (1986). *Applied strategic planning: A how to do it guide.* San Diego: University Associates.

Rice, D.M., and Rosen, M. (1991). Direct-care staff: A neglected priority. *Mental Retardation*, 29(4), iii–iv.

Robbins, S.P. (1990). *Organization theory: Structure, design and applications.* Englewood Cliffs, NJ: Prentice-Hall.

Rowe, A.J., Mason, R.O., Dickel, K.E., and Snyder, N.H. (1989). *Strategic management: A methodological approach* (3rd ed.). Reading, MA: Addison-Wesley.

Rowitz, L. (1991). Leadership in mental retardation. *Mental Retardation, 29*(3), iii–iv.

Rubinstein, M.F. (1975). *Patterns of problem solving.* Englewood Cliffs, NJ: Prentice–Hall.

Schein, E.H. (1972). *Professional education.* New York: McGraw-Hill.

Schon, D.A. (1983). *The reflective practitioner: How professionals think in action.* New York: Basic Books.

Segal, M. (1974). Organization and environment: A topology of adaptability and structure. *Public Administration Review, 20,* 212–220.

Skrtic, T.M. (1987). An organizational analysis of special education reform. *Counterpoint, 8,* 15–19.

Smull, M. (1989). Crisis in the community. Unpublished manuscript. Baltimore: University of Maryland at Baltimore.

Stogdill, R.M. (1974). *Handbook of leadership: A survey of theory and research.* New York: Free Press.

Weiss, N.R. (1990). Positive behavioral programming: An individualized functional approach. In J.F. Gardner and M.S. Chapman (Eds.), *Program issues in developmental disabilities: A guide to effective habilitation and active treatment* (2nd ed.). Baltimore: Paul H. Brookes.

Zeithaml, V.A., Parasuraman, A., and Berry, L.O. (1990). *Delivering quality services: Balancing customer perceptions and expectations.* New York: Free Press.

7

□ □ □
□ □ □
□ □ □

Collaborative Teamwork in Training and Technical Assistance: Enhancing Community Support for Persons with Disabilities

Beverly Rainforth, Michael F. Giangreco,
Pamela D. Smith, and Jennifer York

INTRODUCTION

Interdisciplinary teamwork has long been seen as a necessary element of effective services for persons with disabilities (e.g., Whitehouse, 1951). In 1962 the President's Panel on Mental Retardation identified the need for professionals serving persons with mental retardation to

Acknowledgment: Preparation of this chapter was supported in part by funds from: Grant #HO25F10008 from the U.S. Department of Education, Office of Special Education Programs awarded to the University of Vermont, Center for Developmental Disabilities; Grant #G0087C3061 from the U.S. Department of Education, Office of Special Education Programs awarded to the Kentucky Department of Education, Exceptional Children Services, and conducted by the University of Kentucky, Interdisciplinary Truman Development Institute; and Grant #90DD0204 from the U.S. Department of Health and Human Services, Administration on Developmental Disabilities awarded to the University of Minnesota, Institute on Community Integration.

The opinions expressed herein are solely those of the authors and do not reflect the position or policy of the U.S. Department of Education or the U.S. Department of Health and Human Services.

be trained to work in teams, and for that training to be provided in settings where services are exemplary (Long Range Task Force, 1976). When the President's Panel recommendations were translated into legislation creating the University Affiliated Facilities on Developmental Disabilities (UAFs), the UAF mission was defined in terms of training, services, technical assistance, and research that were interdisciplinary in nature. Thus an interdisciplinary focus became recognized legally as a feature surrounding exemplary services for children and adults with developmental disabilities.

The Long Range Task Force on University Affiliated Facilities defined *interdisciplinary training* as a process that "promotes the development and use of a basic language, a core body of knowledge, relevant skills, and an understanding of the attitude, values, and methods of participating disciplines" (1976, p. 11). The task force also asserted, in 1976, "Today the state of the art has substantially progressed so that defined interdisciplinary training objectives, core courses, and well-articulated team practicum experience exist in many of the current UAF programs" (p. 11). The outcome was services involving professionals from many disciplines who shared reports and recommendations, recognized the important contributions of others, and generally coordinated services with team members. Unfortunately, the services themselves typically were provided in isolation from one another, resulting in overlap, fragmentation, or even incompatibility. This chapter (a) examines a collaborative team approach that extends beyond the traditional interdisciplinary model to be more consistent with current best practices in services for people with disabilities, (b) discusses the training and technical assistance efforts needed to promote adoption of a collaborative team approach, and (c) presents examples of these training and technical assistance activities through three University Affiliated Programs.

A COLLABORATIVE TEAM APPROACH

As early as 1969, federal and private nonprofit agencies funded projects to develop a more integrated model of service provision for children and adults with disabilities; this model eventually was termed "transdisciplinary" (Hutchison, 1978). The defining feature of the transdisciplinary approach is the process of "role release" that enables team members to cross discipline boundaries and use methods traditionally associated with other disciplines (Lyon and Lyon, 1980). Conceptualization of the model recognized that (a) the knowledge, skills, and roles associated with any one discipline overlap with the other disciplines and (b) many members of a team can develop competence in using specific strategies with specific children or adults in specific situations. All members of the transdisciplinary team are expected to participate in teaching their teammates, learning from their teammates, and providing services that incorporate their new learning.

In effective teams, then, role release is a reciprocal process among all team members, not a unidirectional process emanating from "specialists." It is particularly important that parents and others who have frequent contact with the person with disabilities teach other members of the team. Teams often designate a parent, professional, or paraprofessional as the primary interventionist for a child or adult with disabilities, reducing the number of people and isolated services to which the child or adult must respond. The team integrates the strategies from the component disciplines, designs a comprehensive intervention plan, and teaches the primary interventionist the specific skills from each discipline, as needed to implement the plan.

The team continues to support the primary interventionist through ongoing supervision, problem solving, program design and modification, and retraining. While the transdisciplinary approach established an important framework for team members from multiple disciplines to improve coordination and consistency of their services, a weakness was that services continued to be provided in isolated settings and nonfunctional contexts: medical centers, segregated schools, laboratory classrooms, therapy rooms, and so on. Furthermore, while team members agreed to a shared set of goals, the goals still might be addressed in isolation from one another.

During the same time frame, educational teams established a model for "integrated therapy" in which students with disabilities received intervention in the routine activities and natural settings where skill improvement was most desirable (Sternat et al., 1977). While the model did not specify the use of a transdisciplinary approach, providing integrated therapy has proven to require role release for effective implementation. For example, the routine of eating lunch in the cafeteria involves (a) walking to, from, and through the cafeteria; (b) manipulating materials such as lunch tickets, trays, and eating utensils; (c) making requests; and (d) interacting with other children and adults. Whether the team chooses the physical therapist, speech-language pathologist, or another team member to teach this routine to a child with multiple disabilities, input from several disciplines may be needed to assess the student's performance within the context of this routine and design an appropriate instructional plan.

When teams fail to coordinate and combine the interventions from the various disciplines, fragmentation results. By default, frustrated students and their families may take on this coordination function, with varying degrees of success. Even when families are very skilled in this type of coordination, often it is more supportive for the entire team, including the student and family, to work closely during assessment, program planning, instruction, and program evaluation.

Effective implementation of the transdisciplinary and integrated therapy models requires collaboration among professionals from many disciplines, paraprofessionals, children and adults with disabilities, and their families. To emphasize the need for collaboration, "collaborative teamwork" is now used to refer to service provision that combines the essential elements of the transdisciplinary and integrated therapy models (Giangreco, York, and Rainforth, 1989; Rainforth, York, and Macdonald, 1992; York, Rainforth, and Giangreco, 1990). Rainforth, York, and Macdonald (1992) defined the characteristics of collaborative teamwork in educational settings as follows:

1. Equal participation in the collaborative teamwork process by family members and the service providers on the educational team.
2. Equal participation by all disciplines determined to be necessary for students to achieve their individualized educational goals.
3. Consensual decision making about priority educational goals and objectives related to all areas of student functioning at school, home, and in the community.
4. Consensual decision making about the type and amount of support required from related services personnel to achieve student goals.
5. Attention to motor, communication, and other embedded skills and needs throughout the educational program and in direct relevance to accomplishing priority educational goals.
6. Infusion of knowledge and skills from different disciplines into the design of educational methods and interventions.
7. Role release to enable team members who are involved most directly and frequently with students to develop the confidence and competence necessary to facilitate active learning and effective participation in the educational program.
8. Collaborative problem-solving and shared responsibility for student learning across all aspects of the educational program.

Although this list is framed around educational programs, the characteristics are equally valid for medical, vocational, community living, and other support services for children and adults with disabilities.

Defined in this way, collaborative teamwork supports implementation of current best practice in the field of disabilities in at least three ways. First, collaborative teamwork is consumer-centered. The consumer, family members, and friends are equal partners with professionals. Collaborative teamwork is a means to facilitate the supports that enable people with disabilities to exercise freedom and control over their lives, rather than a way to surround "clients" with "experts" who will make good decisions on the clients' behalf. Interdisciplinary teams traditionally have consisted of specialists who have expertise not shared with others; collaborative teams consist of partners who have specialized knowledge or skills that some teammates do not possess *yet.*

Members of collaborative teams constantly strive to share information to facilitate achievement of each person's goals. Rather than start with identification of a person's deficits and problems, the collaborative team acquires its focus by learning about who the person is, what his or her goals are, and what barriers to achieving those goals he or she has encountered. From this framework, the consumer, family members, friends, and professionals collectively determine the priorities that guide the team's efforts. Because each team member possesses unique abilities and knowledge, all members of the team share equally in responsibility for developing effective services and overcoming barriers.

Second, collaborative teamwork was conceptualized to improve coordination and relevance of services for people with disabilities. Rather than assemble a team of fifteen to twenty professionals, which is overwhelming and inefficient, a small core team that can address priority needs is identified. The small core team develops a coordinated plan for assessment that avoids duplication and gaps. Rather than professionals conducting their respective assessments independently, members of the core team often conduct part or all of their assessments together, enabling them to compare perspectives of the same events, to integrate those perspectives, and to expand their understanding of the consumer's abilities and the impact of his or her disabilities. Rather than each of the disciplines writing a separate assessment report and making separate service recommendations, the core team writes one report in which observations, conclusions, and recommendations are integrated. The team, including the consumer, family members, and friends, determines how decisions will be made about setting priorities, planning intervention strategies, and evaluating outcomes.

It may not be possible for teams to make every decision together, so consensus about a *process* for decision making is essential. For example, one team may meet to discuss priorities; another may not meet but members may give the team leader feedback on proposed priorities, another team might agree that family members make the final determination. Once priorities are set, rather than each discipline independently planning interventions and periodically reporting back to the team, the collaborative team designs a comprehensive plan that incorporates strategies from all needed disciplines. The appropriate core team members combine their strategies into a multifaceted approach and teach the primary intervention-ists (e.g., consumers, family members, teachers) how to use the combina-tion of strategies. Collectively, the core team evaluates the effectiveness of services to achieve the consumer's goals, seeks solutions to problems, and modifies plans when progress is not satisfactory. Coordination and relevance of services are improved because a small core team collaborates extensively to address shared goals.

Third, traditional interdisciplinary services have been center-based; collaborative teams support services that are community-based. Ser-vices for infants and toddlers with disabilities and their families are based in their homes and/or integrated day care settings. Children and youth with even the most severe disabilities, including complex health care needs, are now educated in integrated preschools and neighborhood schools, in regular classrooms alongside their peers without disabilities (Giangreco and Putnam, 1991; Schaffner and Buswell, 1990; Stainback and Stainback, 1992; Villa et al., 1992). Adults with varied types and degrees of disabilities live and work in the same settings as people with-out disabilities (Kiernan and Schalock, 1987; Mount and Zwernick, 1988; Racino et al., 1992).

Collaborative teams are able to understand consumers' goals, abilities, and needs, and develop appropriate support services because they work with consumers in their everyday settings. For example, a core team con-sisting of a community living companion, job coach, speech-language pa-thologist, and psychologist spent time learning about an adult with severe learning and behavior disorders at both his apartment and his community work site. After determining ways the man experienced stress and rewards in his life, the team developed strategies to teach the man more acceptable ways to communicate preferences, needs, and rejection, to increase his tolerance of demands in daily routines, and to expand the work and leisure activities from which he could choose. The core team made use of an extended team when they needed additional assistance, such as when they sought a psychiatrist's reevaluation of the man's longstanding prescription for high doses of psychotropic medications. This man will need lifelong support for community living, but the quality of his life improved signifi-cantly when his team based themselves in the circumstances of his every-day life.

Collaborative teamwork is defined as a team approach that ensures a consumer focus, support from professionals to achieve consumer goals, thorough integration of services with one another, and provision of services in the community settings where consumers prefer to live, work, attend school, and use their leisure time. This shift away from expert-driven, loosely organized, center-based models is essential to implement current best practices in services for people with disabilities. As best practices evolve, however, it is also essential that our teaming models continue to evolve, and that training and technical assistance activities are reshaped to promote adoption of our most current models.

Characteristics of Training and Technical Assistance to Promote Collaborative Teamwork

Given that collaborative teamwork is more consistent with current best practices than the traditional interdisciplinary approach, what are the characteristics of training and technical assistance to professionals and paraprofessionals that will promote a collaborative team approach? Prior to engaging in role release, each team member needs a strong foundation in his or her own discipline (Patterson et al., 1976), acquired through pre-service training and/or practical experience. Each team member also maintains professional competence through ongoing independent study, continuing education, and consultation with members of one's own discipline.

Team members benefit further from increasing their understanding of the nature and needs of persons with certain types of disabilities, through independent study or coursework, such as is typically offered through University Affiliated Programs on Developmental Disabilities (see, e.g., Karan et al., 1986). The more secure team members feel about the knowledge and skills associated with their discipline, the more comfortable they feel about practicing their discipline in front of others, teaching selected aspects of the discipline to others, learning selected aspects of another's discipline, and contributing to team planning and problem-solving efforts. Working with a collaborative team helps team members see that no one discipline has all the answers (Rainforth, 1985).

A second major area of need relates to interpersonal and group work skills. Fortunately, increasing numbers of children are yearning to work in cooperative groups as a routine part of their educational programs. In the process, they learn to work toward a common goal, elicit and find value in contributions from all members of their work group, negotiate agreements among group members, and present outcomes in a group report for which all members take both credit and responsibility (Johnson and F. Johnson, 1987). Unfortunately, most of today's adults were taught to work in individualistic and competitive goal structures, and lack the skills to work cooperatively (Johnson and R. Johnson, 1987).

Many teacher educators have found that they can teach cooperative learning strategies most effectively by incorporating the strategies into the college classroom. That is, they do not just discuss what cooperative learning is and how interdependence can be structured, but they organize their courses so teachers learn to work in cooperative groups as they learn the course content (Cooper and Mueck, 1990; Johnson, Johnson, and Smith, 1990). Although this may not be the best structure for all college courses, all disciplines would benefit from experience with this approach during their pre-service and in-service training. Similarly, existing teams would benefit from technical assistance that teaches them to use cooperative goal structures through direct experience working in cooperative groups.

A third area of need for training and technical assistance relates to working cooperatively with members of other disciplines. Although there is considerable overlap with needs related to group work, this area deserves special attention due to the structures and rewards inherent in universities. Most pre-service and in-service programs related to disability services address the topic of teamwork. Unfortunately, it is almost always a single faculty member representing a single discipline who describes the process to a largely unidisciplinary class. Diversity in class makeup can be increased somewhat by advertising availability of courses as electives for students in other programs, by cross-listing courses with other departments, by recruiting students directly through class presentations, and indirectly through associations among faculty who serve as student advisors in other departments. Ensuring diversity requires a structure that fits already compact program requirements.

Increasing the diversity of a class is a relatively simple issue, however, when compared with modeling collaborative teamwork for the class through strategies such as team teaching. Most university faculty members are appointed to a single department, in which they have responsibilities for teaching, research, and service. The demands and relative importance of these activities vary considerably among departments, however, so faculty members from different departments who try to share a responsibility equally (e.g., for a team-taught course) do not necessarily share equally in rewards. Issues such as who gets how much credit for a course and how to allocate planning time often become insurmountable barriers to team teaching, even within a department.

Furthermore, faculty members typically earn rewards based upon contributions to their department's agenda and needs, so efforts to work with faculty in other departments often are thwarted. Fortunately, some departments have found creative solutions to these problems, devising flexible structures to support collaborative efforts. In other cases, formal structures such as externally funded projects or the umbrella of a University Affiliated Program have provided the impetus and support for interdepartmental collaboration. A shared commitment by specific faculty members seems to be the primary determinant of whether collaboration will occur in universities, however (Rainforth, 1985).

Practicum experiences may offer opportunities for students to observe and practice collaboration with team members from various disciplines, but most clinical sites continue to offer less desirable models: center-based services provided by unidisciplinary or multidisciplinary teams. This situation might be remedied most effectively by establishing "model" programs that demonstrate the best practices discussed earlier in this chapter. Achieving "model" status usually requires both an agency commitment to change and technical assistance from professionals and paraprofessionals who describe, demonstrate, and guide adoption of practices associated with collaborative teamwork. As better models are established at practicum sites, students are more likely to seek out employers and colleagues who will support collaborative teamwork and replication of other best practice experiences.

The fourth and final area of need for training and technical assistance relates to specific programmatic strategies that will enable team members to implement the best practices discussed earlier in this chapter. For example, current and potential members of collaborative teams would benefit from learning to use the following types of strategies:

1. Personal Futures Planning (O'Brien, 1987) or McGill Action Planning (Vandercook, York, and Forest, 1989), to envision a desirable future as defined by the consumer, as the first step in identifying barriers, goals, and services and supports needed to achieve goals.
2. Ecological inventory, to identify priority environments, activities, and embedded skills, to identify demands and opportunities available in priority environments and activities, and to assess consumer performance (Brown et al., 1979; York and Vandercook, 1991).
3. Team planning and program development, to establish goals, objectives, and instructional procedures that reflect input from all relevant disciplines on the collaborative team (Giangreco, Cloninger, and Iverson, 1993; Rainforth, York, and Macdonald, 1992).
4. Block scheduling and other organizational structures that support flexible services in community settings, rather than traditional episodic interventions in clinical settings (Rainforth and York, 1987; York, Rainforth, and Wiemann, 1988).

Rainforth and colleagues (1992) provide a more extensive discussion of these and other strategies useful for collaborative teams in educational settings.

When the goal of training and technical assistance is to increase collaborative teamwork in consumer-driven, community-based services for persons with disabilities, it is most appropriate that the training and technical assistance processes exemplify those attributes.

ACTIVITIES THAT PROMOTE COLLABORATIVE TEAMWORK

There are numerous organizations that might provide training and/or technical assistance to assist teams and team members to adopt a collaborative team approach in consumer-driven, community-based services for persons with disabilities. These include state and local education agencies, public and private nonprofit agencies for persons with disabilities, hospitals and rehabilitation centers, and institutions of higher education. The examples of training and technical assistance activities presented here come from University Affiliated Programs for Persons with Developmental Disabilities (UAPs), which are charged with this type of responsibility, and which they often fulfill through partnerships with the organizations identified above. Undoubtedly there are other UAPs and organizations engaged in exemplary activities that are not described here.

The examples presented in the following sections are intended to reflect an array of training and technical assistance activities involving professionals from a variety of disciplines whose services support children and adults with a variety of needs in a variety of community settings. Examples are drawn from the UAPs at The University of Kentucky, the University of Minnesota, and the University of Vermont. Rather than run clinics and other university-based services, these UAPs focus on increasing the capacity of local organizations and agencies to meet the needs of children and adults with developmental disabilities in the community.

The first section provides an overview of the University of Minnesota's pre-service programs for professional preparation in developmental disabilities. Because relatively few professionals have participated in programs of this type, however, there remain extensive needs for on-the-job training and technical assistance to community service providers. The second section describes a statewide systems change project at the University of Kentucky, which provides training and technical assistance to local education agencies serving students with severe disabilities. The third section describes the work of a team at the University of Vermont, which provides ongoing support to local education agencies throughout the state. Although each of these UAPs sponsors other activities that promote collaborative teamwork, space does not permit complete description of all activities. Additional information is available from the author affiliated with each UAP.

University of Minnesota, Institute on Community Integration

There are four philosophical underpinnings for the design and implementation of training at the Institute for Community Integration: (a) integration or inclusion of individuals with disabilities into typical family, school, community, and work life; (b) an ecological perspective in determining strengths, challenges, needs, and resources for service provision; (c) family- and consumer-centered services and supports; and (d) collaboration that extends across disciplines (interdisciplinary) and agencies (interagency).

Too frequently, professionals who will be involved in the lives of persons with developmental disabilities and their families graduate from pre-service programs to the real world of practice without a solid foundation in these philosophies. At the University of Minnesota, students from a variety of disciplines receive preparation that establishes these underpinnings through two broad approaches to pre-service training: (1) designing comprehensive programs of study and (2) infusing disability information, usually in the form of short teaching modules, into existing survey courses in departments across campus. This section presents brief descriptions of both approaches to training as used by the Institute on Community Integration.

Interdisciplinary Studies in Developmental Disabilities Certificate Program

This sixteen to twenty-four-credit program offers interdisciplinary training for educators, human service professionals, health professionals, community members, and other interested individuals. Initiated in 1987, the program was designed to enable students from a variety of majors on campus to take a specialized course of study in developmental disabilities. Increasing numbers of people who are not in degree programs at the University of Minnesota have enrolled in the certificate program. Many are practicing professionals in the field who enroll for continuing education. Others are seeking information about careers in developmental disabilities. Students enrolled in a degree program find that the certificate program is flexible enough so they can pursue the certificate as a complement to their major area of study.

Central to the design and delivery of the program are elements that promote understanding of and opportunities to experience collaborative teamwork. Reflected in two core courses, these elements include

- Students from a variety of disciplines with diverse experience and perspectives enrolled simultaneously in both core courses
- Heterogeneous small group and cooperative learning instructional formats
- Structured learning opportunities to reflect and write about personal and professional applications of information
- Two instructors (faculty member and graduate student) serving as the core instructor team, who are joined by community service providers, agency personnel, family members, and individuals with developmental disabilities for the majority of sessions
- Specific content area instruction about effective communication among team members and about various models of teamwork (e.g., multi-, inter-, and transdisciplinary models; medical versus educational perspectives)

Three levels of training are offered in the certificate program.

Level 1: Foundational concepts and knowledge. This level focuses broadly on the characteristics, needs, and capacities of persons with developmental disabilities and their families as well as on contemporary philosophy, practices, and issues. Two courses at this level are required for all program participants. The first, Contemporary Services for Persons with Developmental Disabilities, is a three-credit survey course that addresses the characteristics of individuals with developmental disabilities and the etiology of disabilities. Also discussed are historical and current perspectives on issues related to promoting independence, productivity, and integration in home, school, work, and community life across the life span.

The second required course, Family-Professional Planning for Persons with Severe Disabilities, focuses more specifically on family aspects of services and supports, with emphasis on strategies (e.g., Personal Futures Planning, McGill Action Planning System) to promote collaborative planning and implementation. Special aspects of family-professional cooperation during preschool, transition to adulthood, and post-school life are discussed.

Level 2: Specialized knowledge and skills acquisition. At this level, students can select from among a wide range of courses to acquire knowledge and skills focused on intervention, research, or policy. Coursework at this level includes approved electives in special education, family social science, nursing, public health, communication disorders, educational policy and administration, recreation and leisure, physical education, social work, vocational education, and other fields.

Level 3: Demonstration and application of skills. The focus of training at this level is to provide students with opportunities to apply their knowledge and skills through an individually designed learning experience in intervention, research, or policy activities. For students enrolled in a degree program, staff from the Institute on Community Integration work with advisors from the students' major department to design a field experience that meets the requirements of both the major department and the Interdisciplinary Certificate Program.

Students have reflected positively on the Interdisciplinary Certificate Program in course evaluations and at completion of the program. They have noted particular satisfaction with perspectives gained from interacting with students from diverse academic backgrounds and experiences, speakers with disabilities who were self-advocates, and speakers who worked in the field of developmental disabilities in a variety of capacities.

Specialized Pre-service Training Sequences

There are several specialized training sequences that represent collaborative pre-service training efforts between discipline coordinators in various academic departments and faculty and staff of the Institute on Community Integration. The training sequences are designed to promote an interdisciplinary and developmental disabilities theme at the pre-service level. Included are sequences in the areas of early intervention, social work, recreation/leisure, adapted physical education, general education, special education, school psychology, augmentative communication, and transition and employment. The program design for most areas includes the training provided in the Interdisciplinary Studies in Developmental Disabilities Certificate Program, with the courses for Level 2: Specialized Knowledge and Skill focused on the respective content areas. Several specialized pre-service training sequences are described below. As noted earlier in this chapter, interdisciplinary arrangements in university training programs are challenging and usually reflect commitments by specific faculty members in addition to the presence of supportive structures. Therefore, faculty affiliations with diverse schools and departments are noteworthy.[1]

Interdisciplinary leadership training program in early intervention. The program trains students from eight academic programs to provide leadership in research and training of persons to work with infants, toddlers, and preschoolers who may be at risk for or have developmental delays, and their families. Students from different discipline orientations go through their training as a cohort group, learning about each other's disciplines and how to work together as an effective collaborative team.

Secondary transition specialist training program. This program focuses on teaching vocational and special educators to enhance secondary education and employment opportunities for students with severe disabilities and their transition into the workforce.

Training of therapeutic recreation students in community integration. This program prepares therapeutic recreation specialists to facilitate inclusion of children and youths with severe developmental disabilities in recreation programs across home, school, and community settings.

Developmental disabilities rotation in pediatrics. Initiated in the summer of 1991, this one-month rotation is required of all pediatrics residents. In addition to clinical education and practice at a children's hospital, the rotation incorporates parent/family and community agency components. The parent/family component includes instruction provided by parents of children with developmental disabilities and extended interactions with families in the contexts of their own choosing. The community agency component includes discussions with Institute on Community

---

[1]The authors thank the following people for information about the Specialized Pre-service Training Sequences at the University of Minnesota: Scott McConnell, Ph.D., and Mary McEvoy, Ph.D., Department of Educational Psychology, directors of the Interdisciplinary Leadership Training Program in Early Intervention; Jim Brown, Ph.D., Department of Vocational Technical Education, and David R. Johnson, Ph.D., Institute on Community Integration, directors of the Secondary Transition Specialist Training Program; Stuart J. Schleien, Ph.D., and Leo H. McEvoy, Ph.D., School of Kinesiology and Leisure Studies, directors of Training of Therapeutic Recreation Students in Community Integration; Peter Blasco, M.D., and Robert Blum, M.D., Ph.D., Department of Pediatrics, directors of the Developmental Disabilities Rotation in Pediatrics; and Brian Abery, Ph.D., Institute on Community Integration, coordinator of Community Service Training Program.

Integration staff in order to provide an overview of community services and observations/interactions with community service providers in integrated school, recreation, or work environments. Emphasized throughout the community agency component are ways that physicians can support families by connecting them with community resources.

Community service training program. This program provides high school and college students with information about the field of developmental disabilities and related career and community support opportunities. The two main components of this program are weekly seminars and community-based recreation opportunities. In the seminars, students acquire basic knowledge about disabilities, awareness of similarities between persons with and without disabilities, understanding of the roadblocks to making friends that face many people with disabilities, and ways to remove or minimize barriers to friendships. In the community-based component, partners are matched and specific community environments and activities are identified by conducting inventories of activity interests and of personal relationship interests (e.g., preference for a large network of acquaintances versus a small network of close friends). Once partners with shared interests are matched, they are assisted to access community environments and supported to participate and interact in the environments. Because partners might not continue their association after the one-year commitment, emphasis is placed on supporting the person with a disability to establish networks that will continue if the partner leaves.

University of Kentucky Interdisciplinary Human Development Institute: Kentucky Systems Change Project

The Kentucky Systems Change Project is a five-year project funded by the U.S. Department of Education, Office of Special Education Programs, and conducted by the Interdisciplinary Human Development Institute, the University Affiliated Program at the University of Kentucky. The project is operated in collaboration with the Kentucky Department of Education, Division of Special Learning Needs. The goals of the Kentucky Systems Change Project include:

1. Movement of students from segregated to integrated educational placements
2. Enhancement of educational programs for students in integrated placements

3. Dissemination of best practices to policy makers, administrators, parents, and teachers statewide
4. Development of state-level policies and practices to enhance integrated educational opportunities

The focus of the project is to facilitate increased integrated educational opportunities for students with severe disabilities through two levels of systems change: (1) at the state level, including policy changes and statewide personnel preparation needs and (2) at the local level, to develop policies and programs that facilitate the provision of quality integrated educational programs for students with severe disabilities in local school districts. To facilitate systems change at the state level, the project identifies barriers to the provision of integrated educational programs and implements strategies to remove or overcome these barriers, working closely with the project's statewide advisory board, composed of consumers, parents of children and youth with severe disabilities, representatives of state agencies serving infants/toddlers through adults, local school district personnel, representatives from institutions of higher education, and representatives of protection and advocacy.

The project works with selected school districts across Kentucky to improve their educational programs and provides extensive in-service training and on-site technical assistance to administrators, teachers, related services personnel, and parents in these districts. Outcomes to date include (a) movement of 165 students with severe disabilities from segregated schools to age-appropriate, regular school campuses and the subsequent closing of four segregated special schools; (b) provision of systematic, regularly scheduled community-based instruction to 78 percent of students with severe disabilities in participating classrooms; (c) integrated educational opportunities for all students in participating districts, including full-inclusion models in selected programs; and (d) development and dissemination of five major documents statewide and nationally. The following paragraphs highlight project activities aimed at provision of integrated educational programs, exemplify how collaborative strategies were included in these activities, and discuss the subsequent outcomes of these efforts in Kentucky.

Twenty school districts have participated in the Kentucky Systems Change Project, with training and technical assistance designed to meet the needs of the individual school district and staff. Strategies that facilitate collaboration across disciplines and agencies are incorporated into all technical assistance and training activities, with primary emphasis on integration of students with severe disabilities. A project staff member with expertise in special education serves as the change facilitator for each district. This person (a) conducts on-site interviews, observations, and program evaluations (Kleinert, Smith, and Hudson, 1990); (b) works with district personnel across disciplines to develop the district technical assistance plan; (b) works with district-wide teams composed of educators and related disciplines who work with students with severe disabilities; (d) works with school-based teams on collaborative assessment, problem solving, and interventions; (e) works with district-wide Integration Task Forces in districts that are moving students from segregated special schools to integrated neighborhood schools; (f) coordinates all technical assistance and training activities; and (g) monitors the effectiveness of project efforts within the district, with particular emphasis on individual student outcomes.

The change facilitator provides on-site training to teams composed of educators, administrators, and related services personnel. In addition, collaborative planning processes are used to promote input from all team members for making decisions and resolving district-wide issues. This approach is used (a) to promote ownership of both the planning process and the products of implementation and (b) to model and teach collaborative planning and decision making, to empower team members to continue their efforts over time. In the course of the project, several products were developed and used to support training activities, as described below.

The project staff developed *The Quality Program Indicators Manual for Students with Moderate and Severe Handicaps* (Kleinert, Smith, and Hudson, 1990) to determine technical assistance needs and to document changes in programs for students with severe disabilities in local school districts. The manual's components include (a) integration, (b) functional curriculum, (c) systematic instruction, (d) community-based instruction, (e) transdisciplinary services and integrated therapy, and (f) vocational instruction and transition plans. Each component includes a checklist of the quality indicators for that component with a description of each of the indicators. The manual has been used for program evaluation and training purposes and serves as a descriptive document to define and describe programmatic best practices and how to implement these in local programs/classrooms.

Strategies that promote collaborative teamwork are incorporated into all sections of the manual, with the sections on integration, functional curriculum, transdisciplinary services and integrated therapy, and vocational instruction and transition plans incorporating the most emphasis in collaborative strategies. For example, the integration section contains indicators or teacher behaviors that promote collaborative planning for integrated activities and role release of skills to regular education teachers and other school staff to empower them with knowledge, skills, and confidence required to work with students with severe disabilities within the general school environment. The section on functional curriculum focuses on designing functional curriculum that is student and family driven, and uses ecological inventory to determine a single set of discipline-free goals and objectives involving related disciplines to embed basic skill instruction in the context of functional, age-appropriate activities. This approach lays the foundation for ongoing collaboration with related team members to implement and utilize discipline-specific strategies taught to other team members to promote attainment of a single set of goals and objectives for individual students.

These processes are described more extensively in *Curriculum Planning Process and Model Local Catalogs for Students with Moderate and Severe Disabilities* (Hudson and Kleinert, 1991), also developed by the project for training local school district teams. The section on transdisciplinary services and integrated therapy emphasizes collaborative teamwork strategies such as conducting collaborative assessments, block scheduling, embedding basic skill instruction and discipline-specific objectives, service delivery based on student educational outcomes and provided in natural settings, integrated discipline strategies and adaptations, consultation with and training of other team members, team meetings and communication, and implementation issues. The section on vocational instruction and transition plans includes collaborative teamwork in the transition planning process involving the student, family members, school staff, adult agency personnel, and others.

One of the most significant barriers to integrated education of students with severe disabilities identified by the project's statewide advisory board was programmatic integration of related services. The project answered this need in two ways. First, the project developed an implementation manual entitled *Integrating Related Services into Programs for Students with Severe and Multiple Handicaps* (Smith, 1990). The process of planning and reviewing the document embodied collaborative teamwork with equal participation by family members, related discipline representatives, and service providers from across Kentucky.

The document emphasizes the rationale for adopting a transdisciplinary team model of service provision and addresses specific strategies to implement transdisciplinary teaming and integrated related services, including (a) block scheduling; (b) collaborative assessments; (c) embedding related services objectives and basic skills; (d) integrated service provision, integrated adaptations and discipline-specific strategies; (e) consultation, training, and role release; (f) information exchange and team meetings; and (g) administrative and implementation issues.

The document initially was used to train teams, including parents, from school districts in the Kentucky Systems Change Project. A team, consisting of a special educator, physical therapist, occupational therapist, speech-language pathologist, principal, and specialist in dual sensory impairments, provided training and used cooperative learning and group problem-solving activities to further model and demonstrate the benefits of collaborative teamwork to participants. On-site technical assistance and consultation assisted project school districts to implement this service model at the local level. Districts that have implemented integrated related services have gone from an interdisciplinary model with isolated or "pull-out" therapy services to a collaborative team process that includes ongoing communication, regularly scheduled team meetings, student- and family-centered consultation and team problem solving, and services that focus on each student's educational outcomes.

Implementation has been most successful at the local level when all planning, development, implementation, and evaluation activities have been done in a collaborative effort where local team members share equally in the process. Thus, collaborative teamwork not only has benefits in the provision of quality services for individual students, but is a necessary tool in implementing the process.

Another statewide barrier to quality integrated educational programs was the lack of appropriate communication programming for students with severe and multiple disabilities. Most speech-language pathologists had received limited training in appropriate programming for these students and did not feel competent or confident when working with these students and other team members. Communication "systems" or strategies were nonexistent for many nonspeaking students or were limited to laminated boards that contained a few photographs depicting students' basic needs (e.g., eat, drink, bathroom use, TV/toy/music, and so forth) or needs on community-based instruction (e.g., ordering in a fast-food restaurant). Communication programming was not viewed as an integral aspect of every activity in every setting across the student's day. In response, a two-day in-service training workshop was developed and conducted in five different geographical areas of Kentucky, training a total of ninety speech-language pathologists, with many participants representing school districts involved in the Kentucky Systems Change Project.

The workshop concentrated on three areas: (1) designing communication programming, including assessment of communication functions and ecological strategies, identification of communicative intent of aberrant behaviors, strategies for expanding students' communicative repertoire, incidental language instruction and techniques for promoting communication in natural contexts, and provision of instruction in integrated school and community settings; (2) designing augmentative systems with particular emphasis on no-tech and low-tech systems including symbol or calendar shelves, communication boards and booklets, use of endless loop tapes with a tape recorder, eye gaze frames/E-trans, construction of single switches for use with battery-operated devices; and (3) consultation and collaboration with families, classroom teachers, and other team members.

Training was provided by a team of special educators and speech-language pathologists from the university and the community who have extensive knowledge and skills working with children and youth with severe and multiple disabilities. The team used group problem-solving and cooperative learning activities to increase participants' involvement in training and their skills in working with others. An additional session was held for directors of special education and other administrative and supervisory staff to increase awareness related to the workshop content and to foster administrative support for integrated and collaborative service delivery.

Subsequent on-site consultation and ongoing technical assistance was provided to districts in the Kentucky Systems Change Project to assist in implementation. Implementation has been most successful in districts that focus on implementation of integrated related services and collaborative teamwork in the provision of integrated programs. The content of the communication workshop was compiled into a training manual entitled *Communication Programming for Students with Severe and Multiple Handicaps* (Smith and Kleinert, 1991) and distributed to workshop participants, numerous speech-language pathologists across the state, and directors of special education in all school districts in Kentucky.

To achieve the goal of integrated education for students with severe disabilities, the project has sponsored several other training activities that embody collaborative teamwork and/or specific programmatic strategies that promote collaborative efforts. Training participants typically include district- and/or building-level teams composed of special education and regular education teachers, principals, directors of special education, related services personnel, and parents from selected districts in the Kentucky Systems Change Project. The strength of conducting training in a team format cannot be emphasized enough. The benefits are realized through both change in individual team members' behavior and changes in their ability to work together as a team to promote systems change at the local level and have maximum impact on improving the quality of programs for individual students and their families.

The Kentucky Systems Change Project's Statewide Advisory Board formed a committee to develop a plan for changes needed in pre-service training programs in special education and related disciplines. The committee consists of representatives from special education programs at the five major state universities in Kentucky. At the University of Kentucky, project staff also work closely with the Director of Pre- service Training at the Interdisciplinary Human Development Institute (IHDI) to infuse information about integrated education and collaborative teamwork in both the core curriculum and in related coursework in education, social work, psychology, and medicine. Through the committee and IHDI pre-service training, changes include (a) using project products as required or supplemental readings in related coursework, (b) using cooperative learning strategies and collaborative teamwork to teach the course content, (c) incorporating collaborative teamwork with other disciplines in related coursework and practicum experiences, and (d) developing model programs as practicum sites close to each campus that exemplify best educational practices and encourage students to practice collaborative teamwork.

University of Vermont, Center
for Developmental Disabilities:
State of Vermont I-Team

The State of Vermont I-Team was established in 1975 to provide local education teams, consisting of families, educators, and related service providers, with technical assistance and training in provision of quality education for students with intensive educational needs. Originally funded by the U.S. Department of Education, the I-Team is now funded by the Vermont State Department of Education's Family and Educational Support Team and administered through the Center for Developmental Disabilities, the University Affiliated Program at the University of Vermont.

From the inception of the I-Team until recently, the *I* stood for "interdisciplinary." This seemed appropriate because the I-Team consisted of members representing various disciplines (e.g., education, psychology, occupational therapy) who shared information about assessment and services for the children they jointly served. But as time passed, I-Team members recognized that the label "interdisciplinary" did not accurately reflect the changing nature of the community-based services they provided. Because the name "I-Team" was already known to many, the group decided to keep the name but not define the *I*. Their brochure now reads, "State of Vermont I-Team: Providing Intensive Special Education Supports." While it may seem like a small point, the change in name symbolizes the ever-evolving nature of I-Team services and philosophy.

In recent years, changes in the I-Team have reflected the underlying assumptions of collaborative teamwork, assumptions shared both among I-Team members and between I-Team members and consumers of I-Team services. Members of the I-Team provide collaborative assistance to local educational teams and school districts; this represents a shift away from the expert consultation models that were more predominant in the past. Current I-Team services are based on collaborative consultation and problem-solving efforts, facilitated jointly by I-Team members and members of student individual planning teams. This evolution is consistent with philosophical and programmatic advances occurring nationally (e.g., special education as a service not a place, service flexibility, services in integrated environments, consumer empowerment, family-centered services). The I-Team actively promotes increased demonstration of current exemplary practices in education, as outlined in Table 7-1 (Fox and Williams, 1991). The goal is to ensure that every student has opportunities to pursue meaningful and valued life experiences. The I-Team supports the principle that all children are best educated in their local educational setting.

TABLE 7-1   Best Practice Statements

School Climate and Structure

1. The school's philosophy statement and objectives are developed by administrators, staff, students, parents, school board members and other community members and reflect the school's commitment to meeting the individual needs of all students in age-appropriate regular education and community settings.

2. The school's climate is established by administrators, staff, students, parents, school board members, and other community members and promotes respect for individual differences among students, encourages the development of positive self-esteem, establishes high achievement expectations for all students, and encourages the development of caring personal relationships among students and staff.

3. The school's code of conduct for students and staff is established by administrators, staff, students, parents, school board members, and other community members, emphasizes possible behavior, is applied in a consistent, fair manner, and takes into account the unique needs of individual students.

(continued)

TABLE 7-1   Best Practice Statements *(continued)*

School Climate and Structure

4. The school provides ample opportunities for students, staff, administrators, parents, school board members, and other community members to be recognized for their accomplishments, including helping others.

5. The general roles and responsibilities of all school staff (including contracted staff, such as an occupational therapist or psychologist) relative to providing instruction and support to all students are clearly delineated by administrators, staff, students, parents, school board members, and other community members.

6. The school's professional development process is developed by administrators, staff, students, parents, school board members, and other community members and includes in-service training, regularly scheduled observations with feedback, technical assistance, peer coaching, and mentoring.

7. The school's instructional support system (e.g., classroom-based model for delivering support services, teacher assistance team, individual student planning teams, special education pre-referral process, volunteer system) is developed by administrators, staff, students, parents, school board members, and other community members and is available to all students and staff.

Collaborative Planning

8. The school provides opportunities for staff, students, family members, and community members to become proficient at functioning in a collaborative manner (i.e., share responsibility and resources, make decisions by consensus, use a structured meeting agenda format, rotate team roles of facilitator, timekeeper, and recorder).

9. The school provides time during school hours for instructional support teams (e.g., individual student planning teams, teacher assistance teams, teaching teams) to meet and for individual team members to monitor services and to provide timely consultation, support, and technical assistance to families and staff.

10. For students with intensive needs in basic skill and/or social skill areas or who are challenged by their gifts and talents, individual student planning teams are convened that are responsible for the development and implementation of all aspects of the student's educational program (e.g., student goals, student schedules, procedures to address learning/behavior/management issues, transition plans, strategies to support the student and his or her teachers and family).

TABLE 7-1   *(continued)*

Collaborative Planning

11. Individual student planning teams consist of the student, family members, the student's general class teacher(s), and other appropriate persons based upon the student's needs (e.g., principal, Chapter I teacher, music teacher, physical therapist, one or two of the student's peers, teaching assistant, special educator, social worker, representatives of community agencies, family advocates).

12. The individual roles of each student planning team member, including related service providers and other consultants, are specified by the team and are supportive of the educational needs of the student.

Social Responsibility

13. The school facilitates the development of social responsibility and self-reliance by promoting student participation in volunteer organizations and activities (e.g., community service activities, peer tutoring/mentoring activities, student government, participation in decision making about important school or community issues).

14. The school's curriculum provides structured opportunities for students to learn about and appreciate individual differences among people.

15. The school's curriculum provides structured opportunities for students to develop appropriate social skills (e.g., making friends, cooperating with others, sharing, listening, avoiding fighting) that include frequent practice during school, home, and community activities.

16. The school provides opportunities for all students to participate in age-appropriate school-sponsored extracurricular activities (e.g., field trips, sports teams, clubs, dances, assemblies, student government).

17. For students with intensive needs in the social skill area, an individual program for increasing social skills is developed that includes (a) assessment of current skills in identified home, school, and community settings; (b) identification of adaptations and support needed to function in those settings; (c) procedures for working with school staff and families to incorporate social skill training and/or practice into school and family routines.

Curricular Planning

18. The school's curricula are developed by teachers/staff, students, parents, administrators, and community members and identify age-appropriate content (e.g., language arts, math, history, social/emotional,

(continued)

TABLE 7-1   Best Prectice Statements *(continued)*

Curricular Planning

arts, health) and process-oriented (problem-solving and collaboration skills, study skills) goals and objectives that promote meaningful participation in age-appropriate activities in home, recreational, educational, work, and other aspects of community life, set a high standard of excellence, and address the needs of all students.

19. A variety of age-appropriate nonschool instructional settings (e.g., day care settings, the student's home, local stores, and job sites) are available to students and matched to individual needs for learning new skills or for generalizing skills to new settings.

20. The process for identifying curriculum content for an individual student with intensive needs in basic skill and/or social areas includes an analysis of the student's skills and interests and of the age-appropriate activities, skills, and adaptations needed for the student to function in specific home, school, work, recreation, and other community settings.

21. Objectives for students with intensive needs in basic skill and/or social areas specify criteria that include performance in the student's home, school, and other age-appropriate community settings.

22. Students with intensive needs in basic skill and/or social areas have paid work experiences in integrated community settings prior to leaving school.

23. The system for monitoring the progress of students with intensive needs in basic skill and/or social areas includes (a) indications of level of independence on identified skills/activities; (b) indications of environments in which those skills/activities have been demonstrated; (c) an annual summary; and (d) post-school follow-ups for purposes of program improvement.

Delivery of Instructional Support Services

24. Instructional support services and staff (e.g., Chapter I, special education, speech and language, guidance, peer tutoring) are incorporated into ongoing school and community activities.

25. The decision to pull any student out of ongoing school or community activities to receive support services is a team decision based upon documentation that the student's needs could not be achieved through the use of supplementary aids and services in the classroom. This decision is not based upon staff preferences.

26. For students with needs (e.g., counseling, community-based training, medical care) that cannot be met through ongoing activities, pull-out is

TABLE 7-1 *(continued)*

Delivery of Instructional Support Services

scheduled during activities that the team determines to be lowest priority for the student.

27. The delivery of instructional support services (e.g., consultation, training, technical assistance, cooperative planning with support staff, team teaching with support staff, support staff delivering direct services in the classroom, release time for planning, access to instructional support teams) includes support to teachers, teaching assistants, volunteers, and other direct instructional staff.

Individualized Instruction

28. The school provides all students with opportunities to set personal goals and to plan, with parents and teachers, how their goals will be addressed during the school year.

29. The school provides opportunities for all staff to become proficient at previewing instructional activities, giving clear written and verbal directions, checking for student understanding, and giving students constructive feedback and positive reinforcement.

30. The school provides opportunities for all staff to become proficient in using a variety of instructional methods (e.g., cooperative learning, whole language, peer tutoring, drill and practice, incidental teaching, computer-assisted instruction), matching methods to individual student needs, and incorporating methods into ongoing activities.

31. A variety of instructional groupings (e.g., small group, large group, multi-aged groups, cooperative group, individual instruction) are available to all students and matched to individual student needs.

32. A variety of instructors (e.g., teachers, teacher assistants, same-age peer tutors, cross-age peer tutors, peer mentors, volunteers) are available to students and matched to individual student needs.

33. The school provides opportunities for all staff to become proficient at using a variety of instructional materials (e.g., real items, photographs, drawings, worksheets, textbooks, audiovisuals), at matching materials to individual student needs, and incorporating materials into ongoing activities.

34. The school provides opportunities for all staff to become proficient at teaching several different goals from the same curriculum area through a single group activity (e.g., during a group math activity some students may be led in addition while others are learning counting or one-to-one correspondence).

(continued)

TABLE 7-1 Basic Practice Statements *(continued)*

Individualized Instruction

35. The school provides opportunities for all staff to become proficient at teaching goals from different curriculum areas through the same group activity (e.g., during a group social studies activity some students may have a primary goal of learning the social studies content while others have primary goals of learning language or communication).

36. The school provides opportunities for all staff and students to become proficient at identifying a variety of ways students can acquire or demonstrate skills/knowledge (e.g., signing, writing, typing, gesturing, oral tests or reports, art displays, taped presentations), matching them to individual student needs, and incorporating them into ongoing activities.

37. For each lesson currently being taught, there is a written instructional program or lesson plan that is available to all direct instructional staff.

38. Student progress is monitored and analyzed on a regularly scheduled basis.

39. Decisions to modify instructional groupings, methods, or materials are based upon measures of student progress.

40. A current schedule of daily student activities that describes what is being done, when, and with whom, is available and readily accessible.

Transition Planning

41. There are procedures for facilitating the smooth transition of all students from one educational setting to another, and from school to post-school life.

42. A written plan for transitioning each student with intensive needs, including gifted students from one educational setting to another is developed and implemented in advance of the move (e.g., six to nine months).

43. For high-school-aged students with intensive needs, a written graduation plan for transition to post-school life (e.g., employment, education, recreation, residential) is developed and implemented well in advance of the transition (e.g., at age fourteen) and reviewed annually.

Family-School Collaboration

44. The school provides families with the freedom to visit the school and to communicate regularly with school staff on topics important to both the family and the school.

45. There is information available to families that assists them to access informal support networks and connect with community resources (e.g.,

TABLE 7-1 *(continued)*

Family-School Collaboration

day care programs, recreation programs, counseling, respite care, vocational rehabilitation, mental health).

46. The school provides families with opportunities for consultation, training, and follow-up from school staff to maximize their children's development in home and other community settings.

47. Families are included in advisory, decision-making, and advocacy activities of the school (e.g., advisory committees, curriculum committees, development of the school philosophy and climate, school planning teams, staff development committees).

48. Families are included in the decision-making process to determine the high-priority educational needs of their children, and how and where (school, home, or community settings) their children will be taught.

49. Instructional planning includes procedures for assisting families to incorporate instruction and/or practice of skills into ongoing home and community activities.

Planning for Continued Best Practice Improvement

50. A plan for improving best practice–based services within the school is developed every three to five years by a school planning team consisting of administrators, staff, students, parents, school board members, and other community members.

51. The school's plan includes (a) a review of the school's goals and the extent to which goals and best educational practices are achieved; (b) an examination of services offered by the school and how they relate to student, family, and community needs; (c) follow-up measures of students' performance in the next school setting or post-school settings; and (d) guidelines for improving best practices.

52. The school planning team meets periodically to monitor progress on implementing the school's plan and to make necessary adjustments in activities and timelines for achieving the plan.

53. The school's plan and subsequent reports of progress in implementing the plan are disseminated to parents, school district staff, and community members.

54. There is a periodic evaluation of the planning process by school staff, students, parents, community members, and persons from outside the school (e.g., staff from other schools, colleges and universities, state and local government).

Source: Reprinted with permission from Fox and Williams (1991).

Students who reside in Vermont and require special education services to meet their educational needs may be referred for I-Team services by anyone on the student's local educational team or by the special education administrator. Historically, the primary populations served by the I-Team included students with severe, profound, or multiple disabilities, including those identified as deaf-blind. Recently, I-Team services have been expanded to include students with serious emotional disturbance who are transitioning into their local schools from more restrictive settings (e.g., residential facilities) or those who are at imminent risk of being removed from their general education placement.

Traditional eligibility for I-Team services has meant the student had a categorical disability label as well as the need for special education. In this context, special education means specially designed instruction, above and beyond what is typically available in the general education classroom. Of course, what is typically available in general education classrooms varies widely. In 1990, Vermont's Special Education Reform Act 230 was signed into law. Act 230 was designed to increase the capability of general education teachers, thus reducing the need to label students in order for them to receive appropriate instruction in general education classes. In part,

> Act 230 is based on the premise that all schools must begin to pursue a comprehensive system of education services that will result, to the maximum extent possible, in all students succeeding in the regular education classroom. It is hoped that one day only a small percentage of students will need to be labeled "disabled" in order to access "special" education because all teachers will be trained and have the necessary resources to teach all children in the regular classroom [Vermont State Board of Education, 1990].

This means that in some school districts where teachers are prepared to teach heterogeneous groups, students previously labeled "disabled" may no longer be so labeled and the accommodations they formerly received only through referral for special education services will now be part of what is typically available through general education.

This fundamentally changes not only the concept of eligibility for special education and I-Team services, but also changes the context of services to increasingly less restrictive environments for all types of students. A large portion of current I-Team activities are directed toward supporting the education of students with disabilities in general education classrooms. Whereas I-Team members traditionally provided technical assistance and training to special education personnel, they are increasingly providing supportive services to general education personnel.

The I-Team consists of a core group of specialists who are based at the Center for Developmental Disabilities at the University of Vermont. Historically, the Core I-Team has consisted of a coordinator who is an educational consultant, an occupational therapy consultant, a physical therapy consultant, and a communication consultant. The Core I-Team added a dual sensory impairment specialist in 1987, followed by a clinical psychology consultant and family resource consultant in 1990. Core I-Team members provide services statewide within Vermont. Consistent with the concept of services and supports that are community-based, five I-Team regional offices were established in 1978 and 1979. From 1979 to 1988 each I-Team region was staffed with a full-time educational consultant. In 1988 a part-time therapy consultant (either OT or PT) and a part-time family resource consultant were added to each region. Each regional family resource consultant is a parent of a child with a disability. Regional team members provide services to Vermont schools within their geographic region, each having approximately a dozen Vermont Supervisory Unions.

I-Team services for a designated student, family, or school are coordinated by the I-Team Regional Educational Consultant who draws upon Core I-Team members as needed. The consultation, technical assistance, and training provided by the I-Team are highly individualized. Examples include (a) off-campus university courses on topics of regional interest; (b) in-service training; (c) current literature and other information resources (e.g., I-Team newsletter); (d) on-site collaborative consultation; (e) assistance with service delivery planning; (f) consultation to related service providers; (g) family support services; (h) information and referral; (i) transition planning; and (j) ongoing assistance. I-Team services are documented through a referral and permission packet, a general service plan, and specific action plan.

As noted previously, the I-Team is funded by the Vermont State Department of Education's Family and Educational Support Team and administered through the Center for Developmental Disabilities at the University of Vermont. This link between the state education department, the university, and the field creates opportunities for efficient statewide dissemination of information and innovations as well as the development of a shared philosophical framework among the various constituencies in the state. The I-Team also serves as a conduit for other UAP-administered initiatives. For example, exemplary approaches developed and tested through federally funded grants on topics such as statewide systems support, early childhood programs, and services for students with deaf-blindness are disseminated to the field, in part, through the I-Team. This creates an ongoing mechanism for teams in rural areas to have access to the most recent innovations in the field.

I-Team members are an integral part of personnel preparation programs at the University of Vermont. All I-Team core members have faculty appointments commensurate with their educational credentials and experiences (i.e., lecturer, assistant professor, associate professor). One graduate course, Physical and Developmental Characteristics of Learners with Disabilities, is taught by three I-Team members from different disciplines. Two other graduate courses, pertaining to communication and applied behavior analysis, are taught by an I-Team core member. I-Team members regularly guest-lecture in many other special education graduate courses and in classes in other departments (e.g., physical therapy) at the University of Vermont. I-Team members also supervise practicum students in integrated early childhood settings. Involvement of I-Team members in personnel preparation provides ongoing opportunities to model collaborative teamwork among professionals trained in different disciplines.

Throughout its history and development, the I-Team has changed in order to respond to changing consumer needs and to accommodate the emerging vision of Vermont's Education Goals, listed in Table 7-2 (Vermont Department of Education, 1990). The location of services for students with disabilities has shifted from special classes and other separate environments to increasingly integrated sites, most notably general education classrooms in neighborhood schools where students with all types of disabilities receive special education supports. Correspondingly, the adults who receive I-Team assistance have changed from primarily special education personnel to increasing numbers of general education personnel and families.

I-Team membership has changed to include more disciplines and to include a family service component. I-Team services, formerly provided by one core team from one central location, are provided by increasingly

TABLE 7-2   Vermont's Education Goals

Goal 1: Vermonters will see to it that every child becomes a competent, caring, productive, responsible individual and citizen who is committed to continued learning throughout life.

Goal 2: Vermonters will restructure their schools to support very high performance for all students.

Goal 3: Vermont will attract, support, and develop the most effective teachers and school leaders in the nation.

Goal 4: Vermont parents, educators, students, and other citizens will create powerful partnerships to support teaching and learning in every community.

---

decentralized regional and local teams. I-Team consultation has shifted from expert consultation, in which team members advised local service providers, to collaborative consultation, in which interested parties work together as equals. The I-Team's continued importance as a mechanism to promote educational quality for students with disabilities in Vermont has been predicated on its ability to change in ways that are consistent with an increasingly inclusionary vision of people with disabilities.

CONCLUSION

Collaborative teamwork is now recognized as an essential component of effective services for persons with disabilities. Collaboration is fundamental to providing services and supports that truly respond to consumer needs, which is predicated on including consumers as equal members of their own planning teams and ensuring availability of appropriate services in the community. Three University Affiliated Programs for Persons with Developmental Disabilities offered examples of collaboration (a) among universities, state agencies, and local service providers; (b) among providers of training and technical assistance; and (c) among members of local educational teams for students with severe disabilities. Examples illustrated how trainers and technical assistants both model collaborative teamwork and use strategies such as cooperative learning and group problem solving so trainees can experience collaboration themselves as they learn about collaborative teams for students with severe disabilities.

REFERENCES

Brown, L., Branston-McLean, M.B., Baumgart, D., Vincent, L., Falvey, M., and Schroeder, J. (1979). Using the characteristics of current and subsequent least restrictive environments in the development of curricular content for severely handicapped students. *AAESPH Review, 4*(4), 407–424.

Cooper, J., and Mueck, R. (1990). Student involvement in learning: Cooperative learning and college instruction. *Journal on Excellence in College Teaching, 1,* 68–76.

Fox, T., and Williams, W. (1991). *Best practice guidelines for meeting the needs of all students in local schools.* Burlington: University of Vermont, Center for Developmental Disabilities.

Giangreco, M.F., Cloninger, C.J., and Iverson, V.S. (1993). *COACH: Choosing options and accommodations for children.* Baltimore: Paul H. Brookes.

Giangreco, M., and Putnam, J. (1991). Supporting the education of students with severe disabilities in regular education environments. In L. Meyer, C. Peck, and L. Brown (Eds.), *Critical issues in the lives of people with severe disabilities* (pp. 245–270). Baltimore: Paul H. Brookes.

Giangreco, M., York, J., and Rainforth, B. (1989). Providing related services to learners with severe handicaps in educational settings: Pursuing the least restrictive option. *Pediatric Physical Therapy, 1*(2), 55–63.

Hudson, M., and Kleinert, H.L. (1991). *Curriculum planning process and model local catalogs for students with moderate and severe disabilities.* Lexington: University of Kentucky, Interdisciplinary Human Development Institute.

Hutchison, D. (1978). The transdisciplinary approach. In J.B. Curry (Ed.), *Mental retardation: Nursing approaches to care* (pp. 65–74). St. Louis: Mosby.

Johnson, D.W., and Johnson, F. (1987). *Joining together: Group theory and group skills* (2nd ed.). Englewood Cliffs, NJ: Prentice-Hall.

Johnson, D.W., and Johnson, R.T. (1987). *Learning together and alone: Cooperative, competitive, and individualistic learning* (2nd ed.). Englewood Cliffs, NJ: Prentice-Hall.

Johnson, R.T., Johnson, D.W., and Smith, K.A. (1990). Cooperative learning: An active learning strategy for the college classroom. *Baylor Educator, 15*(2), 11–16.

Karan, O., Brandenburg, S., Sauer, M., Yoder, D., Mathey-Laikko, P., Villarruel, F., and Dolan, T. (1986). Maximizing independence for persons who are developmentally disabled: Community-based programs at the Waisman Center University Affiliated Facility. *Journal of The Association for Persons with Severe Handicaps, 11*(4), 286–293.

Kiernan, W.E., and Schalock, R.L. (1987). *Economics, industry, and disability: A look ahead.* Baltimore: Paul H. Brookes.

Kleinert, H.L., Smith, P.D., and Hudson, M. (1990). *The quality program indicators manual for students with moderate and severe handicaps.* Lexington: University of Kentucky, Interdisciplinary Human Development Institute.

Long Range Task Force on University Affiliated Facilities (1976). *The role of higher education in mental retardation and other developmental disabilities.* Washington, DC: Association of University Affiliated Programs for the Developmentally Disabled.

Lyon, S., and Lyon, G. (1980). Team functioning and staff development: A role release approach to providing integrated educational services for severely handicapped students. *Journal of the Association for the Severely Handicapped, 5*(3), 250–263.

Mount, B., and Zwernick, K. (1988). *It's never too early, it's never too late: A booklet about positive futures planning.* St. Paul, MN: Metropolitan Council.

O'Brien, J. (1987). A guide to life-style planning. In B. Wilcox and G.T. Bellamy (Eds.), *A comprehensive guide to The Activities Catalogue* (pp. 175–189). Baltimore: Paul H. Brookes.

Patterson, E.G., D'Wolf, N., Hutchison, D., Lowry, M., Schilling, M., and Siepp, J. (1976). *Staff development handbook: A resource for the transdisciplinary process.* New York: United Cerebral Palsy Associations.

Racino, J.A., Walker, P., Taylor, S., and O'Connor, S. (1992). *Housing, support, and community: Choices and strategies for adults with disabilities.* Baltimore: Paul H. Brookes.

Rainforth, B. (1985). *Collaborative efforts in the preparation of physical therapists and teachers of students with severe handicaps.* Unpublished doctoral dissertation, University of Illinois at Urbana-Champaign.

Rainforth, B., and York, J. (1987). Integrating related services in community instruction. *Journal of the Association for Persons with Severe Handicaps, 12*(3), 190–198.

Rainforth, B., York, J., and Macdonald, C. (1992). *Collaborative teamwork for students with severe disabilities: Integrating therapy and educational services.* Baltimore: Paul H. Brookes.

Schaffner, C.B., and Buswell, B.E. (1990). *Opening doors: Strategies for including all students in regular education.* Colorado Springs, CO: PEAK Parent Center.

Smith, P.D. (1990). *Integrating related services into programs for students with severe and multiple handicaps.* Lexington: University of Kentucky, Interdisciplinary Human Development Institute.

Smith, P.D., and Kleinert, J.O. (1991). *Communication programming for students with severe and multiple handicaps.* Lexington: University of Kentucky, Interdisciplinary Human Development Institute.

Stainback, S., and Stainback, W. (Eds.) (1992). *Curriculum considerations in inclusive classrooms: Facilitating learning for all students.* Baltimore: Paul H. Brookes.

Sternat, J., Messina, R., Nietupski, J., Lyon, S., and Brown, L. (1977). Occupational and physical therapy for severely handicapped students: Toward a naturalized public school model. In E. Sontag, J. Smith, and N. Certo (Eds.), *Educational programming for the severely and profoundly handicapped* (pp. 263–287). Reston, VA: Council for Exceptional Children.

Vandercook, T., York, J., and Forest, M. (1989). The McGill Action Planning System (MAPS): A strategy for building the vision. *Journal of the Association for Persons with Severe Handicaps, 14*(3), 205–215.

Vermont Department of Education (1990). *Vermont's education goals.* Montpelier, VT: Author.

Vermont State Board of Education (1990). *Special education reform: Act 230.* Information Curricular. Montpelier, VT: Author.

Villa, R., Thousand, J., Stainback, W., and Stainback, S. (1992). *Restructuring for caring and effective schools.* Baltimore: Paul H. Brookes.

Whitehouse, F.A. (1951). Teamwork, an approach to a higher professional level. *Exceptional Children, 18*(1), 75–82.

York, J., Rainforth, B., and Giangreco, M. (1990). Transdisciplinary teamwork: Clarifying some misconceptions. *Pediatric Physical Therapy, 2*(2), 73–79.

York, J., Rainforth, B., and Wiemann, G. (1988). An integrated approach to therapy for school-aged learners with developmental disabilities. *Totline, 14*(3), 36–40.

York, J., and Vandercook, T. (1991). Designing an integrated education for learners with severe disabilities through the IEP process. *Teaching Exceptional Children, 23*(2), 22–28.

8

□ □ □
□ □ □
□ □ □

Shifting Roles of Parents and Families

Bonnie Shoultz and Patricia McGill Smith

PARENT AND FAMILY ACTIVISM
SHAPING THE FUTURE

Over the past fifty or more years, parents and other family members of people with disabilities have assumed or been pressed into many different roles, both in their relationship to their family members with disabilities and in regard to the parts they have played within the disability service system. This system, which once essentially ignored the family or actively sought disruption of family ties, has come to view people with disabilities as members of families, and recognizes families as having expertise, wisdom, and rights in regard to the needs of their family members and the services they encounter. Today, progressive professionals acknowledge that well-informed family members, including their members with disabilities, will change the shape of services in the near and

Acknowledgment: Preparation of this chapter was supported by the U.S. Department of Education, Office of Special Education and Rehabilitative Services, National Institute on Disability and Rehabilitation Research, through Cooperative Agreement No. H133B00003-90 awarded to the Center on Human Policy, School of Education, Syracuse University.

The opinions expressed herein are those solely of the authors, and no official endorsement by the U.S. Department of Education should be inferred.

more distant future. This change has come about because parents and other family members have actively sought changes in the relationship between themselves and the rehabilitation system.

Ann and H. Rutherford Turnbull (1990) explore some historical and current roles of parents in a chapter that summarizes the ways in which the role(s) of parents of a child with a disability have been and are currently viewed by professionals and researchers. They describe eight major roles that parents have assumed or been expected to assume: "parents as (a) the source of their child's problems, (b) organization members, (c) service developers, (d) recipients of professionals' decisions, (e) learners and teachers, (f) political advocates, (g) educational decision-makers, and (h) family members" (p. 2). The Turnbulls view some of these roles as having been pressed upon parents, usually mothers, by professionals, and point out that others were assumed by parents in response to negative professional perceptions and/or lack of appropriate services.

It would not be difficult to identify other roles imposed on or assumed by parents and other family members since the beginnings of what we now call the disability services, or rehabilitation, system. Rather than describe the specifics of each role, we will use the phrase *parent activism* to encompass the broad range of activities that parents and family members do as political advocates, systems change agents, service developers, teachers, educational decision makers, and visionaries. This phrase also describes the motivation behind these activities—parents and other family members are actively committed to making changes in public policy and in the behavior of human service systems toward them and their family members with disabilities.

Parent activism includes active engagement in pressing for justice, involvement, and information for themselves and their family members with disabilities. It came about because parents saw not only that people with disabilities were too often neglected and abused, but that they as family members were also vulnerable to being treated in these ways. Many parents have also objected to how their family members were made into clients of a segregated and professionalized system rather than citizens of a community, and viewed as deficient and incapable of benefiting from ordinary opportunities available to others. A small but vocal minority of parent activists has consistently advocated for continued segregation, in the form of institutionalization, of people with disabilities, but their groups are overshadowed by the much larger movement we refer to as the parents' movement.

In this chapter, we often use the word *parent* even though *family* appears to be the most preferred term today. Most of the activists over the history of this movement have been parents, and of those a large majority have been mothers. We agree that inclusive terms like *family* are desirable, because there are many nonparent family members who have contributed and who will do so in the future, and because in any given family no member is more important than another. On the other hand, inclusive terms sometimes hide important realities, including the role and gender of the players. In the case of the parents' movement, most of the active players have been and still are mothers. Therefore, we will often use *parent* or even *mother* when these terms are more appropriate than *family*.

Another inclusive term we frequently use is *professional.* In our usages, *professional* means "any person who receives pay to provide services to a person with a disability," regardless of whether the person has achieved professional status through a process of academic training. This usage recognizes the power and authority of members of the various professions, but it also acknowledges the fact that power and authority, though to varying degrees, are held by any provider of service. It recognizes that services are often delivered through hierarchical structures or systems—school districts or medical bureaucracies, for example—in which the people receiving services have traditionally occupied the bottom rung. In our usage, the term professional is not meant to be a term of judgment. It is inclusive for the same reason that parent encompasses many types of family members: It allows us to talk about very broad categories of people whose lives and work are dependent on each other.

BELIEFS AND VALUES OF ACTIVIST FAMILY MEMBERS

The major way in which family members, mostly parents, have expressed their activism has been through the creation of organizations. Most of their organizations can be said to belong to a huge movement, made up of hundreds of thousands of people. The history of this movement, typically known as the parents' movement, is discussed in the next section. Before we discuss its history, however, we will describe some of the current values and beliefs motivating the movement.

The parents' movement appears to be finding a common stand on many issues that impact on the relationship between parents and professionals. First, the movement promotes the value of people with disabilities—that is, people with disabilities are spoken of as having value, as contributors to the family and society, and as people with strengths and gifts. Second, people with disabilities are viewed as having the same rights as others, including the right to the same quality of life as anyone else. Third, the movement promotes the full inclusion of people with disabilities into all aspects of community life. Fourth, the movement has adopted the perspective that societal attitudes and practices, not disability, cause most of the disability-related problems encountered by people with disabilities and their families. Finally, the movement promotes the idea that well-informed and well-supported parents are the best experts on their children, and are the most able to support and inform other parents.

In these ways, the parents' movement (as does the broader disability rights movement, which of course includes many professionals) speaks against the commonly held beliefs that disability is a tragedy and a burden, that disability causes enormous problems for the individual, the family, and society, that special services staffed by specialists are needed for people with disabilities, that families are inadequate for meeting the real needs of people with disabilities, and that people with disabilities can be nothing more than service recipients.

The latter beliefs were, and too frequently are still, upheld in professional training and practice. Research was conducted in areas such as "parent as cause of or contributor to the disability," "family burden," and the rate of divorce in families with a disabled child, and frequently confirmed that parents had a high degree of pathology, families were excessively burdened, and there was a high rate of divorce. Research conducted in special settings confirmed that special settings were needed. Professional training taught these and many other negative beliefs, and professional decisions were based on them. The public agreed with these beliefs and accepted what professionals prescribed as proper for people with disabilities.

It appears that parents of children with disabilities were subjected to a version of the broader societal process identified by Lasch (1977) as the professional appropriation of parenthood. This process, he says, began in the early twentieth century, when professional disciplines began to acquire authority over societal concerns such as education, health, crime, poverty, and many other areas of community life. With professionalization, increased attention was focused on areas once viewed as personal or communal responsibilities, such as child rearing. Parents of children with disabilities were likely, because of the messages that professionals had expert knowledge about their children, to feel the need to consult professionals and thus were even less able than other parents to avoid the professional system's net.

The parents' movement grew out of parents' resistance to commonly accepted professional practices such as parent-blaming, institutionalization, and denial of medical treatment to people with disabilities and to the patronizing attitudes and beliefs underlying these practices.

THE PARENTS' MOVEMENT: A BRIEF HISTORY

The early parents' movement (beginning in the 1950s) was begun by parents, mostly mothers, of children with disabilities (Dybwad, 1990). These parents, whether their children were at home or in institutions, began to reach out to each other through newspaper ads and by word of mouth to encourage formation of small local groups that could provide mutual support and advocate for better services. The members of these groups began to connect with people in other localities, to form statewide and national organizations of parents. One such organization, the National Association for Retarded Children (NARC, now named The Arc), is probably representative. NARC developed in response to the lack of alternatives for children with mental retardation, especially in the community, and created, through the efforts of its members, mechanisms by which such programs would be developed. It also spearheaded campaigns to improve the many public institutions housing children and adults with mental retardation in the 1950s and 1960s.

Once viewed as problems and as discountable by the disability professional community, parents fought for and won respect, power, and a place of equality within that community. We believe their use of the gender-neutral word *parent* and their general avoidance of *mother* was deliberate. First, *parent* is inclusive, and acknowledges that both mothers and fathers can be active workers for the cause, even though most of the activists are mothers. Second, it avoids the double devaluation that oppresses mothers of children with disabilities. The mothers, who have always done most of the work in the home and in the movement, can borrow the authority of the fathers as they deal with the professionals and bureaucrats that shape their children's services. Because their work seems to belong to all parents, however, the achievements of the mothers as women have been rendered invisible by this ploy.

In many cases, parents operated the early community services themselves until funding could be ensured—but brought in professionals (typically male) when money was available. The professionals are widely seen as having "taken over" this first wave of parent activity. The parents themselves initially saw professionalization as a solution to the lack of services, and tried to maintain parental input, if not control, through membership on boards of directors of agencies serving people with disabilities. For example, many local and state Associations for Retarded Citizens require their boards to have a majority of parent members. Therefore, as professionals moved into and took over the new services that parents had developed, the parents maintained some authority.

In the late 1960s and early 1970s, many parents (again, mostly women) began to question the relevance of the major disability organizations to the pressing needs of parents. Though these organizations were parent-led, they typically focused on the rights of and services for people with mental retardation. Parents were usually expected to serve these organizations, not to get direct support from them. New organizations, focusing more on support, education, and advocacy for parents, began to form. We call this phase of parents' activity "the new parents' movement."

Several factors distinguish the organizations that make up the new parents' movement from those in the earlier parents' movement. First, they tend to cross disability lines, including parents whose children have any type of disability though this is not always the case. The older organizations are disability-specific. Second, the names of these organizations typically include the word *parent* or *family*, as in Parent Advocacy Coalition for Educational Rights, Parent-to-Parent Programs, or Federation of Families for Children's Mental Health. The names of the older parent organizations usually reflected the disability category itself, as in United Cerebral Palsy Association.

Third, the mission statements, values, and activities of these organizations are much more likely to target parents or families. That is, parents' rights and needs are emphasized, information and training on topics of interest to parents are provided, and these organizations see themselves as existing to support and nurture families, not just the person with the disability. While some parent organizations recognize the child as a potential client, others focus their efforts almost exclusively on parents and families, and view the child with the disability as benefiting if the family is well supported and educated as to positive options for the child.

A fourth difference is that women have, for the most part, maintained control within the new parents' movement. Men hold few, if any, of the leadership positions. This difference is rarely mentioned, however.

Additionally, the women in the new parents' movement worked successfully to develop a funding stream and programs that ensure parent control of the new parent programs. A federal set-aside within the U.S. Department of Education's Office of Special Education Programs, established in 1982, provides funding for "Parent Training and Information Centers (PTIs)." This money has grown throughout the past decade to the point where there are now PTIs in every state, with some states having more than one. These programs target the educational system and provide training and information on parents' rights in special education. Many of the original programs—those funded more than ten years ago—have diversified their funding base to the point of having become multimillion-dollar agencies employing scores of people, almost all of whom are parents.

Women head all of the large PTIs, and women predominate throughout the network of PTIs. Mothers of children with disabilities used the networks they had built across the country, first to establish this funding stream and later, as the available amounts increased, to encourage each other to apply.

A small group of parent leaders worked with federal officials to develop a second federal funding source to provide technical assistance to parent groups that wished to apply for funds or, having secured PTI funding, wished to improve their administrative skills and develop greater expertise in the areas where they were expected to provide services to parents. This second funding source allowed several of the oldest and largest centers to form the Technical Assistance to Parent Programs (TAPP) network, which provides annual national and regional conferences for PTI staff and gives assistance with administrative tasks such as developing accountability systems for the money spent and people served. All of the TAPP leaders are women.

THE WORK OF PARENTS IN PARENTS' ORGANIZATIONS

Several categories of paid and/or volunteer work, essential to the operation and growth of parents' organizations, can be identified. *Parent support* includes outreach to new parents, listening, facilitating, informing, connecting parents with services as well as with other parents, advocating for better services for individual families, and modeling (through introducing them to one's own family, showing them that a family with a member who is disabled can be healthy and happy, and that that member can contribute to the family and grow personally). *Systems advocacy* includes work to change the systems that serve people with disabilities and their families, such as giving testimony to legislators or in public hearings, political organizing around specific issues, efforts to change professional attitudes and practice, meeting with human service decision makers, learning about negotiation strategies, learning about how each system works and the rights family members have within each system, preparation and implementation of strategies and tactics to achieve one's goals, and working with groups to accomplish all of the above.

Educating includes development of materials and provision of training for parents, professionals, and the public. *Managing* includes the many activities necessary to sustain organizations, such as planning, budgeting, documenting, working with boards and committees, and recruiting, training, and supervising staff and volunteers. *Networking* can include many types of connecting activities, all of which have the purpose of bringing family members of people with disabilities, especially mothers, into loosely organized networks that can provide support, assistance, and guidance to their members, and that can draw upon their members when systems changes are needed and/or when funds must be raised to support parent activities. Networking also includes finding like-minded professionals, administrators, legislators, and others, and forging ties with them for mutual support and utilization. *Learning* is a kind of work that includes learning about the disability of one's own child, learning about other disabilities, learning about progressive attitudes toward disability, and learning about support, systems advocacy, and networking. It is a basis for all the other work these parents do.

Some Meanings of the Work

As mentioned here, much of the work of these parents is resistance work. It is the work of activists who are trying to change many segments of society, and it is work that is based on and emanates from their personal experiences with the public, with professionals, and with bureaucratic systems. All of their work—the parent support, systems advocacy, educating, networking, learning, and managing—resists the status quo. For the parents who do it, it is energizing; like other forms of resistance work, it gives hope, lifts the burdens of everyday life, and provides an antidote to despair (Garland, 1988; McAllister, 1991). Without their work, professionals and bureaucracies would have almost absolute social control over these parents (Traustadottir, 1991), as they do over parents who have not yet been reached by or caught up in the movement (Kalyanpur and Rao, 1991; Traustadottir, Lutfiyya, and Shoultz, 1994).

At the same time, this movement has been profoundly liberating for family members and for children with disabilities. Largely because of its agenda and the values these parents espouse, most children with disabilities are now living with their families and going to public schools. Many of their mothers, having been introduced to a new world of professionals and services, and having been obliged to engage in unanticipated amounts and types of caring work, have accepted and often embraced the lifestyles into which they were thrust with the diagnoses of their children. And many of them say they have developed into people they never would have been. Many have become leaders who are making changes at the state, national, and even international levels.

Work within the parents' movement represents a nontraditional occupation. It is work that the parents who do it have created, for a number of reasons, and that they do as a result of having had children with disabilities.

Especially in its paid form, it did not exist until the parents, mostly mothers, made public the particular experiences of oppression they and their families had endured because their children had disabilities. At the same time, it expresses traditionally feminine qualities such as caregiving, connecting, facilitating, supporting, and relating.

PARENTS AND PROFESSIONALS: PARTNERS OR ADVERSARIES? THE NEED FOR CHANGE IN PROFESSIONAL PRACTICE

Parents who have been influenced by and influential in the parents' movement believe that many aspects of professional practice must change. First, parent organizations want professional training to change. They take for granted that professional training must cover the particular field of expertise of a profession. Parents expect physicians to know how to diagnose and treat illnesses and chronic medical conditions, physical therapists to be current on physical therapy techniques, and teachers to know how to teach students.

However, parents in the parents' movement generally believe that professional training—at universities and on the job—must be enhanced in a number of ways, to increase understanding of people with disabilities and the issues surrounding them. Many parent organizations have arrangements with local universities, hospitals, and agencies, where they regularly present to classes or provide in-service training sessions on these issues. For example, a family support service in New Hampshire has a "physician's respite" program. In this program, residents of the Department of Pediatrics at Dartmouth Medical School take care of families' children (all the children in the family, not just those with disabilities) while the parents go out for the evening. When they return, the parents and the residents talk about issues within the family, and the residents are led to see the child with the disability as a child and family member first. While these types of exposure may not be sufficient to change deeply held beliefs, parent organizations see them as steps toward sensitization of professionals.

Additionally, there are a number of parents of people with mental, physical, and developmental disabilities who have written books that provide a parent perspective for a professional audience (e.g., Hatfield, 1990; Moise, 1980; Turnbull and Turnbull, 1990). Some of these parents are on university faculties and/or have received professional training that informs their written work, and have as their mission the reformation of professional training (Turnbull and Turnbull, 1977, 1985; 1990) and practice.

Second, activist parents want professionals to be aware of and admit to the limits of their knowledge. Medical professionals, for example, are likely to be as prone as the average citizen to think of disability as a tragedy for children and their families, to recommend approaches based on their own subjective value systems rather than on the available knowledge in the disability field, and to be insensitive or distant in their reactions to children and their families. In regard to individual children, parents often find that they have more expertise than trained professionals in dealing with their child's medical needs (even to the point of being better able to suction the child, deal with the child's feeding tube, understand that something is medically wrong, and so on). Therefore, they demand to be heeded as they give medical and other information about the child.

Educational professionals, especially administrators, are often operating under "old" models for providing special education services and are unaware of "new" approaches such as inclusive education. In many places, administrators and teachers appear unaware of their responsibilities under federal law covering education for children with disabilities, and of parental rights under this law. In regard to individual children, teachers often are seen as unwilling to listen to, learn from, or work with the parent. Parents have many horror stories about things that happen, to the detriment of the child, when teachers do not heed them.

Third, these parents do not accept the traditional professional-client model (Schon, 1983) for their relationships with professionals. Instead, they want a relationship that they call by many different names: equality, partnership, alliance, teamwork. In this type of relationship, the parent and the professional listen to and learn from each other, equally. The professional also recognizes the parents' rights in regard to treatment and educational approaches and methods, such as the right to be informed of the various options (if they are guardians of the person with the disability), to object to professional decisions about the child, and so on. The parent recognizes the professional's technical expertise.

The professional and the parent work together to develop ideas about the child's program or treatment, valuing each other's expertise and judgment. They arrive at jointly agreed-on decisions about the child, and how to work together to implement them. Another partnership relationship is when parents and professionals work together as allies to advocate on behalf of a particular person or a group of people who are similarly situated.

Not all parent leaders in the parents' movement believe in the partnership vision. Some are concerned that the rhetoric of partnership, especially when it is initiated by professionals, is a ploy by professionals to co-opt parents and separate them from the more radical, advocacy-oriented parents who want fundamental changes in how services are delivered.

HOW PARENTS CREATE CHANGE

Parents in the parents' movement differ on how parents can change professional practice. Many believe in an incremental approach, whereby change is created step by step and place by place, working with individual professionals a few at a time. This approach may also include workshops and conferences for parents and professionals that promote a new vision—for example, of school inclusion for students with disabilities. This approach tends to emphasize development of positive relationships with professionals rather than adversarial ones. Parents who promote this approach are typically aware that there are dangers in collaboration, including co-optation or domination by professionals. They may have different beliefs than the professionals—hence a need for diplomacy—but their experience has been that they have gotten what they wanted by using this approach. Often, parent organizations provide training in strategies for bringing about change in this manner.

Other parents believe in or feel they are forced into more militant approaches, typically when they have run into serious resistance to the changes they have proposed or when a professional, especially someone working within a bureaucracy such as a school district, has demonstrated unwillingness to follow laws and regulations. Their tactics might include appearances and testimony at public meetings, appeals of decisions, publicity over practices they feel are harmful or illegal, lawsuits, organized public inquiries, complaints to federal or state oversight agencies, and many others.

It is evident that parents, whether on behalf of their own child or through an organization, develop and use strategies to create change for students with disabilities. Further, a major purpose of the parent organizations is to empower an ever-increasing number of parents to advocate for themselves, to have the skills and knowledge required to bring about needed changes and to get what they think best for their child, and to join with other parents to create changes in systems and in professional practice within those systems.

THE "GOOD" PROFESSIONAL

Parents seem to have a fairly consistent vision of how a "good" professional should behave, regardless of the profession involved. As mentioned before, the good professional would listen to and respect parents, would work in alliance with parents, and would take as well as give in discussions about the child's needs (see Biklen, 1988).

Educators and other helping professionals who fall in the "good" category have the same characteristics. They are helpful, they seek the parent's input, and they behave as if this relationship is a partnership. Parents describe these people as unusual, as people willing to buck the bureaucracies within which they operate. In talking about systems, it is not uncommon for parents to say something like, "If you're lucky enough, or persistent enough, you will find someone who will go above and beyond the requirements of the job, and will work with you to get what you need." This is another way of saying that bureaucratic systems do not apparently require their professional employees to practice in ways that parents would label as good, and may even hinder good practice.

Accompanying this observation is the view, held by many parents as well as other critics (e.g., Larson, 1977; Noddings, 1984), that bureaucratic organizations are self-perpetuating systems that function to meet internal needs (such as "efficiency," internal power relations, and following "the book" of regulations) rather than for client benefit. The "good" professional knows how to work the system to make good things happen for families.

THE ROLE OF PARENTS IN CHANGING PROFESSIONALS: WHAT IS AN EFFECTIVE PARENT?

At the same time, parents take some credit for the relationships they have with "good" professionals. Parents who describe good professionals will typically also describe their own behavior with these professionals. They talk about the strategies they use to shape professional practice, or about how their behavior influences that of the professionals in their lives, as much as (or even more than) they discuss the good professional's behavior. Apparently, they believe that good professionals are made, and that they as individual clients have something to do with the making.

Parents have definite and sometimes contradictory ideas about how to be effective in creating change. Many believe it is ineffective to take an angry or militant or "you-owe-it-to-me" approach. Parent organizations often provide training on assertiveness, negotiation, and communication skills for parents who are dealing with professionals and systems. They seem to view effective parents as able to work with people, even people they don't particularly like, willing to be "open and honest" about what they want and what they think, as willing to give as well as take, and as aware that creating change is a long-term process. Several parents also attribute success to their willingness to follow up on every commitment that is made by professionals.

PARENTS WHO ARE ALSO PROFESSIONALS

There are now many parents who are also professionals. Some were professionals before their child was born or diagnosed, and others became professionals afterward. A special category of "professional," the parent who is paid to work within the parents' movement, is described below. Parents who are professionals in some aspect of disability work (medicine, education, child development, agency management, and so on) are frequently but not always associated with the parents' movement, and have often gone into professional training as a result of their experiences with their child and their contacts with the movement. An excellent book, *Parents Speak Out*, edited by Ann and H. Rutherford Turnbull (1985), explores the perspectives of these parents on the professionals they have encountered. Many of their accounts are passionate and offer blistering denouncements of professional behavior toward themselves and all parents. Many parent professionals have made a commitment to creating change in how professionals practice in relation to people with disabilities and their families.

THE "PROFESSIONAL PARENT"

A growing number of parents receive salaries for their work in the organizations that compose the parents' movement. The phrase *professional parent* is sometimes applied to these parents, and often carries a negative connotation. As one such mother says, "You begin as a volunteer, but when you leap over from volunteer to professional, often beginning with small amounts of pay for discrete tasks, there can be a guilt trip for receiving money for this work. You're supposed to be doing it because you care, and if you're paid you must be doing it for the money, not out of caring." The roles get confused: Is this a parent, a professional, or some combination of both? From the parents' point of view, there is a "taint" of professionalism. If a parent is paid to do parents' work, she must be like the professionals. Compounding this is the notion that women should work for low pay and few benefits, especially when their work is related to a situation in their own family. Professionals, too, sometimes discredit the "professional parent," seeing her as someone whose perspectives have less validity than unpaid parents and, often simultaneously, as a threat. If such a parent develops too much polish, she is suspect.

The negative implications connected to receiving pay for this work are diminishing, however. There are many more parents who are employed part- or full-time within the movement, and parents are now getting paid for their involvement in more types of activities. Parents now may be paid for participation on advisory committees, they are more likely to have their expenses paid to go to meetings and conferences, and there are new mandates, such as the Interagency Coordinating Councils mandated for early intervention programs under Part H of the Individuals with Disabilities Act, that include payment for parents' expenses. As parents are increasingly treated more like professionals in this respect, they and the professionals have come to view this issue somewhat differently: pay is now more frequently viewed as a sign that parents' work is valued and valuable.

PARENTS' ACTIVISM ON LEGISLATIVE ISSUES

Today, many federal and state laws and priorities are demanding the focused attention of the organized parent organizations, which work with others to design and pass legislation, oversee its implementation, and influence the regulatory and funding processes. Following are a few of the federal initiatives of the early 1990s, with short descriptions of areas in which parents and family members are included.

- *The Individuals with Disabilities Education Act of 1989* (IDEA) reauthorized the Education for the Handicapped Act, which mandates a free, appropriate education for all students with disabilities. IDEA added parent training for parents of children from birth to five years of age to the earlier mandate that parents of school-aged children have access to such training, added stronger outreach to racially and culturally diverse families, mandated formation of a Federal Interagency Coordinating Council, and added other parent rights to those given parents under P.L. 94-142.
- *Rehabilitation Act Amendments of 1992* (P.L. 102-569) included new requirements for family member involvement in the vocational rehabilitation process. The language in IDEA relating to Parent Training and Information Centers was incorporated into the act, requiring that basic information on the rehabilitation system must be provided to family members, including support to family members, training on how to negotiate these systems, and bridging the gap between the transition services mandated in IDEA (in which parents are to play an important role) and the services in the Rehabilitation Act. Training is to emphasize that parents have a specific role to play

in the rehabilitation process, that their role is ancillary, not controlling, recognizing their son's or daughter's choices. Outreach to unserved, underserved, and minority populations must be described in each state plan. Each state must establish a State Vocational Rehabilitation Advisory Council, which will include parents and people with disabilities along with professionals. For the first time, parents and other family members are specifically recognized in the legislation that funds the vocational rehabilitation system.

- *The Americans with Disabilities Act of 1990* (ADA), enacted by Congress on July 26, 1990, has received national attention. The implementation of the ADA relies heavily on well-trained and aware parents and people with disabilities. Federal funds were granted to a consortium of parent organizations to operate a project to train family members about the requirements of the ADA.
- *The Administration on Developmental Disabilities* (ADD) periodically establishes new sets of priorities for funding of federal and state projects. In the last years of the Bush administration, empowerment of consumers and families was an ADD priority. A number of projects to promote empowerment were funded at the federal level, and states were required to emphasize consumer and family empowerment as well.
- *The National Institute on Disability and Rehabilitation Research* (NIDRR), a major part of the U.S. Department of Education's Office of Special Education and Rehabilitative Services, funds hundreds of research projects, including Research and Training Centers that focus on various disabilities. Consumer and parent involvement in advising these projects, assisting with the design of research, and as employees or consultants with these projects, was mandated in 1991.

IMPLICATIONS FOR THE FUTURE

Parents and other family members will become increasingly sophisticated in their understanding of the service systems to which they must turn for assistance. Parents and family members from traditionally marginalized groups such as low-income and/or non-European-American families will become more active, as well. The whole family, not just parents, will become more involved as activists, and their sophistication will be exhibited in ease of maneuvering the systems and in the changes these systems will undergo due to their influence. Knowledgeable families will insist on being supported, not served, in settings that include everyone, including people with disabilities, and will have an increasingly influential impact on legislation that affects them and their family members.

Today, more than ever, the concept of "power-sharing" is mentioned and sometimes explored by writers in the disability field. By *power-sharing* they tend to mean that those who have traditionally had the power will or should voluntarily share it with family members and people with disabilities. Power in this sense includes decision-making authority, command of resources, the ability to influence other powerful people, and control over the supports one uses. It is a concept that is closely allied to the "support" concept. Another possibility, less likely, is that power struggles will become more intense as the parents' movement grows in power and dynamism, with each of the many sides battling to hold on to the power they have.

Increasingly, the diversity of families will be recognized and embraced. Parents' organizations today fully recognize the differences between families, and are calling for a similar recognition by professional and provider organizations. In the future, as more diverse families join and participate in the parents' movement, their causes will come to the fore. Professional organizations will be faced with a growing demand for culturally competent services, and will need to develop creative strategies (such as subsidizing professional training for low-income, culturally and linguistically diverse workers) for meeting this demand.

Parents' organizations are beginning to broaden their scope and identify cross-cutting issues that affect other disenfranchised groups, such as the lack of safe and affordable housing or the low employment rate for marginalized groups, as much as they affect people with disabilities. Alliances between these groups, formed to tackle specific issues, can have a larger and more long-lasting impact than can the parents' organizations by themselves, because they can address some of the larger systemic issues that exist.

People with disabilities are growing in strength and sophistication too. In the past, parents and parents' organizations have made decisions and influenced legislation and services in ways today's adults with disabilities object to. In the future, parents' organizations will have to negotiate with organizations of adults with disabilities as legislative and policy changes are being proposed, just as individual parents must learn to negotiate or turn over the decision making to their son or daughter with a disability. Parents' organizations may play a support role in regard to some issues, such as independent living, that affect the lives of adults with disabilities, and may negotiate their role in regard to other issues, such as personal assistance services. Most important, they and the professional organizations must view adults with disabilities as equals, if not as taking the lead, in the battle for adequate support for all people with disabilities in the community.

We believe that many of these projections will be reflected in federal policy and regulations over the next decade. We also believe that the role of professionals will continue to shift, vis-à-vis families, to a support role in which professionals will apply their talents and expertise in the service of ends that families and people with disabilities have chosen.

REFERENCES

Biklen, D. (1988). The myth of clinical judgment. *Journal of Social Issues, 44*(1), 127–140.

Dybwad, R. (1990). *Perspectives on a parent movement.* Boston: Brookline Books.

Garland, A.W. (1988). *Women activists: Challenging the abuse of power.* New York: Feminist Press.

Hatfield, A.B. (1990). *Families as allies in treatment of the mentally ill.* Washington, DC: American Psychiatric Association.

Kalyanpur, M. and Rao, S.S. (1991). Empowering low-income black families of handicapped children. *American Journal of Orthopsychiatry, 61*(4), 523–532.

Larson, M. (1977). *The rise of professionalism: A sociological analysis.* Berkeley: University of California Press.

Lasch, C. (1977). *Haven in a heartless world.* New York: Basic Books.

McAllister, P. (1991). *This river of courage: Generations of women's resistance and action.* Philadelphia: New Society Publishers.

Moise, L.E. (1980). *As up we grew with Barbara.* Minneapolis: Dillon Press.

Noddings, N. (1984). *Caring: A feminine approach to ethics and moral education.* Berkeley: University of California Press.

Schon, D.A. (1983). *The reflective practitioner.* New York: Basic Books.

Traustadottir, R. (1991). The meaning of care in the lives of mothers of children with disabilities. In S.J. Taylor, R. Bogdan, and J.A. Racino (Eds.), *Life in the community: Case studies of organizations supporting people with disabilities* (pp. 185–194). Baltimore: Paul H. Brookes.

Note: Both authors are parents of young adults who have disabilities, and both have been active in parents' organizations since the early 1970s. Bonnie Shoultz, who began her work with parents as a professional, is beginning a qualitative research study of mothers in the parents' movement. Patricia McGill Smith began her work with parents after her daughter was diagnosed as having mental retardation, and now leads a major national parents' organization, the National Parent Network on Disabilities.

Traustadottir, R., Lutfiyya, Z., and Shoultz, B. (1994). Community integration: A multicultural approach. In M. Hayden (Ed.), *Community living for persons with mental retardation and related conditions.* Baltimore: Paul H. Brookes.

Turnbull, A., and Turnbull, H.R. (1977, 1985). *Parents speak out: Then and now.* Columbus, OH: Charles E. Merrill.

Turnbull, A.P., and Turnbull, H.R. (1990). *Families, professionals, and exceptionality: A special partnership* (2nd ed.). Columbus, OH: Charles E. Merrill.

9

Multicultural Influences on Rehabilitation Training and Services: The Shift to Valuing Nondominant Cultures

Farah A. Ibrahim

INTRODUCTION

Providing effective services to individuals with disabilities in a pluralistic society implies a consideration of each person's culture. To understand a person's culture, one needs to consider many variables, including race/culture, ethnicity, lifestyle, life stage, gender, and institutional or noninstitutional status (which can be a much more powerful cultural variable than race, ethnicity, and culture combined). Traditionally, professional training and service delivery has focused on knowledge of the domains of rehabilitation, disabilities, and facilitation of a person medically, psychologically, and vocationally. Today, we are moving from fitting people into programs to a more person-centered approach, in which services and supports are built around the person (Dillman, Karan, and Granfield, 1993).

Within this framework the professional assumes a role of facilitator rather than decision maker for a person with disabilities. To truly "facilitate," however, requires clear knowledge of several variables that influence both the service provider and the consumer—cultural identity, beliefs, values, and assumptions; gender; social class; education; lifestyles—as well as the impact of these variables on the parties' relationship. This chapter clarifies the cultural, gender, social class, and lifestyle issues within the context of facilitating choices and opportunities for individuals with disabilities. Approaches to understanding the consumer's culture, influence of the disability, gender, social class, and other topics will be discussed.

Culture is an issue when helping professionals are involved with consumers in cross-cultural, cross-gender, cross-ethnicity, cross-class, cross-lifestyle, or cross-disciplinary encounters. Although disability by itself qualifies as a cultural characteristic separate from race, ethnicity, impact of religion, and educational level, it is usually not considered as such. But, in fact, like so many other cultural characteristics, if one's disability does not fit the characteristics of mainstream culture, it is often considered an aberration. Typically in service delivery and in professional training programs, everyone adopts the "mainstream" or the first world perspectives (McFadden, 1993). Draguns (1991) maintains that training procedures in the past and present provide possibilities for mainstream consumption, that is, middle-class professionals equipped to deal with middle-class consumers.

The result is often cultural oppression for people with disabilities with varied cultures, worldviews, and perspectives (Ibrahim and Arredondo, 1986, 1990). The tendency to focus on the consumer's behavior or disability without understanding the impact of that person's cultural characteristics violates the consumer in many known and unknown ways. In encounters where multiple differences exist between professionals and consumers, a lack of understanding of these variables qualifies as behavior that is "cultural oppression" (Ibrahim, 1993b). The perspectives presented here will broaden conceptions regarding sensitivity and approaches necessary in working with individuals who have many unique characteristics. Effective facilitation demands mutual understanding between the professional and the consumer.

MULTICULTURAL PERSPECTIVE AND RESPECT FOR NONDOMINANT CULTURES

For more than two decades, literature in the helping professions has examined the viability of the available models for the provision of services, specifically because they rest on the values and belief systems of the majority. The United States is a world leader in developing services, strategies, and educational programs to help people with disabilities gain independence, grow in productivity, and become integrated in the community. Most training models have originated in the United States and reflect mainstream American philosophies; now they are being transposed internationally. Unfortunately, these available models systematically deny the realities of non-Western systems of thinking (Ibrahim, 1993b). Further, in the United States these models are insensitive to the needs of people with disabilities who are also immigrants, ethnic minorities, women, and/or who have different lifestyles (AACD [now ACA], 1987; Ibrahim, 1986, 1991; Ibrahim and Arredondo, 1986, 1990).

Demographic projections show that a century from now, the population of the United States will be closer to the world balance: 57 percent Asian, 26 percent white, 7 percent black, and 10 percent people of Hispanic origin. This group may include any of the following races—i.e., white, black, and native indigenous populations (Edmunds, Martinson, and Goldberg, 1990; Ibrahim, 1991, 1992).

The challenge for professional training programs and service providers to people with disabilities is to respond to these national concerns. Although progress has occurred in clarifying the needs of the underserved, to a large extent it has been limited to theoretical formulations and research applications to "minority" segments of the population (Ibrahim, 1991). Unfortunately, these points of view add nothing to the majority assumptions regarding service delivery (Ibrahim and Arredondo, 1990). Instead, a radical shift in perspective is required: the literature and research in multicultural counseling must make a significant contribution to generic helping domains. Rather than view this information as a specific knowledge area, necessary to assist only nondominant cultures, we need to incorporate it in mainstream theories of helping and facilitation (Ibrahim, 1991).

Theorists and researchers have offered three major recommendations to ease the process of multicultural encounters. These include an understanding of worldview (values, beliefs, and assumptions), its impact on identity, philosophy, modes of interaction with the world—including, but not limited to, problem solving, conflict resolution, and decision making (Ibrahim, 1984a, 1984b, 1985b, 1991; Ibrahim and Schroeder 1987, 1990; Sue, 1978; Sue and Sue, 1991); knowledge of specific cultures; and knowledge of culture-specific verbal and nonverbal skills to ease the particular encounter (Sue and Zane, 1987). Additionally, research has addressed many process and outcome variables, most of them limited to counseling and psychotherapy. These include racial similarity/dissimilarity, consumer expectations, match between therapist and consumer, therapist credibility, and attractiveness.

Pedersen, Fukuyama, and Heath (1989) note that research on consumer, professional, and contextual variables yielded mixed results. Recommendations that encourage professionals to be culturally sensitive and to know the culture of the consumer have not proven to be very effective either (Sue and Zane, 1987). Further, culture-specific techniques applied to consumers across cultures, without attention to appropriateness of the techniques to the specific individual, pose a threat of cultural oppression.

Cultural factors in the treatment of ethnic minority consumers have received considerable attention among professionals. Yet services to minority or culturally different consumers remain inadequate. This is due to a lack of bilingual and bicultural professionals, stereotypes and biases that professionals hold, and their inability to provide culturally responsive forms of treatment. The reason for this inadequacy is attributed to professional training models developed for Anglo-Saxon or mainstream Americans (Ibrahim, Stadler, Arredondo, and McFadden, 1986; Ponterotto and Casas, 1987). Further, such training programs typically do not even apply to mainstream populations.

The helping professions are still seeking viable theories and models for training that would prepare service providers to provide valid, effective, reliable, and ethical professional services in a culturally diverse society (Corey, Corey, and Callanan, 1988). The models must have a solid theoretical basis. It is critical that this multicultural nation shift to models of facilitation and training that recognize the pluralism inherent in this society. We must also acknowledge and respond to the democratic principles for which this nation stands. Individuals, in being forced to the margins, suffer intense pain when they realize that a nation that subscribes to such high ideals will not accommodate the needs of those who are different. It is imperative that professionals acquire specialized skills and be sensitive to the culturally different (Brown and Srebalus, 1988).

ASSESSMENT AND INTERVENTIONS FOR PEOPLE WITH DISABILITIES

To begin to truly value nondominant cultures and lifestyles, we need a strategy to evaluate and assess individuals with disabilities, to understand their philosophy of life, worldview, and their modes of coping and problem solving. The proposed multidimensional assessment strategy needs to incorporate the following:

1. Worldview and cultural identity of: the consumer, the family, and significant others
2. Stage of identity development: cultural and gender perspectives
3. Disability status and its impact on the consumer, his or her family, and on societal expectations

These three dimensions must be considered in the cultural milieu of the persons with disabilities. Since the variables are anchored in a cultural context, it is appropriate that they be considered from the perspective of culture.

U.S. Culture and Disability

Before attempting to clarify the consumer's worldview and cultural identity, it is essential to understand disability in this society. In the United States, people with disabilities have gone through many transitions in the last two hundred years. Funk (1987), in reviewing the changes in treatment of people with disabilities from the founding of the nation until the second decade of the twentieth century, characterizes the movement as "from attic to warehouse" (noted in Gartner, Lipsky, and Turnbull, 1991, p. 39). Gartner, Lipsky, and Turnbull (1991), in an excellent review of culture and disability, note that in most circumstances those who are disabled (versus the "temporarily able") are seen as less attractive, unable to work, lowest on the economic ladder, unable to learn (less intelligent), and so on. They stress that the most negative impact of these cultural perceptions is on the self-concept of people with disabilities, and the limits it puts on their potential, both social and physical. Further, these perceptions limit the potential help people with disabilities can receive, due to the anxiety their disability or disfigurement creates for the helpers, who may be "temporarily" able-bodied.

A natural outcome of growing up in a culture that does not value people with disabilities is the establishment of separate facilities and systems to provide services. Additionally, the culture holds the ideal of being able-bodied. For a person with disabilities, this cultural ideal creates a sense of being less than normal. These attitudinal variables have influenced our expectations of people with disabilities, which tend to support the notion that they are less than normal, and deserve to be treated as sick people, with less expected of them (Gliedman and Roth, 1980). Fine and Asch (1988) support the notion of reframing disability as a "minority" group issue that requires reanalysis in several domains. These domains include the following (p. 19):

1. How the experience of disability is influenced by professionals and how it can be studied by researchers who are nondisabled needs to be assessed.
2. Disability needs to be studied over time and in context, as a socially transforming and changing process, not as a static characteristic of an individual.

3. A social constructivist view of disability enables a reassessment of previously taken-for-granted views of the nature and course of life with impairments.

4. Accepting a minority-group perspective on disability and attending to all aspects of the life space that extend beyond the person with the impairment causes social psychologists to raise new questions for research.

The most critical variable to consider is how being labeled as a person with a disability influences a person's perspectives. It is another layer that separates these consumers from the "norm." Professionals who work with people with disabilities do not necessarily hold positive attitudes toward them (Ibrahim and Herr, 1982). These attitudes and perspectives cannot escape societal values, nor be uninfluenced by the societal context. In the context of the United States, it is also important to recognize that a double-minority status—that is, a person from a nondominant culture who has a disability—carries certain further liabilities, since even if professionals are trained to consider culture/race/ethnicity, gender, age, and so on, it is only as singular variables. The complexity that these and other similar variables involve in combination has been neither adequately researched nor addressed. The remainder of this chapter will attempt to confront the assessment of these variables and their impact on consumers.

ROLE OF VALUES, BELIEFS, AND ASSUMPTIONS IN REHABILITATION WORK

All helping professions are value laden, since training and education occurs in a specific society that imposes its values on the training process. Further, all education socializes professionals to maintain or develop middle-class, mainstream perspectives. This is difficult to escape, since most professionals generally come from middle classes and have a bias toward mainstream assumptions. Controversies regarding the role of professionals' values, and their impact on process and outcome in rehabilitation services, have raged for decades (Patterson, 1989). Some argue that there is a distinction between the theories professionals subscribe to and the personal values they hold (Beck et al. 1979). Others consider this perspective to be impractical and confusing (Cirillo and Wapner, 1986). Most agree that professionals cannot advocate a value position that is free of their personal assumptions or interpretations (Frank, 1973; Strong, 1968). Beutler and Bergan (1991) report that research in the last two decades on value similarity has shown that convergence between the professional's values and the consumer's assumptions helps the relationship and promotes consumer growth and development.

To create convergence or similarity between the professional's and the consumer's assumptions (in spite of the able-bodied/disabled separation), it is important to understand the role of worldview as a mediating variable (Ibrahim, 1991, 1993b). Worldview is a significant contribution of the multicultural counseling literature to the generic fields of applied psychology (Ibrahim, 1984a, 1985b, 1985c, 1991; Sue 1978; Sue and Sue, 1991). This variable mediates knowledge of a specific cultural group and knowledge of culture-consistent and culture-specific techniques applicable to a specific individual (Ibrahim, 1991). Without worldview as a mediating variable, both knowledge of specific cultures and culture-specific techniques can be misapplied, leading to charges of ethical violation and cultural oppression. After clarification of the worldview, appropriate applications of theory and research can take place.

The acknowledgment and acceptance that individual worldviews may vary within a group makes the intervention "person centered," that is, useful and meaningful for the particular person, not only as a representative of a certain racial, cultural, religious, age, or regional group, but as an individual. Without knowledge or the skills to assess and fully understand worldview, the helping professional lacks any alternative but, at best, to apply the information regarding a specific culture to a consumer from that culture—or simply to impose his or her worldview on the person.

This general application of cultural information, or an assumption that the consumer is similar to the counselor, can lead to cultural oppression by forcing an idiosyncratic consumer into a program "slot," where the potential for a mismatch between the person's needs, interests, and capabilities and the environmental demands and expectations is likely. Treating persons as stereotypes of their cultural group violates the person's individuality and may lead to negative outcomes regarding the consumer's perceptions of the helping professional and the field of rehabilitation (Ibrahim, 1993b).

Professionals need a strategy to understand their cultural identity and worldview, and their philosophy of life. This must occur against the backdrop of culture, socioeconomic level, race, age, life stage, ethnicity, gender, and sociopolitical history. If professionals do not understand their cultural identity and worldview, and do not reflect on the multiplicity of factors that have shaped their lives, they will be unable to provide effective services because their cultural assumptions will systematically operate, distracting them from providing meaningful services to consumers.

Worldview and Cultural Identity

To provide ethical services to individuals with disabilities from different cultural backgrounds, nationalities, ethnicities, races, genders, ages, life stages, educational levels, and social classes, the professional must understand his or her worldview and cultural identity, philosophical and psychological assumptions, as well as have knowledge of both the primary and secondary cultural environments that he or she comes from (Ibrahim and Arredondo, 1986, 1990).

According to Sire (1976), our worldview consists of the presuppositions and assumptions we hold about our world. Horner and Vandersluis (1981) assert that since worldviews are culturally based variables, they influence the professional/consumer relationship. Our worldview directly acts on and mediates our belief systems, assumptions, modes of problem solving, decision making, and conflict resolution (Ibrahim, 1991, 1993b).

Sue (1978) defines *worldview* as an individual's perception of his or her relationship with the world, people, and things. Sarason (1984) notes that each of us possesses and is possessed by a worldview as a result of the socialization process. One's worldview influences individual goals and behavior. Worldviews are identified as a critical variable that can enhance or obstruct the communication process (Abramovitz and Dokecki, 1977; Ibrahim, 1984a, 1985b; Ibrahim and Kahn, 1987; Strupp, 1978, Sundberg, 1981).

Sue (1978) originally proposed the idea of worldview based on two psychological theories, locus of control (Rotter, 1966) and locus of responsibility (Jones et al., 1972). This theoretical perspective provided an important tool in cross-cultural encounters. Yet no integrated instrument was developed to assess worldview. Ibrahim (1984a, 1985b) proposed a broader formulation of the construct of worldview based on C. Kluckhohn's (1951) work on value orientations and value emphasis in various cultures. The Kluckhohn framework accounts for both philosophical and psychological dimensions, including beliefs, values, assumptions, attitudes, and behavior of individuals and groups. Kluckhohn (1951) proposed five universal or existential categories that pertain to a general, organized conception of human nature, social relationships, nature, time, and activity. These conceptions he postulated influence human behavior, motivations, decisions, and lifestyles.

The Existential Worldview Theory (Ibrahim, 1984a; Ibrahim, 1993b) is a cognitive-values perspective that uses worldview and cultural identity as mediational forces in an individual's life. The theory proposes that each individual in a professional-consumer dyad be viewed as a unique "cultural entity" (Ibrahim, 1984a), with an emphasis on the individual's "subjective reality" (Triandis, 1972) or worldview (Ibrahim, 1984a). Such a process of self-examination for the professional and focused attention on the consumer's worldview will ease in the development of and establishment of a positive relationship. Further, Ibrahim (1991, 1993b) contends that it can lead to professional-consumer cultural matching based on cultural assumptions and philosophical similarity, instead of basing the matching on some more capricious variables or the simple availability of particular service programs.

In its application, Ibrahim's theory includes the following perspectives: (a) Both the professional's and the consumer's worldview must be clarified. This must include an analysis of both the cultural and gender identity (Ibrahim, 1992) of the parties involved, and implies ethnicity, culture, age, life stage, socioeconomic level, education, religion, philosophy of life, beliefs, values, and assumptions. (b) These worldviews, once clarified, must be placed within a sociopolitical context, history of migration, acculturation level, languages spoken, and comfort with mainstream assumptions and values (Ibrahim, 1985b, 1991, 1993b; Ibrahim and Schroeder, 1990).

The Scale to Assess World View (SAWV) (Ibrahim and Kahn, 1984, 1987) and the SAWV II (Ibrahim, 1993a), based on Kluckhohn's (1951) value orientations and value emphases, have been found to be helpful in clarifying one's worldview. They are clarified by the following existential categories, with the given range of assumptions (Ibrahim, 1991, p. 15):

Human nature: good, bad, or both
Social relationships: linear-hierarchical, collateral-mutual, and individualistic
Nature: subjugate and control nature, live in harmony with nature, accept the power and control of nature over people
Time orientation: past, present, and future
Activity orientation: being, being-in-becoming, and doing

The SAWV has adequate reliability and validity (Ibrahim and Kahn, 1987, Ibrahim and Owen, 1992; Sadowsky et al., in press). The use of the SAWV helps the professional in (a) understanding the consumer's specific worldview, beliefs, values, and assumptions, which have a direct relationship with their cognitive, emotional, social perceptions and interactions with the world; (b) providing an understanding of the consumer's expression and experience of issues and problems; and (c) clarifying the consumer's worldview as compared to his or her primary cultural group, that is, differentiating the consumer from family, primary group, and larger society (Lonner and Ibrahim, 1989). The use of the SAWV as a mediational force eliminates the risk of cultural oppression when applying culture-specific information, knowledge, and skills to counseling, psychotherapy, or training (Ibrahim, 1991).

Cultural and Gender Identity Assessment

The worldview of the consumer must be understood within his or her cultural and gender identity. This incorporates the following variables (Ibrahim, 1992, 1993a):

How gender is conceptualized in the consumer's primary group
- How gender affects the consumer in the familial and primary cultural context

Sociopolitical history

Generation in the United States (group history)

Social conditions experienced by the consumer's group and group status

History of migration to the United States
- How the consumer's group was received and integrated in the United States
- The consumer's own migration history; if an immigrant, voluntary or involuntary immigrant, as with refugees

Religion
- Status of consumer's faith in the United States

Age and its meaning in primary cultural group and the mainstream culture

Life stage, its meaning for the consumer in the primary cultural context, and in mainstream culture

Languages spoken, impact of the philosophies underlying the bilingual or trilingual languages spoken; status or lack of it, due to the language factor

Ability or disability status
- How this is viewed in the consumer's own culture and among mainstream culture
- Is the consumer institutionalized or has the consumer been institutionalized? (assessment of institutionalization's impact on worldview)

The consumer's worldview can be assessed by administering the SAWV or the SAWV II (Ibrahim and Kahn, 1984, 1987; Ibrahim, 1993a). This will provide basic information on how consumers view the world in terms of their values, beliefs, and assumptions. The information provided will yield a primary worldview and a secondary worldview (Ibrahim and Owen, 1992). The four possible worldviews that can be provided by using the SAWV or the SAWV II are Optimistic, Traditional, Here and Now, and Ecological.

After deriving the worldview, the assessment needs to focus on under-standing the cultural identity of the consumer and the meaning of world-view within it. To this end, the Cultural Identity Check List (CICL) (Ibrahim, 1990b, 1993a; Appendix A in this chapter) may be administered. The information gained from the consumer's own statements on the CICL can be used to explore further the variables listed above to understand the person's cultural and gender identity and cultural context. These variables provide information that help clarify values and assumptions within the context of one's life and the history of one's cultural group.

After clarification of the consumer's cultural identity, the professional can work toward developing a relationship with the individual in which both parties feel that they understand the other enough to develop trust. Open sharing of similarities and differences in worldviews between the professional and consumer needs to take place, on the premise that in multicultural encounters the issues of trust and relationship development become very complicated (Beutler and Bergan, 1991). This sharing will enhance the consumer's trust. Further, it will help the consumer under-stand the professional as a person and increase his or her self-knowledge. Eventually, this knowledge can lead to the development of a shared world-view (a composite of the professional's and the consumer's overlapping belief systems).

This shared worldview, according to Torrey (1986), is the basis of highly effective relationships in cross-cultural and intra-cultural encounters. Kelly (1990) also holds that convergence of shared values results in im-proved feelings or functioning for the consumer. The third step is to arrive at goals, create opportunities, and provide needed support that would be con-sistent with the consumer's beliefs, values, and cultural identity. The infor-mation gained also will facilitate the process of communication between the professional and the consumer, because it will help the professional to develop culture-specific modes of communication.

Applications in Rehabilitation

The application of this assessment strategy in rehabilitation involves going beyond the professional-consumer dyad to understand the impact the disability has had on the person, how the person's family addressed the disability (acceptance/nonacceptance), and the impact of this on the consumer's worldview. In rehabilitation work, it becomes essential that the assessment is used as a backdrop to address the following variables: identifying the consumer's issues, deciding on the communication process due to different structures of reasoning and logic, and developing viable outcome goals with the consumer.

Initial Consumer Assessment

The SAWV and the CICL can be used in the initial assessment (Ibrahim, 1984a, 1993a; Lonner and Ibrahim, 1989). The use of these instruments helps in clarifying the beliefs, values, assumptions, and cultural identity of the consumer, by making them tangible and explicit. The information provides a reasonable starting point in a culturally diverse world, since there are very few such assessment measures. The SAWV can also be used to assess the worldview of the consumer's family. This is essential to clarify the consumer's goals and the family's expectations. At this stage, it is critical that some clarity is sought on how the consumer and his or her family coped with the disability, and the impact of the coping style on the consumer's self-expectations and future goals.

The assessments provide information regarding how well the consumer "fits" or does not fit the values, beliefs, and assumptions of his or her primary group, family, and or community setting. They also help in developing an understanding how the worldview of the larger society is assimilated by the consumer, providing a measure of acceleration (Ibrahim, 1991). Worldview assessment also assists in clarifying whether the consumer defines himself or herself objectively or subjectively.

Identifying the consumer's worldview and cultural identity also helps in the assessment of mismatch between individuals and their environments (Lonner and Ibrahim, 1989). This is an extremely complex process in most situations, but with the multiplicity of factors to be considered in multicultural encounters, it becomes extremely difficult.

Lonner and Ibrahim (1989) recommend a three-step process for assisting with the multicultural components of an ecological assessment. This includes (a) understanding the worldview; (b) identifying the consumer's true "norm" group based on an evaluation of the assumptions and cultural outlook of the consumer and the cultural group or groups he or she comes from and identifies with; and (c) using a combination of approaches to clarify the causes of the "mismatch"—direct observation, clinical judgments, and various standardized and nonstandardized assessments may all be required. The key variables again are the worldview and cultural identity. If understood accurately they can increase the probability of a culturally appropriate intervention.

IMPLICATIONS FOR PROCESS AND OUTCOME

Success in helping relationships is highly dependent on the process the consumer experiences. To establish an effective process, one must acknowledge that all helping relationships are essentially a process of interpersonal influence (Strong, 1968). Strong contends that the consumer's acceptance of the professional's assistance depends on the individual's perception of the professional as expert, trustworthy, and attractive. Research in counseling and psychotherapy supports this contention (Atkinson and Carskaddon, 1975; Barak and La Crosse, 1975; Merluzzi, Merluzzi, and Kaul, 1977; Schmidt and Strong, 1971).

Torrey (1986) emphasizes that the consumer has to experience the professional as someone who understands and will be effective in assisting him or her. Basic to this process of interpersonal influence is a shared worldview (Ibrahim, 1984a, 1985b, 1991; Ibrahim and Schroeder, 1990; Torrey, 1986). The most critical task facing the professional in transcultural encounters is the establishment of a shared worldview or a common culture with the consumer (Ibrahim and Schroeder, 1990). This can be accomplished by using the SAWV (or SAWV II) and the responses to the CICL to better understand the consumer's beliefs, values, and assumptions, cultural identity, and ways of problem solving and decision making.

During this process the professional may share his or her personal beliefs, values, and assumptions wherever they overlap with the consumer's in an attempt to create a common cultural world to enhance communication, the relationship, and the support process (Ibrahim and Schroeder, 1990). The goal here is not to minimize or overlook the differences. The process makes the differences explicit and clarifies the outcomes and solutions that may be meaningful for the professional but antithetical for the consumer. This discussion gives the consumer permission to identify and articulate his or her personal perspectives and find solutions within them.

TRAINING AND EDUCATION MODEL TO INCREASE PROFESSIONALS' SENSITIVITY

The need to incorporate multicultural perspectives in applied psychology and rehabilitation is recent (Bales, 1985; D'Andrea, Daniels, and Heck, 1991; Ibrahim, 1991; Ibrahim, Stadler, Arredondo, and McFadden, 1986; Leake, James, and Stodden, Chapter 2 in this book; Ponterroto and Casas, 1987). The Existential Worldview Theory has significant implications for training and education in rehabilitation and applied mental health professions. A major difference between this approach and other models is that it is anchored in a theoretical model, with assessment tools available to operationalize the model, and it has been tested and proven to be effective in increasing consumer-perceived empathy and cross-cultural sensitivity of the professional (Cunningham-Warburton, 1988; Sadlak and Ibrahim, 1986).

In two studies, consumers reported feeling understood and appropriately responded to by professionals, and reported greater satisfaction with professionals trained in using the SAWV and cultural information. Additionally, research supported the contention that professionals trained in using the Existential Worldview Theory and the SAWV would develop a shared frame of reference with consumers (Cunningham-Warburton, 1988; Sadlak and Ibrahim, 1986). Further, this model also incorporates gender differentiation and does not treat people as simply cultural beings. It also considers how gender and cultural identity may interact in the challenges consumers face and the resolutions they will require (Furn, 1986, 1988; Furn and Ibrahim, 1987; Ibrahim, 1991).

This approach uses a cognitive, affective, and skills approach (Ibrahim and Schroeder, 1989). The three aspects of training are not discretely separated; they occur as overlapping stages. The training model ensures that the process and goals established to assist a consumer are consistent with the consumer's assumptions (Axelson, 1985; Brown and Srebalus, 1988; Corey, Corey, and Callanan, 1988). The approach ensures that professionals are clearly aware of their assumptions, and of the consumer's, which simplifies interventions at both the process and outcome levels. The specifics of this professional training model follow.

Awareness and Sensitivity

Prior to the actual training, a need for the training is created among the participants by heightening their awareness of their cultural self. Further, the cultural pluralism of the world and the relativity of human values are explored. A group-dynamics, experiential approach is taken. This is a critically important stage in creating a readiness among the participants to explore themselves and others in the group. The focus of the exploration is on members as cultural entities, and to start hypothesizing about the experience of people who are culturally different from a society or system. Simple exercises that help the participants identify their values and the agencies (family, school, church, and society) that may have influenced them are used. During this stage, the SAWV and the CICL are administered. The participants are encouraged to share information with others in the group, but the sharing is voluntary.

Affective

This component overlaps to a large extent with the Awareness and Sensitivity and the Cognitive stages. It is highly experiential: group exercises are used to explore issues of race, gender, culture, socioeconomic level, educational level, age, life stage, lifestyle, and ability or disability status. The goals here are to help the participants identify their feelings about their cultural identity, gender, age, and so on. Further, the focus is to develop an understanding of what it means to be different, and the many ways that we are similar to and different from each other. A major goal at this stage is to help the participants identify feelings about themselves and others in the group. The participants practice empathic responding skills regarding the differences experienced by the group and others in a specific society.

Cognitive

This component provides information about the history and theories of cross-cultural counseling. The Existential Worldview Theory, along with the SAWV and the CICL, are presented. The participants learn to administer these instruments and learn about using the information in helping relationships (consumer engagement, professional consumer matching, assessment, process and goal development).

Skills

Here the participants are exposed to specific communication skills that would be useful in encounters with people from nondominant cultures. Further, training tapes that explore cross-cultural issues are used to enhance the participant's ability in cross-cultural encounters. In the final sessions, the participants identify case vignettes representing different cultures and role-play the vignettes. The participants give each other feedback, and the instructor also provides feedback.

The model has been tested and is effective, as noted earlier. However, further research is needed to identify how the varied information on cross-cultural training models can be merged to prepare highly effective and sensitive professionals (Ibrahim, 1993b).

CONCLUSION

This chapter presented a model for assessment and intervention and a training model to enhance the cultural sensitivity and knowledge base of professionals working with individuals with disabilities from both dominant and nondominant cultures. The information presented focused on initial consumer assessment and on identifying appropriate processes and outcomes for the consumer based on the information gained from the theory and the assessments. The theory explores issues that are generic to the human condition and issues that clarify the unique beliefs, values, and assumptions of each individual from his or her cultural perspective.

REFERENCES

Abramovitz, C.V., and Dokecki, P.R. (1977). The politics of clinical judgments: Early empirical returns. *Psychological Bulletin, 84*, 460–474.

American Association for Counseling and Development (AACD) (1987). *Human rights position paper*. Alexandria, VA: Author.

Atkinson, D.R., and Carskaddon, G.A. (1975). A prestigious introduction, psychological jargon, and perceived counselor credibility. *Journal of Counseling Psychology, 22*, 180–186.

Axelson, J. (1985). *Counseling and development in a multicultural society*. Monterey, CA: Brooks/Cole.

Bales, J. (1985). Minority testing falls short. *APA Monitor, 16*, 7.

Barak, A., and La Crosse, M.B. (1975). Multidimensional perception of counselor behavior. *Journal of Counseling Psychology, 22*, 456–471.

Beck, A.T., Rush, A.J., Shaw, B.F., and Emery, G. (1979). *Cognitive therapy of depression*. New York: Guilford Press.

Beutler, L.E., and Bergan, J. (1991). Value change in counseling and psychotherapy: A search for scientific credibility. *Journal of Counseling Psychology, 38*, 16–24.

Brown, D., and Srebalus, D.J. (1988). *An introduction to the counseling profession*. Englewood Cliffs, NJ: Prentice-Hall.

Cirillo, L., and Wapner, S. (Eds.) (1986). *Value suppositions in theories of human development*. Hillsdale, NJ: Erlbaum.

Corey, G., Corey, M.S., and Callanan, P. (1988). *Issues and ethics in the helping professions* (3rd ed.). Monterey, CA: Brooks/Cole.

Cunningham-Warburton, P. (1988). *A study of the relationship between cross-cultural training, the scale to assess world views, and the quality of care given by nurses in a psychiatric setting*. Unpublished doctoral dissertation, University of Connecticut.

D'Andrea, M., Daniels, J., and Heck, R. (1991). Evaluating the impact of multicultural counseling training. *Journal of Counseling and Development, 70*, 143–150.

Dillman, J., Karan, O.C., and Granfield, J.M. (1993). *Building relationships: A training manual for those who provide support to people with developmental disabilities*. Storrs: The A.J. Pappanikou Center on Special Education and Rehabilitation: A University Affiliated Program, University of Connecticut.

Draguns, J. (1991). Cross-cultural psychology in 1990. *Journal of Cross-Cultural Psychology, 22*, 6–7.

Edmunds, P., Martinson, S.A., and Goldberg, P.F. (1990). *Demographics and cultural diversity in the 1990's: Implications for services to young children with special needs.* Washington, DC: Office of Special Education Programs, U.S. Department of Education.

Fine, M., and Asch, A. (1988). Disability beyond stigma: Social interactions, discrimination, and activism. *Journal of Social Issues, 44*, 3–21.

Frank, J.O. (1973). *Persuasion and healing* (rev. ed.). Baltimore: Johns Hopkins University Press.

Funk, R. (1987). Disability rights: From case to class in the context of civil rights. In A. Gartner and T. Joe (Eds.), *Images of the disabled/disabling images* (pp. 7-30). New York: Praeger.

Furn, B.G. (1986). *The psychology of women as a cross-cultural issue: Perceived dimensions of worldviews.* Unpublished doctoral dissertation, University of Connecticut.

Furn, B.G. (1988). *Worldviews and gender: Implications for counseling and psychotherapy.* Paper presented at the annual meeting of the American Psychological Association, August, Atlanta.

Furn, B.G., and Ibrahim, F.A. (1987). *The psychology of women: Perceived dimensions of world views.* Paper presented at the annual meeting of the American Psychological Association, August, New York.

Gartner, A., Lipsky, D.K., and Turnbull, A.P. (1991). *Supporting families with a child with a disability: An international outlook.* Baltimore: Paul H. Brookes.

Gliedman, J., and Roth, W. (1980). *The unexpected minority: Handicapped children in America.* New York: Harcourt, Brace, Jovanovich.

Horner, D., and Vandersluis, P. (1981). Cross-cultural counseling. In G. Althen (Ed.), *Learning across cultures.* Washington, DC: National Association for Foreign Students Affairs.

Ibrahim, F.A. (1984a). *Cross-cultural counseling and psychotherapy: Initial assessment.* Paper presented at the annual meeting of the Association for Counseling and Development, March, Houston.

Ibrahim, F.A. (1984b). Cross-cultural counseling and psychotherapy: An existential-psychological perspective. *International Journal for the Advancement of Counseling, 7*, 559–569.

Ibrahim, F.A. (1985b). *Cross-cultural counseling training.* Paper presented at the annual meeting of the Association for Counseling and Development, April, New York.

Ibrahim, F.A. (1985c). Human rights and ethical issues in the use of advanced technology. *Journal of Counseling and Development, 64*, 134–145.

Ibrahim, F.A. (1986). *Reflections on the cultural encapsulation of the APA's Ethical Principles*. Presented in a symposium, chaired by P.B. Pedersen, at the annual meeting of the American Psychological Association, August, Washington, DC.

Ibrahim, F.A. (1990a). *Workshop on clinical applications of the Scale to Assess World Views*. Presented at the annual meeting of the American Psychological Association, August, Boston.

Ibrahim, F.A. (1990b). *Cultural Identity Check List (CICL)*. Unpublished copyrighted checklist. University of Connecticut, Storrs.

Ibrahim, F.A. (1991). Contribution of cultural worldview to generic counseling and development. *Journal of Counseling and Development, 70*, 13–19.

Ibrahim, F.A. (1992). Children's rights in a pluralistic society. *Journal for Humanistic Education and Development, 31*, 64–72.

Ibrahim, F.A. (1993a). *Scale to Assess World View II*. Unpublished copyrighted scale. University of Connecticut, Storrs.

Ibrahim, F.A. (1993b). Existential Worldview Theory. Applications in transcultural counseling. In J. McFadden (Ed.), *Transcultural counseling: Bilateral and international perspectives* (pp. 25-58). Alexandria, VA: ACA Press.

Ibrahim, F.A., and Arredondo, P.M. (1986). Ethical standards for cross-cultural counseling: Preparation, practice, assessment, and research. *Journal of Counseling and Development, 64*, 349–351.

Ibrahim, F.A., and Arredondo, P.M. (1990). Essay on law and ethics: Multicultural counseling. In B. Herlihy and L. Golden (Eds.), *American Association for Counseling and Development: Ethics casebook* (4th ed.). Alexandria, VA: AACD Press.

Ibrahim, F.A., and Herr, E.L. (1982). Attitude modification toward disability: Differential effect of two educational modes. *The Rehabilitation Counseling Bulletin, 26*, 29–36.

Ibrahim, F.A., and Kahn, H. (1984). *Scale to Assess World Views*. Unpublished copyrighted scale. University of Connecticut, Storrs.

Ibrahim, F.A., and Kahn, H. (1987). Assessment of world views. *Psychological Reports, 60*, 163–176.

Ibrahim, F.A., and Owen, S.V. (1992). *Factor analytic structure of the Scale to Assess World Views*. Paper presented at the annual meeting of the American Psychological Association, August, Washington, DC.

Ibrahim, F.A, and Schroeder, D.G. (1987). *Effective communication with multicultural families*. Paper presented at the annual meeting of the Connecticut Association for the Education of Young Children, October, Storrs.

Ibrahim, F.A., and Schroeder, D.G. (1989). Americans can learn to be free of racism and sexism. *Hartford Courant*, March 27, 1989, B11.

Ibrahim, F.A., and Schroeder, D.G. (1990). Cross-cultural couple counseling: A developmental psychoeducational intervention. *Journal of Comparative Family Studies, 21*, 193–207.

Ibrahim, F.A., Stadler, H.A., Arredondo, P.M., and McFadden, J. (1986). *Status of human rights issues in counselor preparation: A national survey.* Paper presented at the annual meeting of the American Association for Counseling and Development, April, Los Angeles.

Jones, E.E., Kanouse, D., Kelly, H.H., Nisbett, R.E., Valins, S., and Weiner, B. (Eds.) (1972). *Attribution: Perceiving the causes of behavior.* Morristown, NJ: General Learning Press.

Kelly, T.A. (1990). The role of values in psychotherapy: Review and methodological critique. *Clinical Psychology Review, 10,* 171–186.

Kluckhohn, C. (1951). Values and value orientations in the theory of action. In T. Parsons and E.A. Shields (Eds.), *Toward a general theory of action* (pp. 388-433). Cambridge: Harvard University Press.

Leake, D.W., James, R.K., and Stodden, R.A. (1995). Shifting paradigms to natural supports: A practical response to a crisis in disabilities services. In O.C. Karan and S. Greenspan (Eds.), *Community rehabilitation services for people with disabilities.* Boston: Butterworth–Heinemann.

Lonner, W.J., and Ibrahim, F.A. (1989). Assessment in cross-cultural counseling. In P.B. Pedersen, J.G. Draguns, W.J. Lonner, and J.E. Trimble (Eds.), *Counseling across cultures* (3rd ed.) (pp. 229-334). Honolulu: University of Hawaii Press.

McFadden, J. (1993). Introduction. In J. McFadden (Ed.), *Transcultural counseling: Bilateral and international perspectives* (p. XII). Alexandria, VA: American Counseling Association.

Merluzzi, T.V., Merluzzi, B.H., and Kaul, T.H. (1977). Counselor race and power base: Effects on attitudes and behavior. *Journal of Counseling Psychology, 24,* 430–436.

Patterson, C.H. (1989). Values in counseling and psychotherapy. *Counseling and Values, 33,* 164–176.

Pedersen, P.B., Fukuyama, M., and Heath, A. (1989). Client, counselor and contextual variables in multicultural counseling. In P.B. Pedersen, J.G. Draguns, W.J. Lonner, J.E. Trimble (Eds.), *Counseling across cultures* (3rd ed.) (pp. 23-52). Honolulu: University of Hawaii Press.

Ponterroto, J.G., and Casas, M. (1987). In search of multicultural competence within counselor education programs. *Journal of Counseling and Development, 64,* 430–434.

Sadlak, M.J., and Ibrahim, F.A. (1986). *Cross-cultural counselor training: Impact on counselor effectiveness and sensitivity.* Paper presented at the annual meeting of the American Psychological Association, August, Washington, DC.

Sadowsky, G.R., Maguire, K., Johnson, P., Ngumba, E., and Kohles, R. (In press). Worldviews of white Americans, mainland Chinese, Taiwanese, and African students: An investigation into between group differences. *Journal of Cross-Cultural Psychology.*

Sarason, S.B. (1984). If it can be studied or developed, should it be? *American Psychologist, 39,* 477–485.

Schmidt, L.D., and Strong, S.R. (1971). Attractiveness and influence in counseling. *Journal of Counseling Psychology, 18,* 348–351.

Sire, J.W. (1976). *The universe next door.* Downers Grove, IL: Intervarsity.

Strong, S.R. (1968). Counseling: An interpersonal influence process. *Journal of Counseling Psychology, 15,* 215–244.

Strupp, H.H. (1978). Psychotherapy research and practice: An overview. In S.L. Garfield and A.E. Bergin (Eds.), *Handbook of psychotherapy and behavior change: An empirical analysis* (pp. 3-22). New York: Wiley.

Sue, D.W. (1978). World views and counseling. *Personnel and Guidance Journal, 56,* 458–462.

Sue, D.W., and Sue, D. (1991). *Counseling the culturally different.* New York: Wiley.

Sue, S., and Zane, N. (1987). The role of cultural techniques in psychotherapy: A critique and reformulation. *American Psychologist, 42,* 37–45.

Sundberg, N.D. (1981). Cross-cultural counseling and psychotherapy: A research overview. In A.J. Marsella and P.B. Pedersen (Eds.), *Cross-cultural counseling and psychotherapy* (pp. 28-62). New York: Pergamon.

Torrey, E.F. (1986). *Witchdoctors and psychiatrists.* New York: Harper & Row.

Triandis, H.C. (1972). *The analysis of subjective culture.* New York: Wiley.

SUGGESTED READINGS

Arredondo-Dowd, P.M., and Gonsalves, J. (1980). Preparing culturally effective counselors. *Personnel and Guidance Journal, 58,* 657–661.

Atkinson, D.R. (1985). A meta-review of research on cross-cultural counseling and psychotherapy. *Journal of Multicultural Counseling, 1,* 138–153.

Banks, W.M. (1972). The differential effects of race and social class in helping. *Journal of Clinical Psychology, 28,* 90–92.

Becker, E. (1973). *The denial of death.* New York: Free Press.

Bergin, A. (1991). Values and religious issues in psychotherapy and mental health. *American Psychologist, 46,* 394–403.

Bradley, V.J., and Knoll, J. (1995). Shifting paradigms in services to people with disabilities. In O.C. Karan and S. Greenspan (Eds.), *Community rehabilitation services for people with disabilities.* Boston: Butterworth–Heinemann.

Carkhuff, R.R., and Pierce, R. (1967). Differential effects of therapist race and social class upon patient depth of self-exploration in the initial interview. *Journal of Consulting Psychology, 31,* 632–634.

Coombs, A., and Snygg, D. (1959). *Individual behavior.* New York: Harper & Row.

Griffith, M.S. (1977). The influence of race on the psychotherapeutic relationship. *Psychiatry, 40,* 27–40.

Ibrahim, F.A. (1985a). Effective cross-cultural counseling and psychotherapy: A framework. *The Counseling Psychologist, 13,* 625–638.

Ibrahim, F.A. (1987). The person-centered approach to peace: Commentary in a cross-cultural context. *Counseling and Values, 32,* 73–75.

Ibrahim, F.A. (1989). Response to psychology in the public forum on socially sensitive research. *American Psychologist, 44,* 848–857.

Rotter, J. (1966). Generalized expectancies for internal versus external control of reinforcement. *Psychological Monographs, 80* (1, whole number 609).

APPENDIX A

Cultural Identity Checklist

Name: _____ Age: _____ Gender: _____

Race: _____ Religion: _____

Please answer the following questions in the most direct manner. This checklist is designed to assist in helping you and the counselor understand your cultural identity. Please respond to the questions as *you really see yourself,* than as others define you. If any of the questions make you uncomfortable, you may not answer them. This information will be held in strictest confidence.

1. What is your ethnic background? Please list ethnicities of both your parents and their parents.
2. Which ethnic group do you think has influenced your values and beliefs the most? Which ethnic group do you identify with personally?
3. In which generation did your family migrate to this country?
4. Was migration a free choice or was it forced?
5. How was your ethnic group received?
6. How has your primary group established itself in this country?
7. What do you know about the sociopolitical history of your primary group in this country?
8. How do you feel about the sociopolitical history of your primary group?
9. What was the socioeconomic status of your family of origin?
10. What is your socioeconomic level?
11. What was the educational level of your father? _____ mother _____?
12. What is your educational level?
13. Is your family monolingual? If your family is bilingual or trilingual, please list the languages they speak, read, and write.
14. Are you monolingual? If you are bilingual or trilingual, please list the languages you speak, read, and write.
15. Do you actively practice your faith and believe in it?
16. What is your birth order in your family of origin? Oldest, middle, or youngest child (please circle).
17. What is your sexual preference? How does your family relate to your sexual preference? How does your cultural/ethnic group relate to your sexual preference?
18. Do you have any disabilities?

Please feel free to add other information that you consider relevant to this checklist.

10

Assessment of
Natural Supports
in Community
Rehabilitation
Services

Robert L. Schalock

INTRODUCTION

There is currently considerable conceptual and practical interest in the use of natural supports as an efficient and effective way to maximize rehabilitation services to persons with disabilities. While the concept of natural supports is by no means new, what is new is the belief that the judicious application of appropriate supports can improve the functional capabilities of individuals with disabilities. This belief is exemplified in the current emphasis on supported employment, supported living, and regular class support systems in education. The importance of supports is that they hold the promise of providing a more natural, efficient and ongoing basis for enhancing a person's independence/interdependence, productivity, community integration, and satisfaction.

The heightened interest in natural supports comes at a critical time in community rehabilitation services. For example, we are now implementing the Americans with Disabilities Act of 1990 (P.L. 101-136), which draws the nation's attention to the forty-three million Americans who have one or more physical or mental disabilities. In addition, as noted throughout this book, the rehabilitation profession is currently experiencing a significant paradigmatic shift characterized by the following:

- A quality revolution, with its emphasis on quality of life, quality enhancement techniques, and quality assurance
- A consumer-referenced goal of personal growth and development, emphasizing choices, decisions, and empowerment
- An increasing need for fiscal and programmatic accountability
- The provision of services in natural environments, based on the principles of real jobs and real homes, communitarianism (Turnbull and Brunk, 1990), and natural supports

The assessment of those natural supports in community rehabilitation services is the focus of this chapter. The chapter's three major purposes include (1) discussing the interrogatories of natural supports; (2) explaining a three-step model for assessing natural supports; and (3) pointing out a number of implications of using natural supports.

THE INTERROGATORIES OF NATURAL SUPPORTS

Natural Supports Defined

Throughout the chapter, natural supports are defined as:

resources and strategies that promote the interests and causes of an individual with or without disabilities, that enable him or her to access resources, information, and relationships inherent within integrated work and living environments, and that result in the person's enhanced independence, productivity, community integration, and satisfaction.

Note the three key aspects of natural supports: (1) They pertain to resources and strategies. (2) They enable persons to access resources, information, and relationships within integrated environments. (3) Their use results in increased integration and enhanced personal growth and development.

Support Functions

The resources and strategies referenced in the definition can be grouped into seven support functions for the purposes of conceptualization and providing the basis for assessment activities. These seven support functions include befriending, financial planning, employee assistance, behavior support, in-home living assistance, community access and use, and health assistance. Representative activities associated with each support function are summarized in Table 10-1.

These functions and associated activities provide the basis for the assessment of natural supports in community rehabilitation services, focusing on those sources of support discussed in the following section.

TABLE 10-1   Support Functions and Representative Activities[a, b]

Support Function	Representative Activities	
1. Befriending	Advocating	Evaluating
	Befriending	Carpooling
	Communicating	Associating
	Supervising	Training
	Collecting data	Instructing
	Feedback	Socializing
2. Financial planning	Working with SSI/Medicaid	Protection and legal assistance
	Advocating for benefits	Check cashing
	Adjusting work benefits	Budgeting
	Assisting with money management	Income assistance planning and consideration
3. Employee assistance	Counseling	Job/task accommodation
	Procuring/using assistive technology devices	Redesigning job/work duties
	Supervisory training	
	Job performance enhancement	
	Crisis intervention and assistance	

(continued)

TABLE 10-1 *(continued)*

Support Function	*Representative Activities*	
4. Behavioral support	Functional analysis Multicomponent instruction Manipulation of ecological and setting events Minimizing the use of punishers	Emphasis on antecedent manipulation Teaching adaptive behavior Building environments with effective consequences
5. In-home living assistance	Personal maintenance/care Transfer and mobility Dressing and clothing care Architectural modifications Communication devices	Behavioral support Eating and food management Housekeeping Respite care Attendant care Home health aides Homemaker services Med alert devices
6. Community access and use	Carpooling/rides program Transportation training Vehicle modification Recreation/leisure involvement	Community awareness opportunities Community use opportunities Interfacing with generic agencies
7. Health assistance	Medical appointments Medical interventions Supervision Med alert devices Emergency procedures Mobility (assistive devices) Counseling appointments	Medication-taking assistance Hazard awareness Safety training Physical therapy and related activities Counseling interventions

[a]Adapted from Googins (1989); Horner et al. (1990); Hughes, Rusch, and Curl (1990); Kiernan and McGaughey (1991); Koehler, Schalock, and Ballard (1989); Meador et al. (1991); Nisbet and Hagner (1988); Powell et al. (1991); Roberts et al. (1991); Schalock and Kiernan (1990); Schalock and Koehler (1988); and Temple University (1990).

[b]The support functions and activities may need to be modified slightly to accommodate persons of different ages.

Sources of Support

Supports can come from a number of sources, including oneself, other people, technology, and rehabilitation services. Examples of each include the following:

- *Oneself*—competencies, the ability and opportunity to make choices, money, and information
- *Other people*—family, friends, coworkers, cohabitants, mentors
- *Technology*—assistive devices, job/living accommodations, behavioral technology
- *Services*—currently available rehabilitation services that are used if the above resources are not available

A two-phase Delphi procedure was completed recently to reach consensus among a panel of twenty-nine nationally known rehabilitation experts regarding the above sources of support. For those not familiar with the Delphi process, it is a systematic method of collecting opinions from a group of experts through a series of questionnaires in which feedback of the group's opinion is provided to the group, until a satisfying consensus emerges. It is a method that allows one to obtain a group's opinion and formulate a group's value judgment (Dalkey and Rourke, 1971; Shefer and Starmsa, 1982).

The task of the Delphi respondents was to identify the most important natural supports within each of the three sources—oneself, other people, and technology. These sources of natural supports are listed in descending order in Table 10-2.

Support Standards

Since the use of natural supports is just emerging in the rehabilitation field, one needs to consider carefully the standards that guide their development and use. This is especially true because, currently, accreditation and licensing/certification standards focus primarily on services that are driven by the individual planning process. The assumption underlying these standards is that current rehabilitation programs should be offered through a structured collaborative teamwork (Rainforth et al., Chapter 7 in this book) program planning process involving different disciplines. There are currently no comparable standards for support programs because support services frequently do not require the level of structure or intensity of typical rehabilitation programs (Pearce, 1990).

TABLE 10-2 Potential Natural Supports Provided by Oneself, Other Persons, and Technology

Oneself	Other Persons	Technology
Social skills	Job coach	Job accommodation
Work skills	Coworker	Transportation
Competencies	Supervisor (employer-paid	Behavioral technology
Communication skills	Family	Natural cues
Motivation/enthusiasm	Friends	Self-management
Accepting supervision and suggestions	Other company employees	Creative job design
Choices	Mentor	Assistive devices
Information	CEO or personnel director	Assessment (data collection)
Self-advocacy	Customers	Employee assistance programs
Money	Attendant	Self-instructional techniques
Appearance	Self-support groups	Size and wealth of employer

However, there is still a need for developing standards to guide the assessment and use of natural supports. Seven proposed natural support standards are presented in Table 10-3.

Although these proposed standards may change over time, they seem reasonable to use at this point to evaluate the presence and quality of natural supports use.

In summary, the current emphasis on natural supports is significantly different from our previous orientation, which focused on external human service agencies providing services to persons with disabilities. The primary objective of the current emphasis is to increase the person's level of integration and personal growth through the use of supports that occur naturally within the person's living, work, and community environments. Thus, as one assesses natural supports in community rehabilitation services, it is important to stress that the primary focus of one's efforts is to interface the person with those resources, information, and relationships inherent within integrated work, living, and recreation-leisure environments. A three-step process for doing so is outlined in the following section.

TABLE 10-3 Proposed Natural Support Standards

1. Natural supports occur in regular, integrated environments.
2. Support activities are performed primarily by persons normally working, living, or recreating within that environment.
3. Support activities are individualized and person-referenced.
4. Natural supports are coordinated through a person such as a support manager.
5. Outcomes from the use of natural supports are evaluated against quality indicators and person-referenced outcomes.
6. The use of supports can fluctuate, and may either be of life-long duration or be needed intermittently during different stages of one's life.
7. Supports should not be withdrawn unless the service provider continues to monitor the person's current and future level of needed support.

ASSESSING NATURAL SUPPORTS

As currently envisioned, assessing natural supports involves a three-step process that includes the following tasks: (1) inventory the natural supports available to the person; (2) determine the discrepancy between needed and available supports and target the needed additional supports; and (3) assess the needed supports. Each step is discussed in the following sections.

Inventory Available Natural Supports

The core concept that should guide the inventory and use of natural supports is lifestyle planning, defined as:

> Bringing together the people whose cooperation is important to the person with a disability, and focusing on the quality of that person's life. The process results in a shared sense of direction and priority that guides the selection of life aim goals within integrated environments, activities, and performance objectives [O'Brien, 1987; Schalock and Kiernan, 1990].

A process, such as the Life Experience Profile summarized in Table 10-4, can be used to capture this core concept and develop jointly the person's life aim goals related to employment, living arrangement, and social/leisure activities. As seen in Table 10-4, the Life Experience Profile can be used to help establish the person's life aim goals through focusing on the following six factors regarding the person's life experiences:

- *Community presence*—the sharing of the ordinary places that define community life
- *Community participation*—the experience of being part of a growing network of family and friends
- *Choice*—the experience of autonomy and decision making
- *Respect*—the reality of having value in one's community
- *Competence*—skills and abilities
- *Satisfaction*—the fulfillment of a need or want and the contentment and happiness that accompanies that fulfillment

A person's life aim goals can be used to organize the first assessment step, which is to inventory the natural supports that are available to the person. The concept that one needs to follow is analogous to looking at one's own environments (living, work, recreation/leisure) and asking, "What are all the supports available to me in that environment?" The intent of Table 10-5 is to facilitate the natural supports inventory.

Note that three tasks are required in reference to each of the seven support functions listed: (1) list the specific natural supports available to the person in that environment; (2) indicate whether the source of support is oneself, other persons, or technological; and (3) specify whether the natural support meets the support standards found in Table 10-3. Once the available supports are inventoried, they are used as part of the support discrepancy analysis described in the next subsection.

Support Discrepancy Analysis

The primary intent of this second step in the assessment process is to determine the discrepancy between needed and available supports. This part of the model is based on considerable work in the area of person-environmental analysis (Schalock, 1989; Schalock and Jensen, 1986), which derives from the principle that the characteristics of persons and environments can be compared and discrepancies identified.

The critical steps involved in the support-discrepancy analysis are outlined in Figure 10-1. The analysis begins with determining the person's needed supports based on the discrepancy between the person's capabilities in regard to his or her job, living, and recreation/leisure environments, and

TABLE 10-4   Exemplary Questions from the Life Experience Profile[a]

Community Presence

1. What community settings does the person use regularly?

2. What other comunity settings would it be in the person's interest to use, or use more independently?

3. What would it take to increase the number of community settings the person uses?

Community Participation

1. With whom does the person spend the most time?

2. Who are the other important people in the person's social network with whom the person spends time occasionally?

3. Who are the person's friends?

4. What would it take to provide more natural support in the person's integrated employment, living, and recreation/leisure environments?

Choice

1. What decisions are regularly made by the person?

2. What would it take to increase the number, variety, and importance of the decisions the person makes?

3. What are the person's strongest interests and preferences?

Respect

1. What are the valued community roles the person occupies?

2. What characteristics about the person's appearance or actions could interfere with receiving value or respect in the community?

3. What would it take to enhance or improve these characteristics to receive value or respect in the community?

Competence

1. What skills has the person developed that help him or her to be perceived as competent?

2. Are any restrictions being placed on the person?

3. Are there any health and/or safety issues that interfere with the person's continuing development?

4. What would it take to increase the person's competence in valued activities?

Satisfaction

1. What evidence exists that the person is satisfied with his or her home life, work life, community life, and relationships?

2. What would it take to improve the person's satisfaction?

[a]Adapted from Schalock and Kiernan (1990).

TABLE 10-5   Natural Supports Inventory Matrix

Support Functions	Specific Natural Supports Available to the Person (List for each)	Source of Support (Check)	Natural Support Meets Support Standards[*]
1. Befriending		Oneself Other People Technology	Yes No
2. Financial planning		Oneself Other People Technology	Yes No
3. Employee assistance		Oneself Other People Technology	Yes No
4. Behavioral support		Oneself Other People Technology	Yes No
5. In-home living assistance		Oneself Other People Technology	Yes No
6. Community access and use		Oneself Other People Technology	Yes No
7. Health assistance		Oneself Other People Technology	Yes No

[*]See Table 10-3.

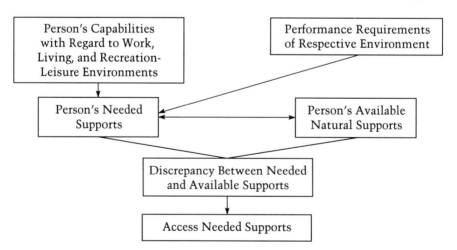

FIGURE 10.1   Support Discrepancy Analysis Model

the performance demands of those environments. Specific strategies for completing such person-environmental analyses can be found in Calkins and Walker (1990); Hughes, Rusch, and Curl (1990); Kregel (1990); Schalock and Koehler (1988); and Schalock, Johnsen, and Schik (1985).

Once the discrepancies between capabilities and performance demands are identified, then one completes a second-level analysis involving the discrepancy between the person's needed supports and those natural supports available within the respective living, work, or recreation/ leisure environment. Table 10-6 presents a table shell that can facilitate this process.

TABLE 10-6   Support Discrepancy Analysis Based on Person-Environmental Analysis and Available Supports

Support Function	Needed Supports Based on Person-Environmental Analysis (List for each)	Available Supports*	Discrepancy between Needed and Available Supports	Targeted Additional Sources of Support (Check)
1. Befriending				Internal (Natural) External (Agency) Personal, other person, or technological
2. Financial planning				Internal (Natural) External (Agency) Personal, other person, or technological
3. Employee assistance				Internal (Natural) External (Agency) Personal, other person, or technological

(continued)

TABLE 10-6   (continued)

Support Function	Needed Supports Based on Person-Environmental Analysis (List for each)	Available Supports*	Discrepancy between Needed and Available Supports	Targeted Additional Sources of Support (Check)
4. Behavioral support				Internal (Natural) External (Agency) Personal, other person, or technological
5. In-home living assistance				Internal (Natural) External (Agency) Personal, other person, or technological
6. Community access and use				Internal (Natural) External (Agency) Personal, other person, or technological
7. Health assistance				Internal (Natural) External (Agency) Personal, other person, or technological

*See Table 10-5.

The first step involves listing, for each of the seven support functions, the supports the person needs based on the discrepancy between the person's capabilities and environmentally based performance demands. These needed supports are then compared to those natural supports that were identified through the environmental inventory (Table 10-5). Any discrepancies between needed and available supports are then identified and become the focus of the third step in the assessment process, namely, targeting and accessing additional supports.

Access Needed Supports

Once the support manager has completed Tables 10-5 and 10-6, the next task is to procure the needed supports. Again, it is important to stress that the primary objective is to access those natural supports occurring within the person's integrated living, work, and recreation-leisure environments. This process is accomplished through one or more of the activities summarized in Table 10-6 (last column) under the heading "Targeted Additional Sources of Support." Note in Table 10-6 the two aspects of the targeting process: (1) whether the focus is *internal*, occurring naturally within the environment, or *external*, provided by a human service agency/program; and (2) whether the source of support is personal, other person, or technological.

There is currently considerable work being done on developing mechanisms for accessing and/or procuring natural supports for persons with disabilities. Although the two models that will be described below come from the supported employment literature, there is no reason to assume that the models are not equally appropriate to the person's living and recreation-leisure environments.

The first model comes from work at the University of Oregon on expanding the role of employers in supported employment (Rhodes et al., 1992). Specific techniques suggested by the authors to expand the role of employers (and thus provide increased natural supports to persons with disabilities) include:

- Extend [supported employment–developed] support techniques such as precise instruction, individualized supervision strategies, job analysis, and self-management strategies to employee personnel.
- Assist company training departments.
- Utilize employee assistance programs.
- Develop the capacity of trade associations.
- Shape the service system to be responsible to employers.

The second model represents a number of optional support persons, whose roles and responsibilities are graduated from internal (to the environment) to external (provided by an outside human service agency). These options, which are discussed in considerable detail in Nisbet and Hagner (1988), are summarized in Table 10-7. The increased emphasis on natural

TABLE 10-7 Community Employment Support Options

Option	Support Person/Role		Responsible to	Agency Role
	Initial	Ongoing		
Job coach	Job coach trains	Coach fades; worker is presumed independent	Agency	Direct: Training and follow-up
Mentor	Job coach trains; supervision is transferred to mentor	Mentor remains on-site, providing support and supervision	Company	Indirect: Matching and support for mentor
Training consultant	Job coach trains with the co-workers and supervisors	Coworkers/supervisor provide support, supervision, and additional training	Company	Indirect: Consultation and stipend
Job sharing	Job coach identifies job sharer, then trains and assists	Job sharer remains on-site	Agency and company	Indirect: Matching: support for job sharer, stipend
Attendant	Attendant trains and assists (may need some assistance from job coach)	Attendant remains on-site at worker's discretion	Worker	Possibly initial training; afterward little or no intervention

Source: Adapted, with permission, from Nisbet and Hagner (1988).

supports should lead to an increase in supports provided by mentors, training consultants, and job sharers.

In summary, assessing and accessing needed supports within one's integrated living, work, and recreation-leisure environments requires both new thinking and different staff utilization patterns. The new thinking focuses on the "naturalness" and potential effectiveness of natural supports; the new staff utilization patterns focus upon a support manager who is competent in completing the three-step assessment process just described. The implications of this new way of thinking are discussed in the chapter's final section.

IMPLICATIONS OF USING SUPPORTS

The concept of supports and their use with persons with disabilities is just emerging in the rehabilitation field. Therefore, the three implications regarding the use of natural supports discussed in this section of the chapter are based on current understanding, and may change over time.

The first implication is that the natural support paradigm is very different from the facility-based service delivery system that characterizes most current rehabilitation programs. The five standards that are listed in Table 10-3 against which natural support programs should be evaluated characterize some of the differences. Other significant differences pertain to

- Assuming the presence and availability of natural supports;
- Focusing on inventory of natural supports and a support discrepancy analysis; and
- Building the capacity of the workplace and community-living environments to integrate persons with disabilities, and to assign value to these persons.

The second implication relates to the emerging technology of support. Bellamy (1990) suggests that the following five features appear critical in a technology of support:

- The technology should blend public and private sources of support in a coherent, manageable model.
- Ongoing support should address assistance needs in all parts of a person's life.
- Models for providing ongoing support should reflect realistic cost constraints.

- Support should enhance opportunities for integration and participation.
- Support should be linked to measures of individual benefits and outcomes.

The final implication of using supports relates to their effect on research. One apparent effect is to increase the call for research efforts in demonstrating whether specific types or levels of support differentially enhance personal and social outcomes for persons with disabilities. Related research would attempt to answer the question "what kinds of supports or support programs employing what kind of persons serving what kinds of needs achieve what kinds of result?" (Roberts et al., 1991). A third effect on research will be to focus considerable efforts on evaluating the costs, benefits, and effectiveness of natural supports.

In that regard, rehabilitation services are currently being buffeted by powerful forces, including recipient empowerment, cost containment, and accountability. These forces are causing us to focus increasingly on the issue of what rehabilitation actually achieves for service recipients, and how those achievements can be identified and measured. In reference to natural supports, the current working assumptions are that their use will increase the person's level of integration and result in improved living, work, and community integration outcomes. The task of evaluation then is to determine whether these assumptions are either supported or not supported. The data sets summarized in Table 10-8 are suggested for use to determine both the short-term effects and longer term effects on person-referenced outcomes from using natural supports.

CONCLUSION

This chapter has summarized the interrogatories of natural supports, a three-step procedure to assess natural supports in community rehabilitation services, and some of the more important implications of using natural supports. Throughout the chapter, the potential of natural supports to provide a more natural, efficient, and ongoing basis for enhancing persons' integration and personal growth was stressed. Natural supports appear attractive to many persons because they are consistent with the current zeitgeist and its emphasis on communitarianism (Turnbull and Brunk, 1990), community integration, and quality of life.

TABLE 10-8 Data Sets to Evaluate the Short-Term Effects and Longer Term Person-Referenced Outcomes from Using Natural Supports[a]

| Short-Term Effects | Longer Term Person-Referenced Outcomes | |
	Measurement Focus	Exemplary Data Sets
• Less or different staff involvement	Independence	Decisions made Competencies/Skills acquired Choices offered
• Attainment of goals and objectives	Productivity	Salary Benefits Occupational history Volunteerism Avocational activities
• Person's (family's) self-assessment on how natural supports are going	Community integration	Physical (same space) Functional (same space and time) Social (interactions with nondisabled) Societal (productive citizens of the community)
• Support provider's assessment of how natural supports are going	Satisfaction	Physical and material well-being Relations with other people Social, community, and civic activities Personal development and fulfillment Recreation and leisure

[a]Adapted from Schalock and Thornton (1988).

REFERENCES

Bellamy, G.T. (1990). Book review. *Journal of the Association for Persons with Severe Handicaps, 15*(4), 261–265.

Calkins, C.F., and Walker, H.M. (1990). *Social competence for workers with developmental disabilities: A guide to enhancing employment outcomes in integrated settings.* Baltimore: Paul H. Brookes.

Dalkey, N.C., and Rourke, K.L. (1971). *Experimental assessment of Delphi procedures with group value judgment.* New York: The Rand Corporation.

Googins, B. (1989). Support in integrated work setting: The role played by industry through employee assistance programs. In W.E. Kiernan and R.L. Schalock (Eds.), *Economics, industry, and disability: A look ahead* (pp. 223–236). Baltimore: Paul H. Brookes.

Horner, R.H., Dunlap, G., Koegel, R.L., Carr, E.G., Sailor, W., Anderson, J., Albin, R.W., and O'Neill, R.E. (1990). Toward a technology of "nonaversive" behavioral support. *Journal of the Association for Persons with Severe Handicaps, 15*(3), 125–132.

Hughes, C., Rusch, F.R., and Curl, R.M. (1990). Extending individual competence, developing natural support, and promoting social acceptance. In F.R. Rusch (Ed.), *Supported employment: models, methods, and issues* (pp. 181–197). Sycamore, IL: Sycamore Publishing Company.

Kiernan, W.E., and McGaughey, M. (1991). *Employee assistance programs: A support mechanism for the worker with a disability.* Boston: Training and Research Institute for People with Disabilities, Children's Hospital.

Koehler, R.S., Schalock, R.L., and Ballard, B.L. (1989). *Personal growth habilitation manual.* Hastings: Mid-Nebraska Mental Retardation Services.

Kregel, J. (1990). *VCU-RRTC computerized consumer/job match.* Richmond: Virginia Commonwealth University, Rehabilitation Research and Training Center.

Meador, D.M., Osborn, R.G., Owens, M.H., Smith, E.C., and Taylor, T.L. (1991). Evaluation of environmental support in group homes for persons with mental retardation. *Mental Retardation, 19*(3), 159–164.

Nisbet, J., and Hagner, D. (1988). Natural supports in the workplace: a reexamination of supported employment. *Journal of the Association for Persons with Severe Handicaps, 13*(4), 260–267.

O'Brien, J. (1987). A guide to personal future planning. In G.T. Bellamy and B. Wilcox (Eds.), *A comprehensive guide to The Activities Catalog: An alternative curriculum for youth and adults with severe disabilities.* Baltimore: Paul H. Brookes.

Pearce, C.K. (1990). Building values into accreditation practices. In V.J. Bradley and H.A. Bersani (Eds.), *Quality assurance for individuals with developmental disabilities: It's everybody's business* (pp. 221–232). Baltimore: Paul H. Brookes.

Powell, T.H., Panscofar, E.L., Steers, D.E., Butterworth, J., Itzkowitz, J.S., and Rainforth, B. (1991). *Supported employment: Providing integrated employment opportunities for persons with disabilities.* New York: Longman.

Rainforth, B., Giangreco, M.F., Smith, P.D., & York, J. (1995) Collaborative teamwork in training and technical assistance: Enhancing community support for persons with disabilities. In O.C. Karan and S. Greenspan (Eds.), *Community Rehabilitation Services for People with Disabilities.* Boston: Butterworth-Heinemann.

Rhodes, L., Sandown, D., Mank, D., Budkley, J., and Albin, J. (1992). Expanding the role of employers in supported employment. In J. Nisbet (Ed.), *Natural supports in the home, school and community*. Baltimore: Paul H. Brookes.

Roberts, R.N., Wasik, B.H., Casto, G., and Ramey, C.T. (1991). Family support in the home: Programs, policy and social change. *American Psychologist, 46*(2), 131–137.

Schalock, R.L. (1989). Person-environmental analysis: Short and long-term perspectives. In W.E. Kiernan and R.L. Schalock (Eds.), *Economics, industry, and disability: A look ahead* (pp. 105–116). Baltimore: Paul H. Brookes.

Schalock, R.L., and Jensen, C.M. (1986). Assessing the goodness-of-fit between persons and their environments. *Journal of the Association for Persons with Severe Handicaps, 11*(2), 103–109.

Schalock, R.L., Johnsen, D.L., and Schik, T.L. (1985). *Employment screening test.* Hastings: Mid-Nebraska Mental Retardation Services.

Schalock, R.L., and Kiernan, W.E. (1990). *Habilitation planning for adults with disabilities*. New York: Springer-Verlag.

Schalock, R.L., and Koehler, R.S. (1988). *Individual assessment/planning guide for home and community living skills*. Hastings: Mid-Nebraska Mental Retardation Services.

Schalock, R.L., and Thornton, C. (1988). *Program evaluation: A field guide for administrators*. New York: Plenum Press.

Shefer, D., and Starmsa, J. (1982). Street lighting projects selection: A rationale decision making approach. *Socio-Economic Planning Services, 16*(6), 245–259.

Temple University. (1990). *The final report on the 1990 national consumer survey of people with developmental disabilities and their families*. Philadelphia: Temple University Developmental Disabilities Center/UAP, Research and Quality Assurance Group.

Turnbull, H.R., and Brunk, G.L. (1990). Quality of life and public philosophy. In R.L. Schalock (Ed.), *Quality of life; perspectives and issues* (pp. 193–210). Washington, DC: American Association on Mental Retardation.

PART III

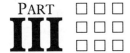

The Changing Roles and Functions of Professionals

In this last part, representatives of various professional disciplines describe how their disciplines are changing or need to change so as to better achieve partnerships with consumers and families within the context of the new paradigm. The authors of the ten chapters in this part represent the disciplines of social work, rehabilitation counseling, communication sciences, nursing, assistive technology, special education, psychiatry, psychology, physical therapy, and therapeutic recreation. In preparing their chapters, each author was encouraged to describe the evolution of their discipline, its conventional and/or characteristic practices, and how these are changing or have changed within the context of the new paradigm.

Although each chapter presents a wealth of information pertinent to its specific discipline, there are at least three unifying themes: (1) shifts from direct service roles to those of facilitators, consultants, or enablers; (2) calls for more collaboration; and (3) emphases on person-centered planning within the natural environments in which people with disabilities live, work, and play. The primary challenge for all professionals regardless of discipline will be to operationalize the values associated with the new paradigm by advancing the options and opportunities available to people with disabilities and their families, without being unduly constrained by conventional organizational and professional practices and policies that run contrary to true person-centered approaches.

In Chapter 11, entitled "The Changing Role of Social Workers," Nancy Weiss, Audrey Leviton, and Mary Mueller describe several philosophical changes in services to individuals with disabilities that have led to more community-based, consumer-driven delivery systems. The authors pay particular attention to the role of social work in both facilitating and reacting to this movement. The new paradigm has been the impetus for numerous changes in the delivery of social work services, as seen in the role of the social worker, the decision-making process, the social worker's relationship to the family, and the locations in which social work services are delivered.

In Chapter 12 William Kiernan and David Hagner outline some of the highlights in the development of the state-federal vocational rehabilitation (VR) program and review the various roles that rehabilitation counselors play in the process of providing rehabilitation services to people with disabilities. They first address the consistencies and inconsistencies present in the VR program as the changes in service delivery and role emerge. They then suggest future directions in light of the paradigm shift. With this shift these authors believe that the focus of VR will move away from its sole emphasis on work and toward participation across work, community living, leisure, and recreational environments, as well as enhancing the quality of life of the individual. They also discuss some of the guiding principles of rehabilitation, its inconsistencies in practice, and some necessary changes as the movement toward consumer empowerment and choice progresses.

In Chapter 13 Stephen N. Calculator describes the shifting paradigm within the context of communication needs of adults with disabilities. Because communication needs are dynamic, he believes they must not be viewed out of context. To him, the new paradigm is a move away from the old therapy settings, in which both the context and the majority of the communication bear little relationship to actual situations or are more important to the clinician than to the individual. The new paradigm represents a move toward practices that look at the extent to which individuals exercise control over their lives and others. Calculator advocates for integrated therapy, where objectives are embedded into daily living and monitored in different natural settings. From his perspective, communication is a means of facilitating an individual's participation and inclusion in new settings and environments.

Mary Musholt believes that the nurse's role in planning for community services and in providing thorough assessments and appropriate interventions is evolving. The shift to community membership and meeting the health care support needs of individuals in their own homes and natural environments present challenges to the nursing profession. The principle of using professionals as consultants fits well into the scheme of the community framework she describes. In Chapter 14 she advocates for the concept of role release, in which the nurse serves as a consultant to others—to professionals, parents, support personnel, or to the consumers themselves—empowering them to take on certain traditional aspects of the nursing role. Although historically nurses have been associated with the care of persons with disabilities, nursing today is not as visible as other disciplines in promoting and designing health care services for people with disabilities who are living in or planning to return to their home environments. A reference list for information on health care needs of adults with developmental disabilities is included at the end of this chapter.

In Chapter 15 Gregory Bazinet addresses the role of assistive technology, its evolution, and its contribution to the enablement of individuals with disabilities. Bazinet argues that those involved in developing the technology must work closely with the individual to try to understand the process and opportunities that he or she hopes to realize through the use of appropriate technology. Through such person-centered planning, focused on fulfilling the needs of the individual, Bazinet believes that appropriate interfaces are more likely to be developed. In this process, visits to the person's natural environment are usually required, to observe the environment and evaluate the individual in the actual setting where accommodations will be used. Bazinet also argues that those who assist in the development or matching of assistive technology should not simply prescribe solutions for the individual with disabilities but instead should plan in a collaborative environment with the individual's unique and focused input. The chapter contains a comprehensive listing of assistive technology resources, including nationwide organizations and rehabilitation engineering centers.

In Chapter 16, entitled "Shifting Paradigms in School Environments: Special Education and the Role of the Educator," Kay Norlander reviews the history of public schools in relation to their services for students with disabilities, and she identifies areas in which education needs to make significant changes describing teacher roles and their preparation in school reform and reorganization. To her, the role of the special educator must be more effectively linked with that of the regular educator, and ways of fostering a shared responsibility must begin in one's training and carry on into professional practice. She believes that fostering effective working relationships between regular and special educators requires that teachers who work with students with disabilities no longer be trained separately from teachers who work with students without disabilities. From her vantage point, not only should regular educators be prepared to accept students with handicaps, but also special educators need to be ready, willing, and able to assist in this effort. From this framework, educators and related service professionals must learn how to deliberate together because it is within the context of joint deliberation and collaboration that there is potential to change the way adults interact in schools.

In Chapter 17, which may have been his last writing prior to his untimely death, Frank Menolascino reviewed the history of psychiatry from the time of Itard's work with Victor, "The Wild Boy of Aveyron," to the present day. He identified the underlying value systems that were prevalent in various periods, as well as the major clinical and programmatic structures that resulted from such belief systems. He also examined the current ideological and subsequent clinical and programmatic shifts that guide psychiatry in its services to individuals with disabilities today. Therapeutic goals today are changing from those of control and compliance to interdependence through mutual change. From this framework the person is seen as an equal and the psychiatrist must become a partner and advocate in the development of an array of community-based options. Menolascino believed that psychiatrists need to take leadership roles in the development of community alternatives. In this capacity, as is true of other disciplines, the psychiatrist will have to counsel and guide staff and parents, teach direct caregivers how to help, oversee long-term community placements, and serve as an advocate for the individual.

In Chapter 18 Harvey Switzky documents the evolutionary process of the shifting paradigm in services to persons with disabilities as regards the changing role of psychologists. As an eyewitness to the changes, Switzky reflects on his own firsthand experiences in the form of a qualitative retrospective case history of the phenomena. He describes the psychologist's role as one that has expanded from mere test giver to educator, interdisciplinary and transdisciplinary facilitator, consultant, administrator, and researcher. In the current era, the role of the psychologist includes a lot of time listening to people with disabilities—their dreams, hopes, fantasies, and plans as they assume more control over their lives. Clearly the psychologist's role has expanded greatly, and to Switzky, the future presents some unprecedented opportunities for those in the profession who are willing and prepared to accept the challenge.

In her chapter on physical therapy, Chapter 19, Ronnie Leavitt traces the historical evolution of this discipline that goes back for centuries. The actual science of physical therapy, however, developed very late, and there were no comprehensive programs for people with disabilities before World War I. In spite of its relative youth, physical therapy is firmly entrenched within the health care system, but the role of the physical therapist is evolving and the functions of therapists are changing. Strongly bound to the roots of traditional medical models, physical therapy is beginning to broaden its scope and focus less on the medical approach and more on a person-centered approach. Leavitt identifies a number of ways in which physical therapists can be very helpful to individuals with disabilities, to parents, school systems, and others. Further, to alleviate some of the acute shortage that exists in the profession, Leavitt also describes ways to utilize physical therapy assistants. With this assistance, physical therapists can extend their roles to perform a variety of functions rather than simply being a direct provider of services. She believes that physical therapists must be prepared to relinquish their traditional roles as primary decision makers and move toward roles that are more consistent with those of consultant to and partner with the natural support systems within the consumer's community environments. From this framework, consumers will be elevated to positions of dominance and decision-making power.

Finally, in the last chapter of this book, Robert Cipriano reviews the history of leisure and recreational pursuits, first of people in general and then of people with disabilities specifically. He examines the traditional role of therapeutic recreation, which emphasized recreation activities and specially designed segregated facilities, and the shift to the contemporary, holistic person-centered-planning approach, in which the recreational therapist functions as an enabler and facilitator rather than as a leader and programmer. From his vantage point, contemporary recreation approaches bring services to people rather than people to services. The traditional notion of offering "program options" in segregated settings gives way to responding to individualized support service needs. Cipriano argues that professional recreators will be assuming subtle roles as facilitators, "connectors," and community resource locators. He believes that such a change is not only new for the recreational person but also includes expectations that families and friends consider active new roles in transportation, problem solving, leisure education, accessibility, and other newly emerging support areas.

11

The Changing Role
of Social Workers

Nancy R. Weiss, Audrey N. Leviton,
and Mary H. Mueller

PARADIGM SHIFTS EVIDENT
IN CONTEMPORARY
PRACTICE

Richard Ferris, former chairman of the board of United Airlines, once said, "The one constant in society today is change." This statement is especially pertinent to the system of services and supports offered to individuals with disabilities. This chapter will describe several philosophical changes in the field of services to individuals with disabilities that have led to a more community-based, consumer-driven service delivery system; we will pay particular attention to the role of social work in both facilitating and reacting to this movement.

In many ways social workers are uniquely qualified to participate in this movement. Historically, social workers have been in the forefront of community organization, social change, and advocacy efforts. In addition, the basic values of social work practice are the same values that have guided the field of disabilities toward a more community-based, consumer-driven orientation. These values include the right to self-determination for individuals and their families; the belief that each individual is innately valued; the belief that individuals are part of systems such as families, neighborhoods, and agencies; and the belief that change can occur at all levels of these systems (Adams, 1971; Glassman, 1991; Hollis, 1964; McFadden and Burke, 1991; Perlman, 1957). This same set of values has become the basis for the principles of normalization and consumer-driven decision making that are the foundation of systems change in the field of services to individuals with disabilities.

As systems within the field of disabilities have evolved, several major paradigm shifts have emerged. Three of these paradigm shifts representing a continuum of change from a more institutionally based, professionally controlled approach to a more community-based, consumer-controlled approach will be described.

The three major paradigm shifts are the following:

1. A shift from specialized, institutional, or clinic-based services delivered in more integrated, community-based settings such as homes, schools, and job sites
2. A shift from professional control in planning and decision making to individual or family control of the decision-making process
3. A shift from treatment of people with disabilities in a manner that does not emphasize their worth to treatment that reflects full integration and normalization or social role valorization

Each of these paradigm shifts has occurred and continues to occur along a continuum. Social workers and agencies may find that their services fall at various points on this continuum of change. Although most social workers aspire to practice in a more consumer-driven fashion, various constraints such as funding, philosophy of the agency, or gaps in services may inhibit their ability to do so. In spite of these constraints, social workers have often been in the forefront in advocating within their agencies to move toward more consumer-driven practices.

In an effort to more fully understand the effects of the philosophical changes on the role of social workers, this chapter will examine these paradigm shifts in greater detail.

Paradigm Shift 1

A shift from specialized, institutional, or clinic-based services to services delivered in more integrated, community-based settings such as homes, schools, and job sites.

The first institution for individuals with mental retardation in the United States opened in 1848. By 1967 the population of individuals in institutions in this country peaked at just under 195,000 (Bruininks et al., 1981). Although since that date there has been a steady decrease in the populations of institutions, in 1988 more than 90,000 individuals with mental retardation still lived in facilities of this kind (Braddock et al., 1990).

Children and adults who did not live in institutions still tended to be served in settings that were isolated, nonintegrated, and clinical in nature. Children with severe disabilities were often denied educational services prior to the passing in 1975 of the Individuals with Disabilities Education Act (P.L. 101-476), formerly called the Education for All Handicapped Children Act (P.L. 94-142). Even after the enactment of that legislation (U.S. Congress, 1990), educational services for children with disabilities were likely to be provided in segregated settings. Children were seldom offered opportunities to participate in schoolwide activities or to learn and socialize with their nonhandicapped peers. Medical and other specialized services for children and adults with disabilities were, and in many cases continue to be, provided in specialized clinical settings. Hospitals and clinics sprang up across the country to provide for the needs of individuals with a wide range of disabilities. Social workers who specialized in working with people with disabilities tended to practice in these segregated schools, clinics, sheltered work settings, or institutions.

Professionals and families have recognized that providing services in people's homes or in settings that are as natural or generic as possible, while still assuring that the specific needs of individuals are met, is a more advantageous approach. While some highly socialized services may still need to be provided in facilities designed specifically to meet the needs of people with disabilities, a wide range of services and supports can, and should, be provided in the natural settings in which individuals and families spend their time.

Providing services to families in their homes is sometimes known as "family support" or "home visiting." One parent described the advantages of the professional coming to her home as follows:

> I like the term "home visiting" because it says several important things to me. First, it says that the interactions occur in my home. Professionals are coming to me on my turf. Secondly, it established the relationship between me and the professional. He or she is a visitor in my home. I am more in control of the interaction. She is here at my initiation to help me in some way that we have mutually defined as something I need or want to have happen [Roberts, 1988].

When social workers meet with the individuals in their homes, at children's schools, at adults' work sites, or even at a local park or restaurant, they are contributing to a more balanced relationship. Services provided in individuals' natural settings help to convey the belief that the social worker and the service recipient are partners in a helping relationship that hinges on the mutual sharing of resources, strengths, and capabilities.

Paradigm Shift 2

A shift from professional control in planning and decision making to individual or family control of the decision-making process.

Historically, decision making regarding what services were needed by individuals with disabilities and their families was strongly influenced by professionals. Individuals with disabilities and, in the case of children, their families, were not always viewed as competent to make decisions that would guide what services were received, in which setting they were offered, and who was to provide the services. Even in simple, daily decisions, individuals were frequently offered no choices and family members often felt excluded.

Many people with disabilities residing in institutions have led lives that were almost totally controlled by others. Decisions such as when to wake up, whether to take a bath or a shower, what to wear, and when or what to eat were often made for them. Decisions were made by professionals regarding where and with whom people would live and the manner in which they would spend their time.

Historically, the literature relating to parents of children with disabilities has often portrayed them as being a possible cause of their children's problems. Therefore, parents were often viewed as unable to make informed decisions affecting their child's treatment and goals (Linz, McAnally, and Wieck, 1989). For example, Bruno Bettleheim, a leading expert in the 1950s and 1960s, "contended that the autistic child's severe withdrawal was a response to the stress created by parental attitudes and feelings. He even advocated 'parentectomy,' institutionalizing the child to replace parents with institutional staff and professionals considered more competent and caring" (Turnbull and Turnbull, 1986). As far back as the eugenics movement (1880–1930), when it was asserted that heredity was the cause of a host of disabilities, parents have been blamed for contributing to their children's mental retardation, physical disabilities, and emotional problems.

It was widely believed that parents couldn't appropriately care for their children with disabilities and that professional services available in institutions were necessary. The policies and procedures of state institutions often prevented parents from being the prime decision makers in the lives of their children. In *Parents Speak Out: Then and Now* (Turnbull and

Turnbull, 1985), Dorothy Avis, a social worker with many years of experience in institutional settings, describes some of these policies:

> Practices within institutions seemed to separate parents from their children. Visiting hours were limited, and sometimes visits were supervised. Permissions were required. It is not too hard to interpret that the child needs protection from the parent—or the reverse.
>
> If, in the past, parents requested a home visit for their child, a social worker made a home study—another test of measuring up that parents had to weather. Old records show refusals of requests for visits because of housekeeping standards and other value judgments. Often the reasons given for refusal were that the child needed further training and time for adjustment. I am still not entirely sure what that meant, and in some instances we might wonder what training was being considered. However, if one had accepted the rationale that only professional people could care for the child, then there must be something (beyond a mere parent's understanding) that was going on that shouldn't be interrupted [pp. 188–189].

This history of attributing blame to the parents of children with disabilities, of separating parents from their children, and of distrusting their capabilities to make decisions that affect their children has presented barriers to the establishment of true decision-making partnerships. As long as families were treated as if their instincts regarding what was best for them as a family, or for their child, could not be trusted, parents understandably approached professionals with feelings of distrust or defensiveness.

The social work profession has made an effort to overcome this perception. Social workers have played leadership roles in promoting a view of individuals with disabilities and their families as being capable of identifying their own needs. Social workers have advocated for families and individuals to capitalize on their own competencies and to take the lead in decision making.

The continuing challenge for social workers, working with individuals with disabilities and their families, is to recognize and promote the abilities of the individuals served. This is best achieved when consumers

- set their own goals and priorities,
- make choices in response to a range of major and minor decisions that affect them,
- determine what services and supports would be helpful,
- obtain and manage the services they receive, and
- set the pace for any services or supports that are received.

This list is easy to embrace in principle but is exceedingly difficult to put into practice. Social workers in this field must strive to support these practices even when they may have misgivings about the choices a family or individual might make. Social workers will need a combination of experience, confidence, and commitment to support individuals and families in their decisions.

Paradigm Shift 3

A shift from treatment of people with disabilities in a manner that does not emphasize their worth to treatment that reflects full integration and normalization or social role valorization.

Normalization was defined by Wolf Wolfensberger (1972) as the "utilization of means which are as culturally normative as possible in order to establish and/or maintain personal behaviors and characteristics which are as culturally normative as possible" (p. 28). Normalization relates to the way social workers and other professionals in the field assist individuals with disabilities to become valued, participating members of their communities. John O'Brien (1980) has developed a model for applying the principle of normalization to service delivery. He suggests measuring the degree to which programs for people with disabilities conform to the principle by examining:

1. *What* the program achieves for those it serves ("personal behaviors, experiences, and characteristics" in the definition):
   - the social competencies people develop,
   - the personal appearance of people in the program,
   - the public image of the people in the program, and
   - the quality and variety of the life options people experience over time.

   This includes choices of living arrangements, educational opportunities, leisure time pursuits, productive work roles, and other opportunities to participate in the lives of natural families and communities.

2. *How* the program accomplishes its objectives ("means" in the definition):
   - the physical settings used in delivering the program;
   - the ways in which people are grouped for various program purposes;
   - the goals of the program;
   - the activities selected to meet program goals, as well as the way they are scheduled;

- the people who provide the program's services and control the program's direction; and
- the language used to describe the program, as well as the people it serves (p. 12).

In 1983 Wolfensberger coined a new term, "social role valorization," which he felt better described the intentions of the original term "normalization." He defined *social role valorization* as "the establishment, enhancement, or defense of the valued social roles of a person or group via the enhancement of people's social images and personal competencies" (Wolfensberger, 1983, p. 234).

O'Brien (1987) also helped to clarify the way in which this new concept could be measured and applied. He suggests that the quality of social roles and life experiences for individuals with disabilities can be measured by observing five related outcomes:

- **Community presence** is the sharing of ordinary places that define community life.
- **Choice** is the experience of autonomy both in small, everyday matters . . . and in large, life-defining matters.
- **Competence** is the opportunity to perform functional and meaningful activities with whatever level or type of assistance that is required.
- **Respect** is having a valued place among a network of people and valued roles in community life.
- **Community participation** is the experience of being a part of a growing network of personal relationships that includes close friends (pp. 177–178).

Many of the services available to individuals with disabilities traditionally have been provided in settings and in ways that devalue these individuals. Recently, several positive changes have occurred. Many individuals who were previously institutionalized have moved into smaller, self-selected, community settings. Individuals have been offered a wider range of opportunities for decision making and self-determination. Families of children with disabilities have been encouraged to take charge of the services offered to their children.

The service system must continue to change in order to conform to Wolfensberger's definitions of normalization and social role valorization. Still needed to a great extent are the following:

- Services and supports that emphasize individual and family strengths.
- A system that supports and enhances the ability of individuals and their families (when appropriate) to make decisions and choices that affect their lives and the delivery of services to them.
- A shift away from fixed and limited expectations of what individuals can achieve to a broader and more challenging view of what may be possible.

- Assistance to individuals with disabilities to broaden their network of friends, community contacts, and generic resources.
- Abandonment of the "continuum" model. That is, the logic underlying service delivery should be shifted from an emphasis on *preparation for* normal living to one of *support in* normal living.
- A shift away from offering programs that have "beds," "placements," or "slots" available toward the development of individualized services that respond to a specific person's or family's wants or priorities.
- A focus on services and supports that *in the view of the recipient* are valuable, meaningful, and desirable.

IMPLICATIONS OF THE PARADIGM SHIFTS ON ASPECTS OF SOCIAL WORK SERVICE DELIVERY

The shifting paradigms in the provision of care to individuals with disabilities have been the impetus for numerous changes in the delivery of social work services. This section examines the effect of these paradigm shifts on the role of the social worker, on the decision-making process, on the social worker's relationship to the family, and on the locations in which social work services are delivered. We will describe each of these areas as they would appear at the two extremes of a continuum: at one end is an institutional, professionally controlled service delivery system; at the other end is a community-based, consumer-driven system. For the purposes of this discussion, the former will be called the *traditional* end of the continuum and the latter will be called the *consumer-driven* end of the continuum. The practices of most social workers are not typically at either end of the continuum but are more likely to be represented at various points along it. Table 11-1 provides an overview of this continuum, along with the challenges facing social workers in moving toward the consumer-driven end.

The Role of the Social Worker

The role of the social worker is multifaceted and can vary greatly depending on the needs of individuals, families, and agencies. The roles of the social worker that have been most affected by the paradigm shifts can be divided into three categories/functions: service coordinator (case manager), advocate, and counselor.

The Role of Service Coordinator

At the traditional end of the continuum, social workers acting as service coordinators assist individuals with disabilities and their

TABLE 11-1 A Continuum of Change: Implications for Social Work Practice

Aspects of Social Work Service Delivery	At the Traditional (Institutionally Based, Professionally Controlled) End of the Continuum	At the Consumer-Driven (Community-Based, Consumer-Controlled) End of the Continuum	Challenges to Social Workers in Moving toward the Consumer-Driven End of the Continuum
1. Role of the social worker Case manager/service coordinator	• Assist individuals with disabilities and their families by making referrals and coordinating services.	• Act as consultants/ trainers to assist individuals with disabilities and their families to obtain, develop, and coordinate services.	• To become knowledgeable in consultation skills.
	• Refer to already existing resources that are rarely integrated into services utilized by the general population.	• Refer to and assist in the development of generic as well as specialized services.	• To expand knowledge of generic and community-based services.
	• Coordinate services for the individual with disabilities and make referrals for other family members when issues arise that impact on the family member with a disability.	• Coordinate services for all family members.	• To be sensitive in addressing the needs of all family members.

(continued)

TABLE 11-1 A Continuum of Change: Implications for Social Work Practice (*continued*)

Aspects of Social Work Service Delivery	At the Traditional (Institutionally Based, Professionally Controlled) End of the Continuum	At the Consumer-Driven (Community-Based, Consumer-Controlled) End of the Continuum	Challenges to Social Workers in Moving toward the Consumer-Driven End of the Continuum
Advocate	• Advocate for individuals with disabilities to receive existing services and resources.	• Join with consumers and other community providers to advocate for systems change.	• To envision a system of services and resources that does not already exist. • To advocate with interdisciplinary and administrative agency staff for the establishment of more consumer-/family-centered policies and procedures.
	• Identify advocacy issues for individuals and families.	• Participate in coalitions composed of consumers and professionals who identify advocacy issues to be addressed.	• To develop skills in community organization and political activism.

TABLE 11.1 (continued)

Counselor	• Provide counseling to parents concerning issues primarily related to the family member with disabilities. Refer siblings and other family members to counseling, as requested.	• Expand counseling to address issues identified by the family that may be unrelated to the family member with disabilities. Provide counseling services to siblings and other family members.	• To advocate within their own agencies to expand counseling services to include all family members.
	• Rarely, identify mental health needs among individuals with disabilities. Provide support and encouragement, but counseling to address mental health needs is seldom offered.	• Identify the mental health needs of individuals with disabilities and provide counseling if requested.	• To learn how to effectively screen for the mental health needs of individuals with disabilities.
2. Process of decision making	• Participate on professional teams that develop plans and recommendations for families.	• Act as consultants to assist individuals and families in team building to assist in the development of plans and recommendations.	• To provide individuals/families with enough information so that the family can make informed decisions.

(continued)

245

TABLE 11-1 A Continuum of Change: Implications for Social Work Practice *(continued)*

Aspects of Social Work Service Delivery	At the Traditional (Institutionally Based, Professionally Controlled) End of the Continuum	At the Consumer-Driven (Community-Based, Consumer-Controlled) End of the Continuum	Challenges to Social Workers in Moving toward the Consumer-Driven End of the Continuum
	• Provide leadership in the decision-making process.	• Support family/individual leadership in the decision-making process.	• To respect and support the choices of families/individuals even when one may believe a different decision may be more effective.
3. Relationship to family	• Assess family functioning and assist families in utilizing recommended services.	• Act as consultants in assisting families to develop and implement a plan for services. Complete a family assessment only if requested.	• To train parents in the skills that will help to make them more successful in developing and implementing service plans.
	• Encourage the team to develop a plan that is sensitive to all family members.	• Provide a range of services (e.g., flexible funds, sibling groups) to all family members.	• To develop skills in negotiation and advocacy to assist in the creation of teams that are supportive of the development and implementation of plans for all family members.

TABLE 11-1 *(continued)*

	• Determine their relationship with families based on the agency's service delivery approach.	• Respect the family's wishes in determining the relationship. Vary their roles based on the unique strengths and needs of each family.	• To develop skills as a consultant, service coordinator, advocate, counselor, and so on and provide only those services that each family requests.
4. Location of service delivery	• Provide services in specialized residential centers, institutions, hospitals, day programs, and so forth.	• Provide services in more generic, community-based settings such as supported living settings, supported employment sites, and in the home.	• To develop new networks with a variety of community providers. This will require increased skills in coordination and negotiation.
	• Assist individuals with disabilities to function more effectively within these settings.	• Assist the individual with disabilities to function more effectively within his or her own home or community.	• To develop skills needed to work more successfully in the home and in other community-based settings.

families by making referrals. These referrals are typically to resources that are designed solely for use by individuals with disabilities and are not integrated into services utilized by the general population. The social worker also makes referrals to services for other family members when issues arise that have a direct impact on the family member with a disability. For example, a social worker employed by a hospital might refer a young child with cerebral palsy to the local United Cerebral Palsy organization for respite care and to a specialized preschool program that would provide needed therapies. The social worker might also refer the child's parents to a community mental health center for marital therapy to assist them in controlling their fighting, which might be having a negative impact on their child's behavior.

At the consumer-driven end of the continuum, a hospital social worker working with this family would take a different approach. The social worker might begin by asking the parents what types of supports, activities, and resources would benefit their child and their family. Instead of the social worker developing a plan based on existing services, the social worker would act as a consultant to assist the family in acquiring the skills necessary to coordinate a plan that meets their family's needs. This plan might consist of not only specialized services from organizations that serve individuals with disabilities (e.g., respite care through the local United Cerebral Palsy organization), but also generic services with or without needed supplemental supports (e.g., regular preschool with teacher training by a physical therapist). The plan might also include newly developed services to address the unique needs of this family (e.g., a parent-organized play group at the neighborhood swimming pool). In addition to assisting the family to develop their plan, the social worker might also offer to assist in obtaining services for other family members (e.g., seeking funding for a summer camp for a brother of the child with disabilities).

These examples illustrate the three major challenges that social workers address in moving from a traditional to a consumer-driven orientation in their role as service coordinators. First, social workers must become more knowledgeable in acting as consultants who assist individuals with disabilities and their families to coordinate a plan that meets their needs. Second, social workers must become more aware of not only specialized services, but also of generic services. Finally, social workers must be able to assist families by becoming more actively involved in addressing not only the needs of the individual with a disability but also the needs of other family members.

The Role of Advocate
Social workers have always advocated for individuals with disabilities to receive needed services. This included advocating for indi-

vidual consumers to receive services through existing resources as well as working with other professionals to develop new services. More recently, the role of the social worker as an advocate has expanded. Social workers have joined a coalition of consumers (individuals with disabilities and their families) and other professionals to advocate for a more responsive service delivery system. The coalitions have actively developed new services and resources, lobbied for increased funding, and encouraged consumer-driven systems change at both local and national levels.

The most salient change in the social worker's role as an advocate relates to the process by which advocacy issues are identified. No longer are issues identified independently by the social worker and other professionals relying primarily on their clinical expertise and experience. Today, advocacy issues are identified by coalitions of consumers and professionals, with individuals with disabilities and their family members in leadership roles.

These changes in the advocacy role present a variety of challenges. Social workers must not only utilize existing resources, but also envision and assist in the development of new service systems. To participate in this systems change, skills in community organization and political activism will need to be developed further. These skills will facilitate the ability of social workers to advocate, both within their own agencies and in the community, for the establishment of more consumer-/family-centered policies and procedures. In the current economic climate, social workers face an additional challenge in advocating not only to maintain services, but also to further develop community-based, consumer-driven systems and services.

The Role of Counselor

At the traditional end of the continuum, social workers, as counselors, provide supportive counseling to parents and to individuals with disabilities. Counseling for parents of individuals with disabilities is designed to assist parents to adjust to their child's diagnosis and to support them in their use of services. Counseling for the individual with disabilities is most often directed at improving the individual's functioning in day programs, school settings, medical facilities, and so on. It may be felt that individuals with disabilities cannot effectively participate in, or benefit significantly from, counseling.

At the consumer-driven end of the continuum, social workers are expanding their counseling role with families to address a broader range of counseling needs identified by parents of children with disabilities. Parents may request counseling for a variety of issues that may or may not be directly related to their child with disabilities (e.g., marital counseling, parents' feelings of anxiety, or depression). In addition, counseling issues of siblings and extended family members are more frequently identified and addressed.

Social workers, along with other professionals, have begun to recognize the tremendous potential of individuals with disabilities. In order to assist these individuals to achieve their potential, social workers are now more likely to address the mental health needs of this population. Social workers are providing counseling to individuals with disabilities and are making referrals to related mental health services when requested. For example, a twenty-five-year-old man with mental retardation who is experiencing feelings of depression previously might have been given support and encouraged to participate in socialization activities. Now, a similar individual would be more likely to receive counseling services, which might consist of support, behavioral recommendations, and insight-oriented therapy. A social worker might also refer the individual to a psychiatrist to evaluate the possible effectiveness of medication in treating the depression.

Social workers providing counseling services face two major challenges. First, social workers need to advocate within their own agencies for the expansion of counseling services to address the many needs of all family members. Second, social workers must refine their skills in screening for and addressing the mental health needs of individuals with disabilities.

Decision-Making Process

The social worker's role in the decision-making process varies at different points along the continuum. At the traditional end, social workers join with other professionals on teams to develop plans and recommendations that they believe will be most beneficial to the individual with disabilities and his or her family. These recommendations are then shared with the individuals and their families, and assistance is provided in accessing and utilizing the recommended services. For the most part, professionals take the leadership role in the process of decision making.

At the consumer-driven end, parents and individuals with disabilities are not only team members but also team leaders. Plans and recommendations often are developed by these consumers, using social workers and other professionals as consultants and facilitators. The role of the social worker is to assist in developing a team that includes consumers in all stages of the decision-making process. The consumer chooses his or her role on the team. This role may vary from being an active observer to being a team leader. For example, a twenty-one-year-old woman with cerebral palsy might choose to be a team leader and schedule an interagency meeting to develop a plan for independent living, including housing and job opportunities. As the team leader, she decides which professionals and family members will attend this planning meeting.

The social workers participation in a more consumer-driven decision-making process presents a major challenge. Social workers who act as consultants no longer determine needs and recommend solutions, but assist consumers in obtaining pertinent information so that individuals and families can make informed decisions. Social workers need to respect and support the choices of consumers even when they, as professionals, may believe that another choice might be more beneficial. Although the clinical experience and expertise of social workers is valuable, they must remember to value the consumers' expertise in knowing what services and resources are needed by them or their families. Social workers should consider ways to better utilize their clinical expertise within a framework of consumer-directed decision making.

Relationship to Family

The social worker's relationship to the family is undergoing many changes. At the traditional end of the continuum, a major role of the social worker is to assess family functioning in order to develop a plan that meets the needs of the individual with disabilities. This assessment helps the team determine how the individual and/or the family can best access and utilize recommended services. The social worker's role is to encourage the team to develop a plan for the individual with disabilities that is sensitive to the needs of all family members. The degree to which social workers are able to advocate for and respond to the needs of families is often dictated by their agencies' service delivery approach. For example, a school social worker might be aware that a family could most effectively take advantage of school services if they were provided in the home. However, if the school system does not offer home-based services, the social worker will need to refer the child to another program or advocate to make the school program as responsive as possible.

At the consumer-driven end of the continuum, individuals with disabilities and their families actively determine the parameters of their relationship with social workers. Based on the unique strengths and interests of each family, the social worker's role might include acting as a therapist, advocate, trainer, provider of information, or service coordinator. In all of these roles, the social worker acts as a consultant in assisting families to develop and implement a plan for all family members, including parents and siblings.

The changes in the social worker's relationship to families present several challenges. Social workers must offer training and support to interested parents to assist them in developing and implementing service plans for their families. In addition, social workers must learn to negotiate and advocate on their teams to create an atmosphere that supports a family-centered planning process. Finally, social workers must develop the range of skills necessary to function in a variety of roles (i.e., consultant, service coordinator, advocate, or counselor) with families.

Location of Service Delivery

At the traditional end of the continuum, social workers provide services in specialized residential centers, institutions, hospitals, and day programs. Within these settings, social workers, as members of interdisciplinary teams, participate in the development of service plans that are implemented by the agency staff. Since services are provided in center-based facilities, social workers spend the majority of their time dealing with psychosocial issues (e.g., social skills, missed appointments, adjustment problems) that relate to the ability of the individual with disabilities to function within these center-based programs.

At the consumer-driven end of the continuum, social workers provide services in more generic, community-based settings such as supported living settings, supported employment sites, and in-home programs. These settings encourage social workers to participate on their own agency's interdisciplinary teams, as well as on consumer and interagency teams and coalitions. As members of these teams, social workers address psychosocial and systems issues (e.g., integration into the community by arranging transportation to neighborhood association meetings and church services, socialization with other workers on the job, and assisting individuals to register to vote) that relate to the ability of the individual with disabilities to function more effectively within his or her home and community.

The increased participation of social workers on interagency teams and coalitions presents a major challenge. Social workers must be more responsive to a variety of community systems. Their responsibilities lie beyond the boundaries of their own agency. To effectively advocate within this new network of community providers, social workers need to continue to develop their skills in coordination and negotiation. A more integrated and collaborative service system has begun to develop as social workers, consumers, and other service providers have engaged in this cooperative planning process.

CONCLUSION

The underlying values of the social work profession (i.e., self-determination, the innate value of the individual, the importance of advocacy and systems change) are essential to the development of a more community-based, consumer-driven service delivery system. As the field of disabilities has embraced these changes, social workers have had the opportunity to take leadership roles in encouraging the development of new policies and programs that incorporate these social work values. The primary challenge for social work has been and will continue to be to operationalize these values within the constraints of agency settings and economic realities. As funding for human service programs becomes more limited, social workers will need to continue to broaden their community organization and advocacy efforts to ensure that the movement toward a more community-based, consumer-driven system continues to thrive.

REFERENCES

Adams, M. (1971). *Mental retardation and its social dimensions.* New York: Columbia University Press.

Braddock, D., Hemp, R., Fujiura, G., Bachelder, L., and Mitchell, D. (1990). *The state of the states in developmental disabilities.* Baltimore: Paul H. Brookes.

Bruininks, R., Meyers, C., Sigford, B., and Lakin, K. (Eds.) (1981). *Deinstitutionalization and community adjustment of mentally retarded people.* Washington, DC: American Association on Mental Deficiency.

Glassman, U. (1991). The social work group and its distinct healing qualities in the health care setting. *Health and Social Work, 16,* 203–212.

Hollis, F. (1964). *Casework: A psychosocial therapy.* New York: Random House.

Linz, M.H., McAnally, P., and Wieck, C. (Eds.) (1989). *Case management: Historical, current and future perspectives* (p. 145). Cambridge, MA: Brookline Books.

McFadden, D.L., and Burke, E.P. (1991). Developmental disabilities and the new paradigm: Directions for the 1990s. *Family Support Bulletin,* 3–5.

O'Brien, J. (1980). The principle of normalization: A foundation for effective services. In J.F. Gardner, L. Long, R. Nichols, and D.M. Iagulli (Eds.), *Program issues in developmental disabilities* (pp. 12–34). Baltimore: Paul H. Brookes.

O'Brien, J. (1987). A guide to life-style planning. In B. Wilcox and G.T. Bellamy (Eds.), *A comprehensive guide to the activities catalog: An alternative curriculum for youth and adults with severe disabilities.* Baltimore: Paul H. Brookes.

Perlman, H.P. (1957). *Social casework: A problem solving process*. Chicago: University of Chicago Press.

Roberts, R.N. (Conference Moderator) (1988). *Family support in the home: Home visiting programs and P.L. 99-457*. Honolulu: Association for the Care of Children's Health.

Turnbull, A.P., and Turnbull, H.R. (1990). *Families, professionals and exceptionality: A special partnership* (2nd ed.). Columbus, OH: Charles E. Merrill.

Turnbull, A.P., and Turnbull, H.R. (Eds.) (1985). *Parents speak out: Then and now*. Columbus, OH: Charles E. Merrill.

U.S. Congress (1990). Public Law 101-476, Education of the Handicapped Act Amendments of 1990—Individuals with Disabilities Education Act.

Wolfensberger, W. (1972). *The principle of normalization in human services*. Toronto: National Institute on Mental Retardation.

Wolfensberger, W. (1983). Social role valorization: A proposed new term for the principle of normalization. *Mental Retardation, 21*, 234–239.

12 ⬜⬜⬜ ⬜⬜⬜ ⬜⬜⬜

Rehabilitation Counseling and the Community Paradigm

William E. Kiernan and David Hagner

INTRODUCTION

Paradigm shifts are not new to rehabilitation. There have been numerous conceptual shifts throughout its history in populations served, outcomes sought, and scope of services delivered. But a consistent theme over the years in rehabilitation has been the focus on the needs of the individual and the inclusion of the person with a disability in the planning process. Care and protection are not the operational concepts of rehabilitation, but rather partnership, planning, and action steps leading to consumer outcomes. The National Council on Rehabilitation (1944) defined *rehabilitation* as the restoration of people who are handicapped to the fullest physical, mental, social, vocational, and economic usefulness of which they are capable. A more practical description of rehabilitation might be the process engaged in by people with disabilities to define individual or person-specific goals, develop action steps to achieve those goals, and identify resources that can be accessed to meet those goals. Such resources may include (a) those internal to the individual; (b) those that naturally occur, such as friends at work, the use of appointment books, or bells for crossing streets; and (c) those provided by a paid support person, such as a rehabilitation counselor (Kiernan, 1991).

The first three sections outline some of the highlights in the development of vocational rehabilitation and review the various roles that rehabilitation counselors play in the process of providing rehabilitation services to persons with disabilities. The next section addresses the consistencies and inconsistencies that are present in vocational rehabilitation as the changes in service delivery and roles emerge. The final section offers some suggestions about future directions for rehabilitation in light of the paradigm shift presented earlier in this book.

A BRIEF HISTORY OF REHABILITATION

Since the passage of the first rehabilitation legislation some seventy-five years ago, the focus of the rehabilitation effort has been upon employment and the provision of services that would assist the person with a disability in finding and holding a job. The Soldier Rehabilitation, or Smith-Sears, Act (P.L. 65-178) was what would eventually become the basis of the federal-state vocational rehabilitation (VR) system. As Fifield and Fifield (1995, Chapter 3, in this book) have noted, there have been shifts over the years from an initial focus on veterans to inclusion of the civilian population and from an exclusive emphasis on *return* to work to the acknowledgment that individuals with disabilities of early onset could benefit from rehabilitation services in order to *enter* work and independent living. With the passage of the Rehabilitation Act of 1973 (P.L. 93-112), rehabilitation services were further extended to address the needs of those individuals who were more severely disabled. Consumer involvement in rehabilitation planning and due process protections for recipients of rehabilitation services were also part of this act. And further, a mandate to federal agencies and federal contractors to provide reasonable accommodation in employing individuals with disabilities was included as Title V of the 1973 legislation, signaling a growing recognition that disability was a civil rights issue as well as a clinical or service issue.

The next major conceptual shift occurred in 1978 with the passage of the Rehabilitation, Comprehensive Services and Developmental Disabilities Amendments (P.L. 95-602). This legislation affirmed that outcomes other than employment could be supported through the provision of rehabilitation services. In 1986, amendments to the Rehabilitation Act recognized supported employment as a legitimate outcome of vocational rehabilitation service delivery. Finally, the passage of the Americans with Disabilities Act (ADA) (P.L. 100-336) extended civil rights protections far beyond the narrow scope of the Rehabilitation Act of 1973 and provided clear recognition of the rights of people with disabilities to nondiscrimination in public access, employment, telecommunication, and transportation.

The history of rehabilitation reflects an evolving awareness that persons who have acquired or been born with a disability can, with assistance and support, be productive and contributing members of society. Table 12-1 presents the major laws relating to the development of rehabilitation and more specifically vocational rehabilitation. It is primarily through the passage of these laws that the discipline of rehabilitation counseling and the definition of the range of rehabilitation services have evolved over time.

TABLE 12-1   Legislative History of Vocational Rehabilitation

Title	Legislation Number	Date of Passage	Critical Features
Soldier Rehabilitation or Smith-Sears Act	P.L. 65-178	1918	• Originated what was to become the federal–state rehabilitation system • Focused on those injured in service and returning to work in civilian world
Civilian Rehabilitation or Smith-Fess Act	P.L. 66-236	1920	• Developed civilian counterpart to P.L. 65-178 • Assisted civilians with non-service-connected physical disabilities to receive job placement and retraining • Established an eligibility program that required clients to meet criteria, which remain essentially unchanged to the present day • Established disability as an impairment to work and expectation that with services an individual can return to work

(continued)

Table 12-1   Legislative History of Vocational Rehabilitation *(continued)*

Legislation Title	Number	Date of Passage	Critical Features
Vocational Rehabilitation Amendments or Barden-LaFollette Act	P.L. 78-113	1943	• Expanded VR services to people with mental illness and/or mental retardation
			• Included services such as medical/physical restoration in addition to vocational training and placement
Vocational Rehabilitation Amendments or Hill-Burton Act	P.L. 83-565	1954	• Authorized expenditures on training staff and creating the first graduate-level rehabilitation counseling programs
			• Created start-up funding for new rehabilitation facilities

Unlike many professional disciplines, rehabilitation counseling has been influenced more by legislation than by the evolution of research findings and clinical practice.

PROFESSIONAL ROLES IN REHABILITATION COUNSELING

Rehabilitation is viewed as a range of services and supports that allow the individual who is disabled to be as independent and productive as possible in the community. Rehabilitation services are diverse and offered by a variety of professionals, including psychologists, social workers, physicians, nurses, physical therapists, occupational therapists, speech pathologists, and rehabilitation counselors. The discipline of rehabilitation counseling reflects the early emphasis upon the need for the expertise of skilled professionals to assist individuals in returning to work.

Rehabilitation counseling as a profession has been eclectic in its service approaches, encompassing a wide array of practices and theoretical orientations and relying often on the support and assistance of many professionals in the development and implementation of a rehabilitation plan. As Barker (1988) noted, rehabilitation counselors have been trained using theories borrowed from counseling psychology, medicine, applied behavior theory, and functional analysis/planning. Competencies in case management, individual and group counseling, career development, vocational assessment, work adjustment, job placement, training and support strategies on the job, and family supports represent only a few of the areas addressed in rehabilitation counselor training programs (Houser et al., 1991).

Beyond the development of competencies, clear principles and values have been postulated as key elements of a rehabilitation approach over the years (Wright, 1980). These concepts include:

1. *Holistic Nature*—A comprehensive view of human problems, that is, recognizing the interrelatedness of all aspects of a person's life.
2. *Self-determination*—The individual is at the center, and *controls* the rehabilitation process.
3. *Societal Contribution*—The belief that each individual has an innate desire to be a productive member of his or her community.
4. *Right to Be Equal*—Full civil and citizenship rights extend to people with disabilities.
5. *Human Spirit*—A belief in the capacity of individuals to persevere and rise above obstacles.
6. *Focus on Assets*—The rehabilitation focus on maximizing strengths as much as remediating deficits.
7. *Motivation for Good*—The belief that individuals are capable of changing and will naturally desire to improve their situation.
8. *Influence of Environment*—The focus of rehabilitation activities on modifying environments as well as developing individual skills.
9. *Intrinsic Value*—A belief in the essential worth of a person, solely by virtue of his or her humanity, independent of social/financial/ educational status, and so on.
10. *Concern for Individuals*—Service provision is based on individual desires and needs rather than categorical groupings or diagnoses.

Shafer (1988) spoke of rehabilitation philosophy as having an orientation toward productivity and self-sufficiency. Bitter (1979) identified three essential principles of vocational rehabilitation: equality of opportunity, a holistic and coordinated service approach, and an orientation toward individuality. The basic concept of rehabilitation counseling has evolved, along with the emphasis of legislation and advances in treatment strategies and technology. The concept of a partnership approach to the implementation of a rehabilitation plan is consistent with the shifting design in the provision of early intervention, education, and adult services. Rehabilitation has and continues to have the opportunity to demonstrate how individuals can (and must) be active and, in most instances, the coordinating member of the team, developing and implementing the rehabilitation plan.

The core principles of rehabilitation, which directly influence practice in the community, are based on underlying assumptions about human behavior and the personal change process. Seven major areas have been identified by Whitehead and Marrone (1986), reflecting (a) the individual in control, (b) productivity as not solely related to employment but to other levels of personal achievement, (c) support being willingly offered and accessible, (d) the rehabilitation process reflecting varying rates of advancement and times of plateau, (e) emphasis upon achieving positive changes, (f) focus on the strengths, assets, and interests of the individual with a disability, and (g) the development of specific and concrete action steps reflecting consumer-specific outcomes.

The principles of the rehabilitation process also reflect a philosophy that focuses on (a) the needs of the individual, (b) the development of a working relationship between the counselor and the individual, (c) the identification of strengths and abilities rather than deficits, (d) the emphasis on compensatory strategies rather than remediation in many instances, and (e) the acknowledgment of the need to both develop individual skills and modify environments, thus looking for optimal fit between the individual and a specific environment. The focus of rehabilitation, and specifically vocational rehabilitation, has been on entry into work. With the shift in the emphasis of services to a more holistic perspective, the focus is now moving toward the individual and his or her participation across work, community living, leisure, and recreational environments, thereby enhancing the quality of life of the individual.

NATURE OF REHABILITATION SERVICES PROVIDED IN VARIOUS SETTINGS

The role of the rehabilitation counselor varies and is influenced by the nature of the setting in which the counselor works and agency or organization by which the counselor is employed. The vocational rehabilitation counselor employed in a state VR agency often provides the following services: (a) determination of the nature and extent of the disability and how it affects the individual's employment potential, (b) assessment of the individual's capacity to enter into or return to employment, (c) identification of the needs for specific skills training at the postsecondary level or in specialized training areas, (d) identification of adaptations necessary to assist the individual to become more independent, and (e) the development of personal skills and supports to allow the individual to function more independently in a community living or independent environment.

The services offered by the state VR agency include assessment, counseling, case management, job development, job placement, and postemployment supports. The rehabilitation counselor employed by the state VR agency often will provide short-term counseling interventions that lead to vocational outcomes. Long-term counseling and supports are not typically offered through the state VR agency.

For the rehabilitation counselor employed in a private community-based rehabilitation service agency, counseling and case management supports are more likely to be delivered on an ongoing basis. Private agencies include hospitals, rehabilitation centers or facilities, outpatient clinics, supported employment agencies, and a variety of other organizations. For persons with developmental disabilities, services may emphasize career exploration, community experiences, individual vocational skill mastery, social skill development, personal adjustment, and/or family supports.

The rehabilitation counselor along with other professionals in psychology and special education often assists the individual and the family in identifying career goals, assessing individual needs, and obtaining community resources that are responsive to those needs. In many community-based not-for-profit rehabilitation service agencies, the role of the rehabilitation counselor may include family supports as well as postplacement and employment services over a multiyear period. In such agencies the range of the services provided is often broader than that offered by the state VR agency, frequently including an emphasis on community living and leisure recreational activities.

More recently the rehabilitation counselor has played a role within private for-profit rehabilitation agencies, primarily in the area of resource or case management. The rehabilitation counselor can assist individuals who have experienced traumatic injury or work-related job injuries in returning to work. The rehabilitation counselor may assist the family and the individual in adjusting to a condition as well as identify potential career opportunities for the individual as he or she returns to employment. Additionally, the rehabilitation counselor may work with the employer, employee assistance programs in industry, or the private practitioner in assisting the person with the disability to return to or adjust to a return to work. Within the private rehabilitation agencies, as in the case of the state VR agency, the area of emphasis for the rehabilitation counselor is a return to employment or an increase in the level of independence for the individual in his or her community setting. In these cases frequently there are insurance issues involved, with the focus of the insurance agency on increasing the level of independence and thereby reducing its financial obligation to the individual who has been injured.

The most recent role for the rehabilitation counselor is one of assisting students with disabilities to make the transition from school into employment. With the passage of the Individuals with Disabilities Education Act (IDEA, [P.L. 101-476]), an increased emphasis is placed on development of vocational or adult living goals while the student is in his or her high school years. This law mandates that the rehabilitation counselor serve as a member of an interdisciplinary educational team that assists the student and family in developing goals directed toward transitioning from school to adult life no later than the student's sixteenth birthday and preferably at age fourteen. The rehabilitation counselor in this role can assist the student, family, and other team members to identify realistic career goals as well as to participate in career-oriented educational programs that will lead to the development of more refined employment and adult life goals. Though currently few rehabilitation counselors are employed in local schools, with the passage of this federal legislation there is a growing awareness that planning for the movement from school to adult life is a long-term process and one that must begin when the student is in the early high school (and some might say elementary school) years.

The role of the rehabilitation counselor in the years to come in the local school may include assisting the student and family members in life planning, working with educators in curricula development, providing individual and group counseling for students with disabilities, working with the student and teacher in job development, and providing family supports. In the future the role of the rehabilitation counselor in the school will at a minimum be one of member on an interdisciplinary transition team.

The scope, range, and duration of the services offered by the rehabilitation counselor vary considerably depending on whether the counselor is an employee of the state VR agency, a community-based rehabilitation agency, a private rehabilitation service agency, or a local school system. However, the core services offered, including assessment, counseling, personal adjustment training, case management, and job placement, are relatively consistent regardless of the place of employment. The rehabilitation counselor is playing an increasing role in developing life plans and identifying strategies to assist people with disabilities to realize their specific goals.

IMPACT OF THE COMMUNITY PARADIGM ON REHABILITATION COUNSELING

While every discipline is ultimately based on fundamental principles, values, and assumptions, rehabilitation has, perhaps more so than many other disciplines, remained conscious and clear about its basic principles, examining and reexamining them at critical points in its history and seeking guidance and meaning from them. One such examination occurred in 1958, for example, when leaders in the field of rehabilitation held a national conference devoted to the principles and assumptions of rehabilitation (Wright, 1959).

Many fundamental principles of rehabilitation are closely aligned with the "new paradigm" in human services, including many of the propositions announced at the 1958 conference. However, several gaps and pieces of unfinished business remain problematic for rehabilitation as it adapts to new realities and changes in other fields. Aspects of rehabilitation that are consistent with and inconsistent with the new paradigm are discussed below.

Consistent Elements

Several elements of vocational rehabilitation support the concepts that have come to be known as the community paradigm in human services. These include participation in the community, flexible service options, partnership with consumers, productivity, and a focus on outcomes.

Participation in the Community

Being a part of the community has been a critical focus of vocational rehabilitation since its inception. Participation in natural community settings and the recovery or attainment of valued social roles for people with disabilities has been viewed as the fundamental purpose of rehabilitation. One premise enunciated at the 1958 conference on rehabilitation principles was that "every person has membership in society, and rehabilitation should cultivate his [sic] full independence" (Malikin and Rusalem, 1969, p. 13). More recently, Livneh (1988) conceptualized the

arenas of rehabilitation as composed of two elements: community participation and labor force participation.

Implied in this community orientation is a fundamental dissatisfaction
with segregated rehabilitation outcomes. For example, placement in sheltered employment, while it is certainly widespread, has tended to be approached as either temporary *in theory* (even though practitioners were
well aware that they were seldom temporary in practice) or as a default
option exercised in the absence of viable alternatives. Two sorts of evidence
support this interpretation. First, continuing efforts to develop service
approaches and alternatives more consistent with the primary focus on
community acceptance, such as community work sites (Gerber, 1979),
work crews (Hansen, 1969), Projects with Industry (Research Utilization
Laboratory, 1976), school transition projects (Riscalla, 1974; Wehman et
al., 1988), and job placement techniques (reviewed in Vandergoot, 1987),
have been an integral part of the rehabilitation tradition. Second, as supported employment strategies emerged in the mid-1980s, which held promise as an important new approach to assisting individuals to achieve
employment in community settings, the rehabilitation program quickly
incorporated supported employment into its service delivery system and
funded a series of state systems change projects. Many rehabilitation service agencies have already shifted focus away from funding services in
segregated settings, and a national trend toward an increasing rate of placement of people with severe disabilities into competitive, rather than sheltered, employment has been under way for several years (Andrews et al.,
1991; McGaughey et al., 1990).

Open-ended, Flexible Service Options

Vocational rehabilitation has not been bound by any one service model or approach, and thus has retained the flexibility to respond to
the needs of individuals with a wide variety of interventions and service
designs. Within the state VR program, federal regulations provide an extra-
ordinarily broad interpretation of vocational rehabilitation services. Any
goods or services that can benefit an individual in terms of employability
are allowable under the program. The design of state rehabilitation agencies as brokers rather than as direct providers of most rehabilitation services has encouraged flexibility in the delivery of services.

Because rehabilitation counseling has historically seen the need to
remain a cross-disciplinary enterprise, it has remained centered on the
needs of people with disabilities, rather than subordinating those needs to
professional self-interest or the dictates of any particular method. Rehabilitation interventions may include counseling, training, education,
behavior change, medical treatment, adaptive equipment, architectural

modification, transportation, or virtually any other service that might be dictated by an individual's rehabilitation plan. Even services to the family of the individual with a disability and such indirect efforts as public education and policy reform are legitimate rehabilitation services (Livneh, 1989).

Ecological Focus
Interventions targeting changes in an individual's physical and social environment are particularly noteworthy from the standpoint of the community paradigm, because they are rooted in an appreciation of disability as a product of an interactional process between individuals and their environment (Hahn, 1991). Rehabilitation has from its inception seen the need to understand the world of work as well as individuals with disabilities, and such topics as theories of work adjustment, job analysis, and labor market analysis are an important aspect of rehabilitation counselor training (Houser et al., 1991).

In 1985 the National Rehabilitation Counseling Association issued a position paper affirming that businesses are clients and consumers of vocational rehabilitation and that serving the needs of the business community is an essential component of vocational rehabilitation (Garvin, 1985). Today, the interactional or ecological (Stubbins and Albee, 1984) perspective includes a recognition that people with disabilities constitute a disadvantaged minority group, in many respects seeking civil rights rather than social services (Hahn, 1991). This perspective is perhaps best exemplified by the Americans with Disabilities Act.

Partnership with Consumers
The practice of counseling has tended to emphasize respect for and equality with consumers. Rehabilitation counseling is a highly individualized process best achieved jointly by the professional and consumer in the context of a personal relationship (Ryan, 1988). Empowerment of consumers has been called the backbone of rehabilitation (Emener, 1991).

While all service planning processes purport to be "client-centered," the participation of the individuals receiving services often amounts to no more than "rubber-stamping" plans developed by professionals (Hagner and Salomone, 1989). Rehabilitation goes further than any other program in requiring, in Section 102 of the Rehabilitation Act, that individual written rehabilitation plans be jointly developed by the counselor and the client. At its best, the rehabilitation planning process involves an equal partnership in formulating goals and designing services.

Emphasis on Productivity

Rehabilitation is rooted in the belief that people with disabilities are capable, productive citizens. As such, it is designed to assist consumers in achieving vocational goals and becoming contributing members of society. In contrast to programs based on dependency and care, rehabilitation has emphasized the productive capacity of citizens with disabilities and the importance of work as a valued role for adults in our society.

Focus on Outcomes

In part because of their strong vocational emphasis, rehabilitation services have always been grounded in specific achievable goals. While the goal formulation process may be difficult for some individuals, and while a variety of circumstances may impede progress toward a goal, rehabilitation never loses its goal focus. This focus encourages accountability for service quality and orients rehabilitation services toward the development of action steps leading to person-specific outcomes.

Inconsistent Elements

As the field of rehabilitation confronts the issues raised by the community paradigm, not all the news is good news. Several inconsistencies remain between aspects of rehabilitation and the new paradigm, including some unresolved internal inconsistencies within rehabilitation that have grown in seriousness as the community paradigm has become a major force for change.

Eligibility Restrictions

Despite the fact that the Rehabilitation Act has required, since 1973, that state VR agencies give priority to serving individuals with the most severe disabilities, vocational rehabilitation services have not consistently been made available to individuals with very severe or multiple disabilities. This inconsistency has been made even more striking by the experience of the supported employment program. This program was designed specifically to accommodate the needs of "individuals who, because of the severity of their handicaps, would not traditionally be eligible for vocational rehabilitation services" (*Federal Register*, 1987, p. 30548), yet the recipients of supported employment services have tended to be those with milder disabilities (Kregel and Wehman, 1989; McGaughey et al., 1990).

In part, restricted availability is due to an eligibility requirement within the VR program. In addition to having a disability that poses a barrier to employment, applicants are required to demonstrate a "reasonable expectation" (34 CFR 361.31(b)) that they can benefit in terms of employability. The term "benefit in terms of employability" is a vague, undefined notion, and there is overwhelming evidence that people with any type or severity of disability can work with the appropriate supports. Yet even though extended evaluations can assist applicants to demonstrate their capabilities prior to a final determination, and even though agencies must conduct annual reevaluations of applicants found ineligible, the VR system continues to view many individuals with severe disabilities as inappropriate for services. Possibly more harmful than formal denials of eligibility—which might be disputed or appealed—is the use of informal practices such as discouraging referrals of people believed to be difficult to serve or failing to successfully serve members of a certain group until referrals eventually stop (Rogan and Murphy, 1991). These practices are clearly out of step with the espoused principles of rehabilitation, but because they are difficult to document, they are therefore difficult to stop.

Deficit Focus

An important distinction in human services is that between categorical programs, designed for a group of people with a particular label, and generic programs, designed to assist anyone who needs the service. Rehabilitation is categorical by its very nature because it is designed exclusively for individuals with disabilities. Services designed around identification of personal deficits tend to exacerbate the differences between service recipients and other citizens and to separate people from one another. A shift to focusing on strengths, capacities, and equal community membership may require that we integrate services to people with disabilities into a broader vision of a diverse society that responds to the human needs of all citizens.

Therapeutic Orientation

Rehabilitation has never fully distinguished itself from a clinical or medical orientation. Terms such as "disorder," "treatment," "diagnosis," "prognosis," and "therapy" abound in rehabilitation literature. They point not only to a deficit-centered view but also to a yearning for professional recognition and "expert" status and, perhaps, for a position of social power legitimized by licenses, certificates, fifty-minute hours, and offices with waiting rooms. None of this helps people with disabilities attain a position of social equality or control over their own lives. Professional disciplines tend to emphasize compliance over self-determination and treat "clients" as passive recipients of expert help. Taken to its extreme, professionalism becomes one more obstacle that must be confronted and challenged as the tenets of the community paradigm are incorporated into the delivery of services for and with persons who are disabled.

Time Limitations and Closure Focus

One of the espoused principles of rehabilitation has been that "Rehabilitation is a continuous process that applies as long as help is needed" (Malikin and Rusalem, 1969, p. 13). But, as has been noted, rehabilitation services delivered through the state VR agencies have traditionally been time-limited. Evaluations of rehabilitation service effectiveness are based on "case closures"—the number of people for whom services have ended because they have been "rehabilitated."

The case closure concept creates an expectation that counselors will not serve individuals over a long period of time. Long-term support needs tend to be either taken as evidence that an individual is not appropriate for vocational rehabilitation services or are seen as some other agency's responsibility. The regulations relating to supported employment call for the identification of a long-term support resource other than vocational rehabilitation if the VR agency is to provide services leading to a supported employment goal and VR views its responsibility as the initiator of the service, not the maintainer of long-term supports in supported employment. Yet, by definition, long-term supports are what the individuals who qualify for this service need. This issue has created significant problems in the development of supported employment services nationally (Kiernan et al., 1988; Shafer, 1988; McGaughey et al., 1990).

As a result of the time-limited nature of the services offered by VR, there has been discontinuity in services to individuals who either do not meet the eligibility requirements of another state agency, as is often the case for persons with cerebral palsy or other physical disabilities, or who must negotiate two different waiting lists to receive services (McGaughey et al., 1991). A second result has been a tendency to restrict many people with disabilities to entry-level jobs. Career development, the process of moving through a progression of jobs as skills increase and interests crystallize or change, is not handled well in a closure-oriented system. People with disabilities experience this as what Chubon (1985) called the "one shot approach" to career development.

The closure focus and eligibility problems of people with severe disabilities are closely related because an emphasis on short-term success may serve to discourage the VR counselor from offering services to people with complex needs. The range of services needed and the length of time required to support individuals with severe disabilities mean that fewer people will be served and "rehabilitated" by that counselor. Since its inception, VR has used the number of persons rehabilitated as a way of documenting effectiveness for legislative and other interested parties. The clear intent of the legislation is to have the VR system respond to the needs of those individuals with the most severe disabilities, yet the practice of utilizing the criteria of number rehabilitated for program justification is inconsistent with this intent. The current case closure concept must be rethought if the VR system is to respond to the needs of individuals with severe disabilities.

Narrow Service Focus

While work is a critical life domain for most adults, it is only one domain of life. Issues related to leisure and recreation, adult education unrelated to a specific job goal, community living supports, and other areas of life may be equally legitimate foci of rehabilitation efforts. The current rehabilitation system is far less equipped to handle these. Compartmentalization leads to further discontinuity, conflicts among multiple agencies, and confusion for both the consumer and the agencies involved. Though legislation has established independent living as a service of VR, this is a separate section of the legislation and is often viewed as entirely separate from VR employment and training services. Having the authority to address the needs of people with severe physical disabilities, as is typically the case in VR service programs, has not led to a more comprehensive approach to the major life domain needs of such individuals. Probably the least addressed service from the perspective of legislative mandates or funding supports is the area of leisure activities and recreational options for people with disabilities. Few if any federal or state agencies support the development of such activities for people with disabilities.

A focus on working-age adults limits the involvement of children with disabilities in rehabilitation. Concerted efforts have been made in recent years to involve vocational rehabilitation in the transition of young adults from secondary school. With the passage of the IDEA legislation in 1990 (P.L. 101-476), the involvement of the rehabilitation counselor in the transition process and the requirement to begin transition planning at least at age sixteen may serve to bring both education and rehabilitation closer together. But career-related education begins early in childhood (Miller, 1989), and children with disabilities may require other services, including supports to the family, in addition to education and transition planning.

Special education, vocational rehabilitation, and vocational education each has its own enabling legislation, eligibility criteria, scope of services, and personnel (Szymanski and Hanley-Maxwell, 1992). As a result, collaboration can be problematic. Some efforts at the federal level, through the

TABLE 12-2   Vocational Rehabilitation and the New Paradigm

Consistent Elements	Inconsistent Elements
Focus on community participation	Eligibility restrictions
Flexible service options	Deficit focus
Ecological focus	Therapeutic orientation
Partnership with consumers	Time limitations and closure
Emphasis on productivity	Narrow service focus
Focus on outcomes	

issuance of Requests for Proposals that require a joint response from the state VR agency and education agency, may serve as a catalyst to future collaborative efforts among agencies addressing the needs of students and adults with disabilities.

This section presented many of the issues and challenges facing the VR system, including concerns about eligibility limitations, scope of services offered, integration of service delivery, and inconsistencies in legislative intent and current practices. Table 12-2 summarizes the areas of consistency and inconsistency in rehabilitation counseling and rehabilitation service delivery with the community paradigm shift in human services. The following section offers some suggestions for the future as the movement toward consumer empowerment, community integration, and whole life needs progresses.

DIRECTIONS FOR THE FUTURE

As was noted earlier in this chapter, there are many areas in which the rehabilitation system is consistent with the focus of the community paradigm shift. It is a system that has historically emphasized identifying and meeting the needs of the individual in a flexible and timely fashion. The role and function of the rehabilitation counselor are those of partner, planner, resource manager, and support to the individual with a disability. Rehabilitation has stressed the need to consider the assets of the individual rather than limitations and to look toward the matching of these assets to the requirements of the environment, a focus on the goodness of fit of the individual and the environment. Yet even though there are several areas of compatibility between VR and the community paradigm, there are, as was also noted earlier, many areas in which there is inconsistency.

The following section offers some thoughts about future directions for rehabilitation given the changing climates in human service delivery.

With the growing recognition that the process of career development and vocational interests is initiated in the early years, the logic of involving rehabilitation counselors in the transition process is strong. The view that the movement from school into adult life occurs at the time of graduation is no longer held by many. The passage of the IDEA legislation points out that transition planning is a multiyear process and that it should focus on not only work but also all adult life activities. In the coming years, the VR system must interact more directly with students with disabilities, family members of those students, and educators. The development of vocationally and adult-oriented curricula at the high school level is essential. From a career education perspective, the emphasis on the development of functional life skills should occur throughout the entire school period. The rehabilitation counselor and the VR system can work with students in identifying areas of career interest, with families in reinforcing and supporting career exploration as a component of the educational plan for their son or daughter, and with educators in the development of curricula that provide career exploration and adult life skill development components.

Transition planning addresses the issue of early planning and intervention. However, if the focus remains exclusively on employment, long-term outcomes will be unnecessarily restricted. There is a need, in addition to the development of annual plans such as the Individual Education Plan (IEP) and the Individual Written Rehabilitation Plan (IWRP), for the incorporation of a longer-term planning strategy that addresses the needs of the whole person. Planning solely for a job will not address the needs for community living or leisure and recreational activities. Though employment in adult years provides a basis of identity, economic independence, and self-esteem, more time is spent each week in other life domain areas.

Comprehensive planning is essential if the goal of the rehabilitation process is one of full integration and inclusion into society. The current fragmented approach leads to partial solutions that often break down because other key areas beyond the job are not in place. When there is no living arrangement, or one that does not support or reinforce the individual in his or her job, and when there are few options to engage in leisure or recreational activities, the purpose of working becomes unclear and on some occasions meaningless. The VR system must broaden its focus to include all life domain areas and work with the individual and his or her natural support resources to assure that there is a balanced and acceptable range of options for persons with disabilities.

The emphasis on meeting the needs of individuals with severe disabilities must be strengthened and expanded. As the provisions of the ADA go into effect and businesses and other institutions become more comfortable with adapting settings and services, many routine reasonable accommodations for people with disabilities will no longer be the responsibility of the VR system. The focus of VR should shift more clearly to that of a resource to facilitate the inclusion of people with the most severe disabilities. We cannot afford to prioritize only those who are the easiest to serve. This will entail a restructuring of eligibility standards, time limitations, and program evaluation mechanisms currently utilized by the VR system.

Work in integrated work settings, inclusion in the regular educational setting, and community living are key components of services for people with severe disabilities. There needs to be a clear focus in rehabilitation upon community integration and inclusion. Segregated services in work, community living and leisure and recreational areas do not reflect the principles of the community paradigm shift, the findings of researchers, or the directives of the consumer empowerment movement. In the future, services will need to be in typical work and community settings where the supports and services are adapted to the individual rather than the individual fitting the service model. Continued utilization of segregated settings where there are lower wages, less opportunities for social interactions with persons who are not disabled, and limited opportunities for career advancement is not consistent with numerous research findings reported over the past ten years (Kiernan et al., 1988; Kregel and Wehman, 1989; McGaughey et al., 1990; Shafer, 1988; Vandergoot, 1987; Wehman et al. 1988). The concept of sheltered work as a legitimate rehabilitation outcome must be reexamined.

The Americans with Disabilities Act, viewed by many as the civil rights act for people with disabilities, reinforces the concept that people with disabilities must be accorded all of the rights and privileges of all citizens. Rehabilitation services must, along with both the spirit and the mandate of the ADA, stress the inclusion of persons with disabilities in all aspects of the rehabilitation process, comprehensive planning, program implementation, selection of service resources, payment of support services, and evaluation of outcomes in light of person-specific goals and objectives. The challenge of the late 1990s will be the full inclusion of individuals with disabilities into planning, implementing, purchasing, and evaluating available services. Consumer empowerment and choice will require that services be tailored to the needs and interests of the individual. Partnership between consumer and rehabilitation counselor will place the consumer in control, with the counselor serving as a resource and support.

To develop more consumer-focused services, some administrative changes in the service system will be required. The adoption of services that reflect inclusion into the community and work settings; the development of payment sources that place monies in the hands of consumers (as in the case of a voucher system for payment); and a greater understanding of the role that neighbors, friends, family members, coworkers, and other naturally occurring supports play in the rehabilitation process are critical for assuring that people with disabilities have opportunities for choice and assume greater responsibility for their life plans.

It is not just the service system that needs to be restructured. The process of preparing personnel who will provide rehabilitation services in the future must also be restructured. The role of the rehabilitation counselor will be one of partner, planner, collaborator, facilitator, and community resource. The skills necessary to fill these roles go beyond traditional counseling and assessment and include resource identification, conflict resolution, lifelong planning, person-environment assessment strategies and identification of natural supports, and consultation with businesses and other generic organizations. Formal academic instruction at the preservice level must prepare the emerging rehabilitation counselor with the skills to be a jack-of-all-trades, a resource to the consumer and family members, and an information source about jobs, community living, and leisure and recreational resources. University training programs must provide functional course offerings and community experiences which will assure that future rehabilitation counselors are able to foster consumer choice and decision making and advocate for and participate in the development of inclusive community services and supports.

An aggressive in-service training effort is also necessary to assist practicing professionals in rehabilitation to adjust their practices to reflect the growing emphasis upon consumer empowerment, inclusion, and integration. For those rehabilitation professionals who have not kept current on the literature or participated in in-service training opportunities, the emphasis on consumer empowerment will be troubling, since this was not the approach that they learned in their pre-service training. Requirements for continuing education credits must be strengthened such that all rehabilitation professionals, regardless of their individual discipline or orientation, will be assisted in adapting their practice to reflect the community paradigm.

Training needs at both the pre-service and in-service levels reflect not just the shift in emphasis as a result of legislative initiatives such as the ADA but also advances in the use of technology (both high and low technologies) to reduce the discrepancies between the interests of the individual with a disability and the demands of work and community settings. Movement away from fixing the person and toward optimizing the fit between the person and the environment will require that the rehabilitation professional understand the work culture, community needs, family dynamics, and social support systems.

CONCLUSION

The role of the rehabilitation counselor is broad in scope and continually evolving with changes in technology, knowledge, and societal values, but maintaining a core focus upon movement of individuals with disabilities into or back to employment. The principles of rehabilitation are largely consistent with the concepts expressed in the community paradigm. Since its inception, rehabilitation has focused on the needs of the individual and the transition of that individual from a dependent to an interdependent role. However, there continue to be inconsistencies in how rehabilitation professionals and systems apply these principles. This chapter has discussed some of the guiding principles of rehabilitation, some of the inconsistencies within rehabilitation, and some of the changes that will need to be made as the movement toward consumer empowerment and choice progresses. The challenge of the late 1990s will be the incorporation of consumer choice, individual planning, community inclusion, and holistic planning for the rehabilitation professional in the years to come. The interaction of the consumer and the community must be addressed simultaneously if a truly comprehensive and effective rehabilitation system is to be developed.

REFERENCES

Andrews, H., Barker, J., Pittman, J., Maas, L., Streuning, E., and LaRocca, N. (1991). National trends in vocational rehabilitation: A comparison of individuals with physical disabilities and individuals with psychiatric disabilities. *Journal of Rehabilitation, 58,* 7–16.

Barker, J.T. (1988). Coordination of efforts between vocational rehabilitation and mental health systems. *Switzer Monograph Series, National Rehabilitation Association,* 48–61.

Bitter, J.A. (1979). *Introduction to rehabilitation.* St. Louis: Mosby.

Chubon, R. (1985). Career-related needs of school children with severe physical disabilities. *Journal of Counseling and Development, 64,* 47–51.

Emener, W. (1991). An empowerment philosophy for rehabilitation in the twentieth century. *Journal of Rehabilitation, 57,* 7–21.

Federal Register (1987). August 14, Vol. 52, No. 157.

Fifield, B. and Fifield, M. (1995). The influence of legislation on services to people with disabilities. In O.C. Karan and S. Greenspan (Eds.), *Community rehabilitation services for people with disabilities.* Boston: Butterworth–Heinemann.

Garvin, R. (1985). The role of the rehabilitation counselor in industry. *Journal of Applied Rehabilitation Counseling, 16,* 44–50.

Gerber, N. (1979) The job worksite: An additional resource in preparing psychiatric clients for job placement. *Journal of Rehabilitation, 45,* 39–41.

Hagner, D., and Salomone, P. (1989). Issues in career decision making for workers with developmental disabilities. *Career Development Quarterly, 38,* 149–159.

Hahn, H. (1991). Alternative views of empowerment: Social services and civil rights. *Journal of Rehabilitation, 57,* 17–19.

Hansen, C. (1969). The work crew approach to job placement for the severely retarded. *Journal of Rehabilitation, 35,* 26–27.

Houser, R.A., Seligman, M., Kiernan, W.E., King, M.A., and Pajoohi, E. (1991). A survey of class time devoted to required core curriculum content areas by RCE programs. *Rehabilitation Education, 5,* 11–18.

Kiernan, W.E. (1991). *Natural supports in the work setting.* Boston: Training and Research Institute for People with Disabilities, Children's Hospital.

Kiernan, W.E., McGaughey, M.J., Schalock, R.L., and Rowland, S.M. (1988). *Employment survey for adults with developmental disabilities.* Boston: Training and Research Institute for People with Disabilities, Children's Hospital.

Kregel, J., and Wehman, P. (1989). Supported employment: Promises deferred for people with severe disabilities. *Journal of the Association for Persons with Severe Handicaps, 14,* 293–303.

Livneh, H. (1988). Rehabilitation goals: Their hierarchical and multifaceted nature. *Journal of Applied Rehabilitation Counseling, 19,* 12–18.

Livneh, H. (1989). Rehabilitation intervention strategies: Their integration and classification. *Journal of Rehabilitation, 55,* 21–30.

Malikin, D., and Rusalem, H. (1969). *Vocational rehabilitation of the disabled.* New York: New York University Press.

McGaughey, M.J., Kiernan, W.E., Lynch, S.A., Schalock, R.L., and Morganstern, D. (1990). *National survey of day and employment programs for persons with developmental disabilities: Results from state MR/DD agencies.* Boston: Training and Research Institute for People with Disabilities, Children's Hospital.

McGaughey, M.J., Kiernan, W.E., McNally, L.C., and Cooperman, P.J. (1991). *Supported employment for persons with severe physical disabilities: Survey of service providers.* Boston: Training and Research Institute for People with Disabilities, Children's Hospital.

Miller, M. (1989). Career counseling for the elementary school child: Grades K–5. *Journal of Employment Counseling, 26,* 169–177.

National Council on Rehabilitation (1944). *Symposium on the processes of rehabilitation.* New York: Author.

Research Utilization Laboratory (1976). *Program models for projects with industry.* Chicago: Jewish Vocational Service.

Riscalla, L. (1974). Could workshops become obsolete? *Journal of Rehabilitation, 40,* 17–18, 36.

Rogan, P., and Murphy, S. (1991). Supported employment and vocational rehabilitation: Merger or misadventure? *Journal of Rehabilitation, 57,* 39–45.

Ryan, E. (1988). The rehabilitation relationship: The case for a personal rehabilitation. In J. Ciardello and M. Bell (Eds.), *Vocational rehabilitation of persons with psychiatric disorders* (pp. 219–227). Baltimore: Johns Hopkins University Press.

Shafer, M.S. (1988). Supported employment in perspective. In P. Wehman and M.S. Moon (Eds.), *Vocational rehabilitation and supported employment* (pp. 55–66). Baltimore: Paul H. Brookes.

Stubbins, J., and Albee, G.W. (1984). Ideologies of clinical and ecological models *Rehabilitation Literature, 45,* 349–352.

Szymanski, E., and Hanley-Maxwell, C. (1992). Systems interface: Vocational rehabilitation, special education, and vocational education. In F. Rusch, L. Di-Stefano, J. Chadsey-Rusch, L. Phelps, and E. Szymanski (Eds.), *Transition from school to adult life* (pp. 153–171). Sycamore, IL: Sycamore Publishing.

Vandergoot, D. (1987). Review of placement research literature: Implications for research and practice. *Rehabilitation Counseling Bulletin, 30,* 243–272.

Wehman, P., Moon, M.S., Everson, J.M., Wood, W., and Barcus, J.M. (1988). *Transition from school to work: New challenges for youth with severe disabilities.* Baltimore: Paul H. Brookes.

Whitehead, C., and Marrone, J. (1986). Time-limited evaluation and training. In W.E. Kiernan and J.A. Stark (Eds.), *Pathways to employment for adults with developmental disabilities* (pp. 163–176). Baltimore: Paul H. Brookes.

Wright, B. (1959). *Psychology and rehabilitation.* Washington, DC: American Psychological Association.

Wright, G. (1980). *Total rehabilitation* (pp. 10–14). Boston: Little, Brown.

13

Communication Sciences

Stephen N. Calculator

As I entered Lakeview Gardens ICF/MR, my eyes darted as I searched for Gladys, a fifty-eight-year-old woman whom I had been asked to evaluate as a candidate for some type of augmentative communication system. I made my way to a large dayroom/living room where several adults sat around a television. They appeared to have little interest in one another, and even less in Oprah's guest that day.

Off to one corner I found Gladys slouched in a chair. She was sitting alone, occasionally glancing at events around her. Staff passing by made it a point to exchange greetings with Gladys, and she consistently returned these overtures with a wave and a smile. However, conversations never ensued with Gladys.

Having reviewed her file prior to my visit, I knew that Gladys was a "mildly mentally retarded deaf woman with congenital right hemiparesis and minimal language skills." Somehow, none of these descriptors seemed useful now as I settled in (with Gladys and her staff) and began the process of delineating Gladys's communication needs.

According to her file, Gladys received her education at a school for the deaf. In fact, she was deemed conversant in sign (American Sign Language [ASL]) upon leaving school, some forty years ago. More recently, she had begun attending sign classes at a local community college with a staff member from Lakeview. A speech-language pathologist had evaluated Gladys and determined that Gladys's signing was *inconsistent*. The team agreed with the speech-language pathologist's recommendations that Gladys needed to be encouraged to relearn and use signs more consistently, as a primary means of communication. Her program included recording instances in which specific elementary signs were necessitated (by events arising in the residence) then conveying expectations and, if need be, modeling in order to encourage Gladys to use the various targeted signs.

In reviewing Gladys's file and speaking with staff, I found out that the instructor of her signing class had taken an immediate liking to Gladys. Staff observed the instructor and Gladys signing quite fluently with one another. The instructor indicated that Gladys had retained much of her skill in ASL. Additional reports said that while attending a baby shower for a deaf friend of the instructor, Gladys once again encountered little difficulty interacting with other guests at the party.

The extent of Gladys's communication handicap became increasingly obvious as my evaluation proceeded. Interviews with staff indicated that, with the exception of her primary care provider, Marian (who was attending signing classes, with the idea of gradually training other staff at Lakeview as well), no one was able to sign with Gladys. Staff reported that they liked Gladys quite a bit, but were at a loss when it came to communicating with her. Other than exchanging small talk, and indicating basic wants and needs, they did not attempt conversing with Gladys, since such actions always resulted in feelings of uneasiness and frustration.

The staff acknowledged Gladys's desire to be out in the community as much as possible and had acted on this need in many ways. However, communication continued to present a major obstacle for Gladys, whether her excursions were for work or leisure. Gladys had recently been "excused" from a foster grandparent position at a local day-care program. Gladys used to be dropped off at this program and then picked up at the end of the day. Day-care staff (none of whom signed) would direct Gladys to assist in various ways during the day. Eventually, Gladys's patience was exceeded: uneasy with the quality of her work, and unable to manage the behavior of several of the children who, over time, found Gladys an easy target for taunting (with no repercussions), she lashed out at a child.

Gladys also participated in various craft classes at a local store. Again, through interview it was determined that Gladys worked independently, and in isolation, in these classes. Interactions with others were limited to receiving basic instructions and receiving feedback on her projects.

Gladys's case is representative of the tremendous need to shift paradigms when assessing the communication needs of adults with disabilities. We must stop looking at communication apart from the contexts in which communication needs arise. We must expand our assessments of communication beyond these adults to include staff, families, others in the community, and so on. We must recognize that communication needs are dynamic: they change at least as rapidly as staff turn over in the different settings in which these individuals live and work.

We can no longer look at communication as a set of static skills. Instead, we must examine communication from an interaction perspective: What types of instruction and strategies would result in enhanced daily interactions for individuals with the greatest variety of listeners in the greatest variety of settings? What types of communication (message content, style, modes of communication, actual messages expressed, and so forth) are required with particular listeners, in particular settings?

Let's return to the case of Gladys. Communication training took a turn at this point. Actual recommendations (from the original report) appear in Appendix A (Calculator, 1988b). As can be seen, the top priorities were to develop a means of communication by which Gladys could interact with a wide variety of listeners. Since ASL was severely restrictive (in light of Gladys's limited current and future access to others who signed), an alternative mode of communication, Amer-Ind (Skelly, 1979), was recommended. This gestural system shares many characteristics (and some specific signs) with ASL, yet the guessability of its gestures by untrained listeners greatly enhances the likelihood of successful communication. Vois Shapes (manufactured by Phonic Ear) was also suggested as a possible means of taking advantage of Gladys's signing skills. This is an electronic communication aid that permits its user to generate an infinite variety of messages (with speech output) by encoding signing features (e.g., location, movement, and hand shape) that correspond to different signs. It was also recommended that attempts be made to tie Gladys into the network of deaf adults (e.g., continue her signing class, correspond with other adults, and so forth).

These recommendations (for Gladys) illustrate several aspects of a shifting paradigm in the area of communication. Additional changes are captured in the edited report on Thomas S. (Appendix B). Principal features of this changing orientation are described below.

COMMUNICATION AS AN ACTIVE PROCESS

As we have moved away from traditional assessment and intervention paradigms toward more functional orientations, we have gained a greater appreciation of communication as a dynamic process. The old "therapy" setting is characterized as one in which messages and topics are typically initiated disproportionately by the clinician, the majority of communication is by the clinician, and the adult remains relatively passive. When the adult does initiate, the clinician often redirects him or her back to the task (the task, of course, being preselected by the clinician). Materials and activities often bear little resemblance to actual events in which adults participate from day to day. Where they do, the context in which they are presented (in therapy) bears little relationship to the actual situations in which they are encountered.

Conversely, when we look at communication as an active process, our priorities shift to questions involving the extent to which adults are active participants in their daily living. To what extent do they exercise control over their lives and the lives of others?

A functional orientation prompts us to examine current and potential opportunities for communication. We look at existing settings relative to the extent to which adults' participation is encouraged and discouraged, either wittingly or unwittingly. The earlier example of Gladys demonstrates a situation in which others' lack of knowledge about an adult's method of communication results in their assuming control over decisions affecting her life.

Speech-language pathologists can be instrumental in identifying participation opportunities and barriers. They can collaborate with other team members to develop communication systems that promote enhanced participation. They can also help to discern (and then meet) training needs among staff (e.g., how to program an electronic communication aid, how to set up a communication board, how to select vocabulary for a communication notebook, how to restructure daily activities so that individuals have more opportunities to make choices and indicate personal preferences).

The effectiveness of communication training (of adults with disabilities, staff, coworkers, family, and so forth) is then examined with respect to functional changes in adults' lives. Are interactions occurring in a greater number of environments, with a greater variety of listeners? To what extent are adults determining where they work, shop, engage in leisure activities, and so forth? How readily do staff and others provide opportunities for adults' input, and how responsive are they to such input? Where problems persist, how can changes in the area of communication contribute to enhanced levels of adult participation?

INTERACTION AS A FOCAL POINT: MISTAKEN FOCUS REVISITED

When our emphasis is on communication as an active process and effectiveness is measured in terms of participation opportunities and success, the methods by which individuals communicate are secondary to the messages, feelings, ideas, and attitudes being exchanged. One method of communication is not intrinsically better than another. While an individual may be capable of learning a more sophisticated means of communication, the need for such learning should be demonstrated (e.g., in terms of its providing access to more messages, more efficiently, with a greater variety of listeners) before such training is initiated. Too many such programs have been discontinued and forgotten when introduced in situations in which individuals (and their listeners) do not see any functional benefits of the more sophisticated means of communication. To the contrary, individuals may point out advantages of a less sophisticated means of communication. Here the speech-language pathologist may play a significant role in identifying training needs (e.g., of staff) in the use of equipment and/or interacting with individuals in ways that promote opportunities for maximal participation. It is an unfortunate reality that some staff may prefer to interact with adults who are passive and have little input regarding their daily care, for example, than individuals who (given the means to do so) actively participate in such decision making.

When our focus is on interaction (rather than a particular method of communication), we are more likely to look beyond communication and consider the events in which communication occurs. The concept of skill clusters is consistent with this theme.

SKILL CLUSTERS

Communication cannot be examined in isolation. We must view communication relative to the contexts that give rise to its usefulness as a means of managing and coordinating our daily wants and needs and, every bit as important as, establishing and sustaining relationships with others.

Guess and Helmstetter's (1986) notion of skill clusters provides a useful construct when attempting to place communication in context. Applying this model to assessment, we might "assess" communication as one of many skills necessary to participate in a particular activity. On the flip side, we might look at communication deficits relative to their impact on limiting an adult's participation in a series of corresponding activities.

When using such an approach, we see dramatic changes in how goals and objectives are written for adults. Giangreco, Cloninger, and Iverson (1990) draw a distinction between discipline-referenced and discipline-free (or environmentally referenced) objectives. These concepts apply nicely to communication goal setting and prioritization of learning objectives. For example, an environmentally referenced plan for Terry, a young woman who works at a local supermarket, might cite the following *team* priorities (specific communication objectives related to each broader priority appear in parentheses):

- Use public transportation to commute to work. (Confirm [by her asking the driver] that she is boarding the correct bus.)
- Work as a bagger. (Appropriately greet customers. Ask customers if they need assistance carrying their bags to their car.)

- Dine in a public restaurant once a week. (Use the menu itself, along with signs and a communication book, to give the waiter/waitress her order. Compliment the waiter/waitress on the quality of service at the end of the meal.)
- Participate on her store's softball team. (Verbally encourage her teammates. Walk up to the batter's box at the appropriate time without any need for reminders from the other players.)

These goals and objectives depart significantly from discipline-specific priorities, such as correct usage of he and she, correct usage of regular plurals, learning five new signs, and requesting clarification 90 percent of the time. The latter objective could conceivably be discipline free. For example, let's say an adult's outbursts at work often occurred when he was given directions that he did not understand and then reprimanded for either goofing off or doing tasks incorrectly. In this situation, the goal might be improved work habits, with the objective being his indicating when he needs clarification, prior to acting out.

Contrast this with a discipline-specific situation in which requesting clarification is targeted not because it interferes with work performance, but because testing has revealed that John, a busboy at the local pizza place, is not using this function of communication despite being developmentally capable of doing so. We may wind up in a situation in which John becomes increasingly frustrated at work, while his speech-language pathologist sits with him for a few minutes of their weekly session and purposely mumbles messages so that John can practice detecting ambiguous messages and requesting clarification. John and staff would be far more supported by the speech-language pathologist's providing John with a means of requesting clarification at work, encouraging staff to probe his understanding of tasks prior to moving on, and teaching them to model appropriate methods of asking for clarification.

Discrepancy Analysis

A popular assessment paradigm that is strongly related to the use of skill clusters employs a procedure known as discrepancy analysis (Brown et al., 1979; Calculator and Jorgensen, 1991; Cipani, 1989; National Joint Committee for the Communicative Needs of Persons with Severe Disabilities, 1992; York and Vandercook, 1991). Here the observer delineates communication skills necessitated in a particular activity or environment. These are best gleaned by observing other "successful" individuals in the same setting, then validating these behaviors (as valued and significant) with staff and others. Next, actual communication skills exhibited by the adult are identified (relative to these needed skills). Where discrepancies arise, instructional needs are thus identified and addressed (e.g., the individual is then taught the skill or an alternative behavior—use of an AAC system) to permit fuller participation in the particular event.

PARTICIPATION AND MEMBERSHIP AS DISCIPLINE-FREE GOALS

Participation is a key term here. The adult who (through intervention) is now able to meet the communication demands associated with a particular setting is felt to be in a better position to actively participate in that same setting. Taking this one step further, our overriding goal (through communication intervention) should always be one of enhancing adults' membership in their communities. Ferguson (1992) argues, "the purpose of all of our interventions, programs, indeed, schooling in general, is to enable all [people] to actively participate in their communities, so that others care enough about what happens to them to look for ways to include them as part of that community" (p. 22).

In developing communication systems, it thus becomes essential that we consider their role in enhancing others' likelihood of including these adults (in community events) and actively pursuing meaningful relationships with them. When developing communication systems, it is essential that the needs and abilities of listeners (particularly naive listeners who are currently unfamiliar with the adult) be considered. When a communication system is so intrinsically complex (in terms of its programming and/or use) that it discourages others from interacting with an adult, its efficacy must be questioned. Many adults have found it useful to have access to a variety of communication methods (high- and low-tech, graphic, manual, aided, unaided, and so on), with the knowledge of when to use one method or another depending on their listeners' needs and preferences, the content they wish to exchange, the setting in which the interaction is occurring, and other factors.

Assess and Teach in Natural Settings

Success of communication training cannot be examined outside of the contexts that necessitated the initial referral. What does it mean when we say that adults are able to produce fifty signs on request, point to a hundred line drawings on a communication display in response to being shown corresponding pictures, or operate an electronic communication display? What does it mean when these individuals, in turn, are unable to explain to their job coach why they are frustrated with a particular task, rely on a personal care attendant to order for them in a local restaurant (despite having pictures corresponding to a dozen or more foods and beverages on their communication display), and continually forget (and are never reminded by others) to bring their electronic aid with them when they go shopping each week?

Through discrepancy analyses and related procedures, we can identify real communication needs in real settings. By addressing these needs in ways that make sense (given the setting), we can effect real changes in the effectiveness with which individuals are able to interact in these same settings. With improved effectiveness of communication, we hope to enhance individuals' standing (and membership) in their communities.

Use Natural Supports

Natural supports may be conceptualized in terms of the various philosophies, policies, people, materials, technology, and curricula (or, for adults, work and home expectations and protocol) that can be used to enable people to be fully participating members in their communities (see Schalock, 1995, Chapter 10 in this book). Generally speaking, it is advantageous to employ the least intrusive supports when attempting to enhance individuals' levels of participation. Thus, supports are optimally identified (and, if need be, developed) among coworkers first. If need be, paid staff might then be called on to provide assistance (particularly those who routinely participate in a given activity with the individual). Most intrusive, relative to communication support, would be direct involvement on the part of a speech-language pathologist.

We must get to the point where we all agree that an adult's ability to communicate effectively with a speech-language pathologist is of no significance. The speech-language pathologist is not someone the adult has chosen to interact with, nor will improved interactions with the speech-language pathologist necessarily enhance the likelihood of successful encounters with others in different settings. The effectiveness of the speech-language pathologist (as a team member) must be measured relative to others' (staff, coworkers, family) enhanced quantity and quality of interactions with adults. It is disconcerting to find situations in which adults have been receiving ongoing speech-language services (for years), yet people with whom they live and work have received little or no training in how to interact effectively with these individuals. We are looking for changes in quality of life, not increased MLU (mean length of utterance, a common way of examining and documenting language growth).

Returning to the notion of membership, it is useful to examine communication in the context of relationships, or failures to establish relationships with others. As communication abilities change, do we find increased levels of acceptance (and involvement) of these individuals in the community? How are others' views of these adults shaped by the latter's communication skills?

Integrated Therapy

The effectiveness of natural supports (e.g., in promoting communication skills) will depend in part on ongoing consultation from different service providers (e.g., the speech-language pathologist). Having identified that an adult would benefit from increased opportunities to make choices, the speech-language pathologist might then consult with a staff member, and together they might develop a communication system that will provide a means for indicating choices. The system will be designed with a particular situation in mind. Its effectiveness (in meeting the adults' needs) is then evaluated regularly by the speech-language pathologist through staff reporting and direct observation in the actual situation (restaurant, grocery store, health club) for which it was designed. The "therapy" objectives of choice making are thus integrated, or embedded into daily living, where they are systematically addressed and monitored in different natural settings. (Recall our previous discussion of skill clusters.)

For integrated therapy to be effective, it is critical that all staff have a clear understanding of their respective roles in enhancing adults' communication skills. Within this model, communication, along with other related services, is viewed as a means of supporting adults, as well as staff and others, to promote their successful inclusion in the community. At this point, teams may find themselves in a quandary as to how such principles apply to adults who presently spend limited time in their communities, and live in settings that further isolate them from those communities. Shouldn't these individuals' programs focus on optimizing their abilities to meet current communication demands? I would respond with a resounding "NO!" When one considers the lack of natural opportunities for communication in many such settings, the limited array of meaningful topics of conversation, the inability of individuals to choose their conversational topics and partners, the extent to which the highly organized and scheduled routines of these settings depart from natural contingencies found in the community—I worry about the extent to which such training hinders desired future interactions for immediate (albeit negligible and often nonfunctional) changes in communication behavior.

IMPLICATIONS OF THE COMMUNITY REVOLUTION FOR COMMUNICATION SERVICES

As services for persons with disabilities are increasingly community based, the role of speech-language pathologists must continue to change in order to assure that their services remain both relevant and effective. Implications discussed in this chapter are summarized below.

Who and How   Speech-language pathologists should continue to evolve toward indirect, transdisciplinary models of service delivery. The client base must be expanded beyond persons with disabilities to encompass families, employers, staff, friends, and others. Communication, along with other related services, needs to be embedded in community instruction and daily living (Calculator, 1988a; Meyer, Eichinger, and Park-Lee, 1987; Mirenda and Calculator, 1992; Mirenda, Iacono, and Williams, 1990; National Joint Committee for the Communicative Needs of Persons with Severe Disabilities, 1992; York and Rainforth, 1989). We can continue to refer to this model as integrated therapy, or we may choose to coin a new expression that divorces the medical connotation and instead conveys holistic approaches to people and the systems in which they function.

As indirect, consultative models of service delivery are adopted, they must not be applied haphazardly. Needs for accountability persist, irrespective of who is providing services and supports. Decision making and teaming need to recruit participation from appropriate parties—this should not change.

What   As we move toward environmentally referenced goals, objectives, and activities, speech-language pathologists must share priority-setting with other team members. Consumers should have major input in such decisions, whether or not they are active members of the team. There will be ongoing needs for speech-language pathologists to develop collaborative/interactive teaming and consultation skills (see Rainforth et al., 1995, Chapter 7 in this book).

Where and When   As communication programs are implemented in natural settings, by a variety of persons, innovative scheduling strategies are called for. Time remains a major obstacle to consultative services. Data-collection strategies that are user-friendly should provide for increased efficiency in carrying out this model.

Speech-language pathologists need to move beyond considerations of skills required in present settings. We must now look at communication as a means of facilitating individuals' participation and inclusion in new settings and environments. Efficacy of communication instruction can be evaluated, in part, relative to the number of places that people have access to, and are welcomed in, as fully participating members.

Why The changes discussed previously here are consistent with best practices (as currently defined) and the ADA and are designed to reverse past practices that have failed to promote participation of people with disabilities in mainstream America. If inclusion of people with disabilities is to occur, paradigms must change to encompass the communities in which these individuals and their neighbors live, work, and play.

REFERENCES

Brown, L., Branston, M., Hamre-Nietupski, S., Pumpian, I., Certo, N., and Gruenwald, L. (1979). A strategy for developing chronological age appropriate and functional curricular content for severely handicapped adolescents and young adults. *Journal of Special Education, 13*(1), 81–90.

Calculator, S. (1988a). Promoting the acquisition and generalization of conversational skills by individuals with severe disabilities. *Augmentative and Alternative Communication, 4,* 94–103.

Calculator, S. (1988b). Teaching functional communication skills to nonspeaking adults with mental retardation. In S. Calculator and J. Bedrosian (Eds.), *Communication assessment and intervention for adults with mental retardation* (pp. 309–338). San Diego: College-Hill.

Calculator, S., and Jorgensen, C. (1991). Integrating AAC instruction into regular education settings: Expounding on best practices. *Augmentative and Alternative Communication, 7,* 204–214.

Cipani, E. (1989). Providing language consultation in the natural context: A model for delivery of services. *Mental Retardation, 27,* 317–324.

Ferguson, D. (1992). Is communication really the point? Some thoughts on where we've been and where we might want to go. In L. Kupper (Ed.), *Proceedings of the Second National Symposium on Effective Communication for Children and Youth with Severe Disabilities: A vision for the future* (pp. 17–35). McLean, VA: Interstate Research Associates.

Giangreco, M., Cloninger, C., and Iverson, V. (1990). *C.O.A.C.H.: Cayuga-Onondaga assessment for children with handicaps.* Version 6.0. Stillwater:

Oklahoma State University, National Clearing House of Rehabilitation Training Materials.

Guess, D., and Helmstetter, E. (1986). Skill cluster instruction and the individualized curriculum sequencing model. In R. Horner, L. Meyer, and H.D. Fredericks (Eds.), *Education of learners with severe handicaps: Exemplary service strategies* (pp. 221–248). Baltimore: Paul H. Brookes.

Meyer, L., Eichinger, J., and Park-Lee, S. (1987). A validation of program quality indicators in educational services for students with severe disabilities. *Journal of the Association for Persons with Severe Handicaps, 12*, 251–263.

Mirenda, P., and Calculator, S. (1992). Enhancing curricula designs. In L. Kupper (Ed.), *Proceedings of the Second National Symposium on Effective Communication for Children and Youth with Severe Disabilities: A vision for the future* (pp. 135–163). McLean, VA: Interstate Research Associates.

Mirenda, P., Iacono, T., and Williams, R. (1990). Communication options for persons with severe and profound disabilities: State of the art and future directions. *Journal of the Association for Persons with Severe Handicaps, 15*, 3–21.

National Joint Committee for the Communicative Needs of Persons with Severe Disabilities (1992). Guidelines for meeting the communication needs of persons with severe disabilities. *Asha, 34* (March, Supp. 7), 1–8.

Rainforth, B. Giangreco, M.F., Smith, P.D., & York, J. (1995). Collaborative teamwork in training and technical assistance: Enhancing cimmunity support for persons with disabilities. In O.C. Karan & S. Greenspan (Eds.), *Community rehabilitation services for people with disabilities.* Boston: Butterworth–Heinemann.

Schalock, R.L. (1995). Assessment of natural supports in community rehabilitation services. In O.C. Karan and S. Greenspan (Eds.), *Community rehabilitation services for people with disabilities.* Boston: Butterworth–Heinemann.

Skelly, M. (1979). Amer-Ind gestural code based on universal American Indian hand talk. New York: Elsevier-North Holland.

York, J., and Rainforth, B. (1989). *Related educational services for individuals with severe disabilities. Report from the Related Services Subcommittee of the TASH Critical Services Committee.* Seattle: Association for Persons with Severe Handicaps.

York, J., and Vandercook, T. (1991). Designing an integrated program for learners with severe disabilities. *Teaching Exceptional Children, 23* (Winter), 22–28.

APPENDIX A

Recommendations for Gladys

Gladys continues to rely on manual signing as her primary means of communication, yet she is severely constrained in what she is able to express, since she is surrounded by people with little or no training in ASL or signing in general. Marian has been committed to developing sign and gradually introducing it to others at Lakeview Gardens. We must now ask whether this plan is feasible, especially in light of future changes of placement, staff turnover, and other threats to program continuity.

Currently, Gladys is forced to resort to simple gestures and other means of communication that rely heavily on other persons' interpretation and creativity in constructing meaning. Typically, Gladys is placed in a passive role (communicatively), unable to initiate messages or ideas unless the context is redundant and predictable enough for listeners to guess at Gladys's meaning and then engage her in a session of Twenty Questions.

1. Introduce Amer-Ind as a means of incorporating Gladys's signing competency, while also considering the need for a gestural system that is far more "listener friendly" than ASL. Amer-Ind consists of 250 concept labels that are equivalent to approximately 2500 English words, since each signal/gesture has multiple meanings. Signs can also be chained together (a process known as agglutination) to create additional meanings. Amer-Ind has been used successfully with people with severe and profound intellectual disabilities as well as with adults with aphasia, apraxia, dysarthria, glossectomies, and so forth. As noted earlier, one of its major selling points is the relative ease with which untrained listeners are able to correctly interpret gestures.

Research by its originator, Skelly (1979), indicated that untrained listeners correctly interpret between 80 and 88 percent of these hand signals. Subsequent research has yielded more conservative estimates: 50 to 60 percent of gestures are guessable when presented out of context to untrained listeners. In context, this figure would of course climb. Considering that the guessability of ASL by untrained listeners has been found to range between 10 and 30 percent, Amer-Ind would permit Gladys to gesture successfully with a broader range of listeners, even without any formal training of listeners.

In addition to their guessability, Amer-Ind gestures are motorically easier to produce (than ASL). This is an important consideration, given Gladys's motor limitations (right hemiparesis). Research has demonstrated that a one-handed version of producing these gestures maintains the previously cited high levels of guessability. The fact that many of the Amer-Ind gestures resemble some of the more concrete/iconic signs of ASL should facilitate Gladys's ability to shift from one system to the other. In general, this system has been found to be acquired/learned more easily (than ASL or Signed English).

A videotape of Amer-Ind gestures is available from Auditec (St. Louis)—I would strongly encourage purchasing this tape to enable Gladys and others to begin learning the gestures. In addition, the various gestures (and methods of introducing them) are covered in Skelly (1979), which I would also recommend purchasing.

2. During my visit, I discussed the potential benefits of an electronic communication aid for Gladys. Specifically, we talked about an easily programmable, portable system with speech output that would enable Gladys to interact with listeners who did not know sign. Two possible systems might be worthwhile pursuing in the future: the Intro Talker (from Prentke Romich) and Vois Shapes (Phonic Ear). I have enclosed brochures for each. The Intro Talker would be of immediate use in that frequently used phrases, words, and expressions could be programmed on the display for use at home and in the community.

Mayer-Johnson Picture Communication Symbols can be used to depict vocabulary. I have enclosed ordering information. (Please note: these pictures are reusable and easily reproduced. They could be used by other adults as well, given that cost is an issue). I would continue to work on reading (at present, Gladys recognizes some letters but does not appear to be able to recognize words) but might approach this more functionally—sight words and common phrases. This is certainly a team decision (as are any actions on suggestions raised in the present report).

Vois Shapes is a greater investment (in money and time) but would provide capability for access to unlimited numbers of messages—if Gladys was able and motivated to use this system. I have enclosed a brochure—perhaps a sales representative would be willing to visit and give a demonstration and/or allow Gladys to rent/lease a unit for a trial period. The value of this device would be dictated by Gladys's knowledge of sign (and thus her ability to program and retrieve messages). Could someone conversant in sign (e.g., Gladys's instructor at the Technical College) explore this option with Gladys?

3. Continue to attend evening signing classes with Marian Walsh. While it is unknown how much new information Gladys may acquire in these classes (her teacher has purportedly found that Gladys already possesses an extensive repertoire of signs), the opportunity to interact with other signers is very important for social and other reasons.

Along these same lines, staff should continue efforts to develop relationships and supports in the deaf community (or at least with one or more individuals). If face-to-face contact is not feasible, perhaps a network of pen pals or the like could be developed to enable Gladys to share thoughts and feelings with others.

4. Present methods by which Gladys communicates include sign/gestures/pantomime, vocalizations, pointing, acting on objects, and several words (e.g., "mother," "home"). Encourage Gladys to speak along with her signs/gestures (or Amer-Ind). In addition, staff should speak concurrent with their signing (this is particularly true for Marian). Not only will this encourage Gladys to attempt oral communication along with her signs, but also will allow observers (other staff) to

hear the meaning of signs that Marian and others are exchanging with Gladys, permitting incidental learning by others.

5. I do not feel it would be asking too much for all staff at Lakeview Gardens to be exposed to Amer-Ind (e.g., by viewing the videotape). These gestures would not only enhance interactions with Gladys, but also may prove to be useful with other residents as well. Perhaps Marian *and Gladys* would be willing to coordinate such training.

6. Prior to going into the community, it would be useful if Gladys and a staff person "practiced" conveying messages that would likely be called for. Set up brief simulations in which Gladys has the opportunity to gesture (or use her communication display) as a prelude to going out. Real props (e.g., menu of the restaurant they are going to) would promote carryover from the home to the community.

Please do not hesitate to call me if I can be of any further assistance in explaining and implementing the above recommendations. I greatly enjoyed my visit with Gladys (and staff) and wish you all success in addressing the tremendous communication needs of this delightful woman.

Stephen N. Calculator, Ph.D.
Consulting SLP

APPENDIX B

Recommendations for Thomas S.

To: Sarah Adams, Case Manager

From: Steve Calculator

Re: Communication consultation on Thomas S.

The purpose of this correspondence is to summarize suggestions and recommendations that I shared with you following my observation of Mr. Thomas S. at his care providers' residence on 12/5/92. The primary purposes of my visit were to provide feedback regarding Thomas's home program, answer questions posed by his care providers, and offer suggestions regarding future program efforts.

1. Thomas is indeed fortunate to have found a highly nurturing and responsive home. His care providers appear to offer a stimulating environment in which Thomas's participation is both encouraged and valued.

2. *Regarding switch use.* Thomas was seen on several occasions between March and May, 1991, by staff from the regional center. A switch was recommended, with a primary purpose of enhancing Thomas's access to the environment (environmental control). While this is certainly an appropriate goal in theory, its usefulness has not yet been explored within his home. Specifically, *how* might switch usage enhance Thomas's independence and quality of life by providing access to an increasing range of objects and activities that Thomas values? This question might be posed to the center (Jan Phillips, SLP, has been involved in previous evaluations) in a request for a follow-up visit to Thomas's home. Specific uses of the switch could be reviewed with Thomas's care providers, along with how switch interface might be carried out. *Please keep in mind: use of the switch is only relevant to the extent that it promotes increased access and active participation by Thomas.*

3. Communication objectives should continue to be integrated into Thomas's daily routines to the greatest extent possible. The goal activity matrix (reviewed during my visit) might be completed by you and Samantha [home care provider] in order to identify specific communication and other objectives that would immediately relate to increasing Thomas's participation in everyday activities. Similarly, the discrepancy analysis (reviewed during my visit) would provide a means of identifying additional program content. As you recall, during my visit we generated several objectives that could be implemented at mealtime (e.g., purse lips and move head away from cup to indicate he is finished drinking, shake cup to indicate he wants more to drink, withdraw hand from an object he does not like, . . .).

4. Between you and Samantha, a dictionary of Thomas's various gestures and vocalizations could be compiled. This would serve as a resource for persons who

wish to interact with Thomas and yet are unfamiliar with him and/or these subtle methods of communication. The dictionary would accompany Thomas on excursions outside the home, visits to the doctor, etc. Be specific, trying to attach one (or as few as possible) meaning to each corresponding behavior. You may even wish to snap photographs of Thomas engaged in corresponding behaviors to accompany your written descriptions. Again, please call if you have questions on how Thomas's dictionary might be constructed. Samantha is a tremendously responsive listener whose abilities [to interpret Thomas's behaviors] should be shared with others.

5. Samantha reported that since Thomas has come to live with her and her husband, he has grown increasingly responsive, alert, and interested in people and events around him. While data to support these contentions were not presented, I can concur that I found Thomas to be highly aware and engaging. More than anything else, Thomas's continued gains in communication and overall growth will hinge on opportunities for participation and experience in and out of his home. The greater the number of settings and people (particularly adults without disabilities) with whom he is involved, the greater continued growth (and quality of life) we can expect for Thomas.

14 ⬜⬜⬜ ⬜⬜⬜ ⬜⬜⬜

Nursing Services

Mary A. Musholt

INTRODUCTION

In the process of supporting individuals as full members of their communities, nurses are challenged to examine their beliefs about safety and protection, human dignity and self-esteem, medical care necessity, and innovative health care interventions. This chapter will address the nursing role in habilitation of persons with disabilities and to a lesser extent the broader area of rehabilitation.

The history of American nursing service to persons with disabilities will be reviewed. Contemporary approaches within nursing practices and procedures will be described. The ramifications for nursing practice of the transformation of services from institutions to community will be explored. Finally, the specific implications of these new trends for nursing education, research, and the development of community-based service models will be discussed.

Tracing the historical evolution of nursing as it parallels philosophical changes pertaining to the needs of persons with disabilities is fraught with perils. Most significantly, confusion exists between the practices of rehabilitation and habilitation nursing. This is partly related to lack of definitional clarity between the two terms. Differences also exist about the reliability and safety of enabling consumer-directed decisions, as well as about the relevance of combining pediatric and adult rehabilitation needs (Selekman, 1991). Because of the unclear boundaries between rehabilitation and habilitation nursing, decisions about the content of this chapter were necessarily influenced by the writer's professional experiences in nursing and developmental disabilities. In the process, relevant insights from both rehabilitation and habilitation nursing have been included.

HISTORY OF AMERICAN NURSING
WITH PERSONS WITH DISABILITIES

In the early history of American nursing, two nursing/social reformers took action that affected the lives of "helpless people," which included people with cognitive and physical impairments. In the early 1860s, Dorothea Dix, often identified as an untrained nurse, pressed for special training for "feeble-minded" children, and because of her efforts governmental money was appropriated to build new buildings where children with cognitive impairments could learn to become useful citizens (Wilson, 1975).

By 1875, thanks to Ms. Dix, most states had public money allocated for institutional care of persons with "mental illness," which included people with cognitive impairments. Ms. Dix believed in the need for quality assurances in places where people were congregated. Along with inspection of care, she established schools to train nurses. As the profession of nursing was evolving during the later nineteenth century, the need to educate nurses became a rallying point in order to improve care and to avoid negligence in institutions (Peppe and Sherman, 1978).

At the same time Ms. Dix advocated for improving the care of people in institutions, another nurse reformer, Lillian Wald, sought to enhance the care of people in the community. Ms. Wald, credited with originating the visiting nurse service, conceived the idea of developing a neighborhood nursing service for the sick poor in New York City in the early 1900s. Based on her belief that "neighborliness" would be more helpful than an attitude of an impersonal paid visitor, Ms. Wald contended that nursing care could be delivered in people's homes by nurses assigned to their neighborhoods, who could thus be personally familiar with them. In addition, Ms. Wald helped inaugurate the first ungraded class for children with physical or cognitive impairments who could not keep up with their schoolmates (Williams, 1967).

In the early twentieth century a variety of people who were considered "dangerous to society" were institutionalized. The majority of care was provided by untrained nurses. During this time, social reformers suggested that if the nurses were professionally educated they might be more willing to provide a homelike environment for the people living in these institutions. Educated nurses, it was felt, would value the humane treatment of those institutionalized.

In the 1950s, just as the principle of normalization was spreading across the Atlantic, nurses in long-term care facilities stressed setting individualized goals, oriented toward maximizing independence, and at the same time making institutions "homelike." In addition, nurses saw the value of a team approach in determining goals and plans.

In the 1950s the value of educating persons with cognitive impairments was identified. The custodial care model was changed to an educational care model geared toward human developmental needs, including personal adequacy, social competency, and economic efficiency (Patterson and Rowland, 1970).

The focus of nursing literature in the field of disabilities in the 1970s was primarily on the care of the child, as well as on nursing care for the child's family (Avey, 1973; Barnard and Powell, 1972; Murphy and Pueschel, 1975). Nursing interventions frequently stressed "behavior modification" (Barnard and Powell, 1972; Whitney, 1966). With an emphasis on serving children and their families, nursing made major contributions to prevention, case finding, and home-based services. In fact, the ultimate aim of early detection was to enhance the development of the child within his or her own community.

In comparison, there were apparently few developments in nursing services for adults with cognitive impairments. As with children, behavior modification was integrated into nursing practice. However, with adults the primary emphasis remained on institutional care.

Especially with children the thrust was toward teaching adaptive life skills. Barnard (1975) argued that nursing's involvement was "vital to the progress in the field since it is life activities which are germane to nursing practice, but represent the crux of the problem for the handicapped and their families" (p. 1702). Unlike most of her colleagues, Barnard stressed providing primary care for individuals with disabilities of *all ages.*

In the late 1970s there were relatively large-scale discharges from institutions—often into communities still unprepared to serve individuals with emotional and cognitive disabilities. Nurses sometimes needed to examine their own attitudes toward disabilities and community integration. And they were challenged to provide holistic interventions and to set realistic objectives that would not compromise families' lives. Parents were recognized as best qualified to work with their infant children, and removing infants from their homes was considered inappropriate (Tudor, 1978).

The specialized role of nursing in the field of developmental disabilities was promoted in "The Standards of Nursing Practice in Mental Retardation and Developmental Disabilities," which was written in 1984 (Aggen and Moore, 1984). In these standards, clinical nursing care included prevention and detection as well as provision of services to clients and families. Nursing practice was further characterized by a "focus on maintenance of positive health and development of skill in daily living, communication, socialization and participation in community life" (p. 1). These standards are in step with other professionals' commitment in the 1980s to provide support where people live.

During the past decade, nursing research has identified minimal information on helping adults with disabilities who are living in the community. Although the philosophical reorientation toward community services was discussed (Steele, 1987), practices supporting this philosophical imperative continue to focus on children and families. In reality, nurses today care for persons with disabilities of all ages and their families in virtually every type of health care setting. And nurses are becoming more active in organizations in the field of disabilities (Nehring, 1991). However, more research and description of nursing practices in the areas of consumer teaching and consumer support are needed to ensure that life in the community is a reality for all people with disabilities and that large institutional living is a practice of the past.

CONTEMPORARY APPROACHES TO NURSING PRACTICE

No single, clear-cut unifying thread can be found in describing contemporary nursing approaches and practices in the fields of rehabilitation and habilitation. A synthesis of these approaches is yet to be developed. Hence, this section discusses a number of different topics: (a) nursing specializations relating to disabilities, (b) differential access to nursing services, (c) the involvement of nurses in preventively serving consumers and families, (d) nursing roles in helping adults in community settings, (e) the development of innovative community-based models, and (f) evolving nursing theory relating to disabilities.

Nursing Specializations Relating to Disabilities

A complicating factor in describing contemporary approaches is determining where to locate nursing practice information. For example, no nursing journal specifically addresses the field of developmental disabilities. This is probably because, at this time, developmental disabilities nursing is too specialized to have its own journal or nursing division within the American Nurses Association. Hence, nurses in the area of developmental disabilities tend to affiliate with a variety of different kinds of organizations. This includes the interdisciplinary American Association on Mental Retardation, the American Association of Neuroscience Nursing, the Association of Rehabilitation Nurses, and other nursing special interest groups such as long-term care or maternal-child nursing groups.

Only in the past three decades has nursing research in the area of neuroscience nursing really grown and added significantly to nursing practice knowledge. Within that research, a definite decline has occurred in chronic care and rehabilitation research. Now neuroscience nursing research focuses on care in the acute care setting (Dilorio, 1990). If this trend continues, nursing practice in the person's natural setting will be based on nursing interventions appropriate for acute care. Nurses will evaluate the effectiveness of generalizing nursing practice from one setting to another.

In the maternal-child nursing literature, several articles per year address issues of improving quality of care in the home setting for children with chronic illness or who are dependent on medical technology (Andrews and Nielson, 1988); issues of consumer and nurse partnership building (Brandt and Magyary, 1989; Feeg, 1987); and issues of sensitivity to parental response (Fraley, 1990; Tasch, 1988) and promotion of community integration (Gleeson, 1987).

The long-term care field and home health nursing literature also address issues in providing health care at home for children with complex needs (Kaufman, Lichtenstein, and Rosenblatt, 1986; Lenihan, 1985; McCoy and Votroubek, 1986). The Pepper Commission recommends that a long-term care system be created that serves individuals who are severely disabled and that, among other conditions, it should allow personal choice of care and setting. Enacting this commission's recommendations would imply more comprehensive services for persons with long-term care needs (Pepper Report, 1991).

Articles regarding nursing practice relevant to the needs of persons with disabilities appear in many types of journals, from public health nursing journals (Benchot, 1984; Hulsman and Chubon, 1989) to general nursing journals (Diehl, 1986; Kimball, 1983; Miller, Steele, and Boisen, 1987). Thus in describing current approaches to nursing practice, one must look in a variety of resources.

Differential Access to Nursing Services

In describing contemporary nursing care for people with disabilities, it is essential to consider the consumer's access to that care. The ratio of nurse to consumer is mandated by federal guidelines in residential settings that participate in the Medicaid program. No guidelines exist for planned nursing involvement for people residing in non-Medicaid-funded programs, including the Medicaid waiver programs. Thus describing nursing approaches for people residing in institutions where federal requirements mandate nursing care will be different from describing nursing approaches where no guidelines exist.

Nursing practice in intermediate-care facilities for the mentally retarded (ICF-MR) is expanding because of the federal requirements, and consequently more emphasis is being placed on establishing standards for nursing practice (Curtis, Begin, and Blinkhorn, 1989). The chronic health needs of persons who live in large state ICF-MRs are complex and require active nursing intervention to monitor these needs; at the same time, nurses are intervening to allow greater participation by individuals in their health care. Emphasis is placed on active treatment as a planned system to ensure that persons receiving the federally sponsored services obtain holistic, transdisciplinary care.

Although nursing care for people in institutions may have more universality because of the federal guidelines that outline nursing responsibility, nursing care for people in the community is much less universal. In fact, great diversity exists regarding professional nursing availability and participation from state to state. As an example, Wisconsin has 53 ICF-MRs, ranging in size from 12 to 600 beds. Minnesota has 334 ICF-MRs, ranging in size from 4 to 500 beds, with the majority of facilities having 6 to 15 beds. In states that elect not to utilize the model of small ICF-MRs, nursing care in the community may well be unplanned and inconsistent. This lack of nursing involvement may be a factor in studies that describe how people with complex care needs fare in the community. Clarification by nurses of the anticipated level of nursing services for people with complex medical needs may be an important factor in assessing the adequacy of generic health care resources and whether a person with a disability may need to return to an institution for health care monitoring. This nursing factor may explain the differences of opinion regarding the studies that are demonstrating adequate or inadequate health care services (McDonald, 1985; Minihan, 1986).

The focus of the description of nursing practice in this chapter is on community-based nursing. It is from this description that nurses can plan and make suggestions that will empower the person with a disability to utilize the general health care system. In one of the few studies on this topic, the generic health care system was judged to be adequate in its provision of health care for adults with disabilities who live in the community (Minihan and Dean, 1990). However, the major health service gap listed in this study pertained to the provision of home health care. The nurse's role in home health care was identified in two ways. First, nurses are needed as direct care providers. Almost 60 percent of clients with home health needs had not had a nurse involved in their care. Second, and more important, nurses are needed as trainers, supervisors, and monitors of lay caregivers.

The Involvement of Nurses in Preventively Serving Consumers and Families

As indicated in the historical overview, nursing leadership in prevention and case finding is well known. Nursing care of children has changed dramatically over the past three decades. Including the family and basing nursing practice within the family setting have been suggested as significant nursing priorities for well over a decade (Steele, 1977). As part of working with families, nurses have been encouraged to allow the patient "to tell it how it is" (i.e., to respond to the patient's perceptions) rather than to depend on tests and objective evidence to decide nursing interventions (Chapman, 1977).

The provision of nursing services to children with disabilities in three different settings was described by Peppe in 1987. In each of these settings—public health department, schools, and rehabilitation centers—nurses provide information to promote and maintain optimal health. Interventions are designed to optimize the child's functional abilities. Thus, in these brief descriptions it is demonstrated that the principles of family-based care and of providing care in the child's naturally occurring environment have been strongly developed in the nursing care of children.

An estimated 17,000 to 45,000 children with chronic illness are candidates for home health services (Pepper Report, 1991). These children and their families use technology that may include respiratory or cardiac monitors, phototherapy, supplemental oxygen, enteral feedings, tracheostomies, intravenous antibiotics, ventilatory assistance including respirators, and renal dialysis (Andrews and Nielson, 1988). And the prevalence rate of children with chronic disabling conditions is increasing. Nursing is challenged to help create effective alternatives to acute care settings for these children. These creative alternatives will need to be cost-effective and self-sustaining.

Flexibility has been demonstrated in supporting families who seek a natural environment for their children with medically complex needs. Unique pediatric in-home care services have been developed. These services allow children who were once dependent on inpatient services to live in their homes (McCoy and Votroubek, 1986). Homelike facilities are being developed that provide constant care, usually provided by a private duty nurse, while allowing children who are medically fragile to be with other children. Some of these facilities are enabling parents to keep their children at home by providing this care during daytime hours. Others provide an alternative to institutionalization for children whose families are unable to care for them at home (Caddell and Donaldson, 1990).

Nurses can be in pivotal positions to facilitate families' adjustments to the birth of an infant with a disabling condition. Families must contend with many disruptions to their family life that result from the care of an infant with complex health care needs. Nurses can promote family health by preventing the development of maladaptive coping patterns and family functioning. Macedo and Posel (1987) provide basic assumptions on which the nursing interventions for families with children who have spina bifida are based. The nurse's ability to respond at times of crisis, such as at the time of birth or at other transition points in the developmental stages of the child and family, is identified as critical in developing a collaborative relationship. This collaborative relationship enhances the family's ability to actively define and solve their health concerns.

Nurse practitioners are especially identified as collaborators with families who have children with disabilities. They can positively support and enhance healthy family function. Knowledge of community referral sources is essential for nurses in order to make appropriate health, education, and social referrals (Yoos, 1985).

Collaboration between community nurses and hospital nurses is still as important in ensuring quality care as Curry suggested in 1978. The collaboration allows for continuity of care, which helps to allay parent fear regarding the community's capacity to respond to emergency medical needs (O'Pray, 1987).

Based on nursing research, parents can be taught self-care activities for their children with disabilities that may help decrease the number of physician visits (Steel et al., 1989). By teaching the family how to manage the child's health problems, nurses contribute to the futuristic model of healthy care delivery that is family centered, community based, and co-ordinated.

In addition, models for service coordination and case management are described that encourage self-advocacy and consumer awareness so that families might be empowered (Kaufman, Lichtenstein and Rosenblatt, 1986; Kirkhart et al., 1988). The passage of Public Law 99-457 establishes case management services for infants and toddlers. Nurses with their skills in patient education, coordination, collaboration, anticipatory guidance, and problem solving have the capacity to serve in this case management role (Davis and Steele, 1991).

Nursing Roles in Helping Adults in Community Settings

The description of nursing practice for adults with disabilities is not as clear as for children. For one thing, care of adults with disabilities has not focused on the care required to support them in their own natural setting. And now that the adult population in the community is increasing and is also living longer, information is lacking regarding the natural history of health changes. Little knowledge exists regarding how to adequately provide care that is health promoting and that optimizes quality of life for adults choosing to live in the community. Thus the community-based health care system is attempting to provide comprehensive care to a group of people for whom they are ill prepared, and for whom care standards are unknown. Further, the limited research to date on assessing the adequacy of community-based care is in conflict. While Minihan (1986) found that the four medical specialty services judged to be required for adults scheduled for community placement could not be located in Massachusetts, McDonald (1985) found that the extensive health care needs of a sample of young adults with severe disabilities were being met.

Lacking sufficient research to base health care decisions on changes that occur in adults with disabilities, nurses utilize functional skill assessment as one tool to assess the significance of these changes. Thus, the nurse's role in monitoring health care status in adults with disabilities can be strengthened by more thorough assessment of daily functional activities. Although functional skill assessment is an important assessment activity in geriatric and rehabilitation health care (Granger, Seltzer, and Fishbein, 1987), it is an unfolding tool in the nursing practice for adults with disabilities. Recent helpful nursing contributions describe the value of comparing functional skill loss as an indicator of health changes in epilepsy (Lannon, 1990) and as a way to facilitate and modify neurological assessments of persons with severe cognitive impairments (Burns and Snyder, 1991).

The Development of Innovative Community-Based Models for Nurses

To date the nursing profession has not assessed the adequacy of community-based health care resources from a nursing perspective. Nurses have, however, been identified with many potential roles in providing services to adults in their natural settings. For one, nurses have been involved in developing service models and in providing primary care. Nurse practitioners in a hospital-based developmental disabilities clinic in New Jersey provide ongoing primary health care (Ziring et al., 1988). A group of nurse practitioners in New Hampshire provide primary care through their private practices (Diehl, 1986). Nurse practitioners from a nonprofit medical practice group in Boston perform evaluations, develop plans of care, evaluate new medical problems, and visit adults who are severely disabled in their homes or in the office (Meyers et al., 1987). These models suggest the value of a relationship with a primary provider who knows the potential needs, assumes responsibility for preventive health care interventions, coordinates health care information, and educates residential support providers in the needed health care interventions.

In addition to the role of primary provider, nurses are valued for their contributions in the provision and training of home health care measures (Crocker, Yankauer, and the Conference Steering Committee, 1987; Minihan and Dean, 1990). Unfortunately, nurses in generic community-based health settings, such as outpatient clinics or public health departments, often lack the necessary information and training to meet the unique health care needs of persons with disabling conditions. Nurses readily identify this lack of knowledge and training. Nurses have written articles that describe terminology used in the disability field and provide a perspective that fosters normalization (Benchot, 1984; Glassman-Feibusch, 1984; Steele, 1987). These authors, however, strongly suggest the need for further networking and sharing of experiences by other nurses who are working with people who have disabilities.

The nurse's role in planning community services and in providing thorough assessments and appropriate interventions is evolving. The issue of quality-of-life differences for adults with disabilities who lived in community settings and those who lived in nursing home settings was addressed in a study in which adults with comparable levels of care were interviewed by nurses. The results from the small convenience sample demonstrate no differences in the report of quality of life. The research was conducted with the premise that nursing interventions could be designed to promote quality of life for adults who were chronically ill and disabled and who were being supported to remain out of institutions. Finding no differences in reports of quality of life, research to further identify specific variables is needed (Hulsman and Chubon, 1989).

Another example of how nurses actively participate in providing community-based services is in the area of mental health services for persons who are cognitively impaired. Nurses in a psychiatric inpatient unit for individuals with cognitive impairments who were effectively treated in the community support deinstitutionalization and increased normalization for all citizens with disabilities. Contemporary nursing approaches were found valuable in supporting these inpatients, but the approaches had to be modified in the following ways. Nurses need to: consider the allied medical needs that accompany specific syndromes, consider the alternative ways of communicating when a person is not able to verbalize, provide close observation of effects of the psychoactive medications, and create new ways to interact with people whose developmental level is complicated by cognitive impairments. Nurses in this unit acted in an education–consultant role in teaching other nurses and community providers (Hodgkins and Monfils, 1985).

The role of the community health nurse in delivering service to adults is a varied one, as reported by Glassman-Feibusch in 1984. The opportunity to practice holistic nursing with consumers over a long period of time may provide groundwork to optimize quality of life on a day-to-day basis. Identified nursing roles included teacher, advocate, coordinator, listener, and friend. Nurses have a relatively independent field practice, as the nurse plans and implements care based on nursing knowledge. Interventions that promote health and that treat diseases are needed.

Shanck and Lubkin (1990) describe interventions and solutions for the practices of rehabilitation nursing that will ensure community participation of persons with rehabilitation needs. Treatment and training are the core of rehabilitation nursing. In fact, it is the training component that makes rehabilitation nursing unique. Based on the premise that home is the best setting, the authors make a number of recommendations. Nurses could collect data to demonstrate that institutions can be avoided or delayed with structured rehabilitation that included teaching and counseling. Hospitalizations may be reduced when the consumer and family are adequately prepared for living in the community. A second intervention that nurses could take would be to conduct research that proves the value of nursing interventions that prevent further disability and promote self-care. Third, nurses are encouraged to ensure that teams function as interdisciplinary rather than multidisciplinary. Nurses could well be the interdisciplinary team coordinators.

Evolving Nursing Theory Relating to Disabilities

Nursing theories to assist nurses in making observations and planning care for people with disabilities have been identified. Hall's threefold conceptualization of how nursing relates to people with post-acute rehabilitation needs placed nurses at the bedside in order to implement a specific rehabilitation philosophy. This philosophy required the nurse, rather than nursing assistants, to work with the patient. This hands-on contact was deemed necessary in order for the patients to determine what their goals are and to work out ways to achieve those goals (Bowar-Ferres, 1975).

Levine's conceptual adaptation theory has been described as one way to help nurses determine priorities in care for post-op patients who are disabled. In particular, Levine suggests that nurses can help patients maintain personal integrity by recognizing their rights and by accepting them the way they are. Identifying patient strengths and enabling persons to make some decisions also were avenues to provide dignity (Benchot, 1986).

In Australia nurses applied Orem's self-care model as a meaningful vehicle for delivery of nursing service to people with disabilities. The principles of normalization, self-advocacy, right to choice, and community participation are supported in Orem's self-care model. This theory assumes that with training and support people may become their own self-care agents. This positive change in the ability for self-care requires a nursing system that can be altered to meet the changing needs of the developing person (Raven, 1988). Orem's theory also provides direction for nursing practice that includes supporting parents who have adolescents with dis-abilities (Tasch, 1988). Nursing theories have been described to enforce the concept that nursing practice over the past fifteen years, especially in rehabilitation and in disabilities, has been designed to reflect the principle that nurses work with rather than direct consumers.

Orem's nursing theory of development of a person as his or her own self-care agent parallels the principle of empowerment in many ways. Em-powering a health consumer implies that information is provided so an informed choice can be made. Functional wellness behaviors enable con-sumers to gain skill in assuming responsibility for their own health.

Steele (1986), for example, evaluated and compared the following well-ness behaviors of forty-six adolescents who have mental retardation with a sample of adolescents who were not identified as disabled: ability to treat minor illnesses, self-sufficiency in monitoring their own physiologic health parameter, substance abuse, sexual history, seat belt use, dental floss use, exercise, and knowledge of relaxation. The most significant difference between the two groups was in the area of exercise. Steele suggests that adolescents with disabilities may require more concerted efforts in assuming responsibility for their own health (e.g., 34 percent were unable to use a bathroom scale). She also encouraged health care providers to be more innovative in teaching independence.

More such research is needed to prove the value of health-promoting skills, which enable persons to maintain themselves in the community. Research is also needed to assess the value of teaching people to utilize their capacities in order to manage their activities of daily living (ADLs) to the best of their ability. Currently, most rehabilitation or restorative pro-grams place greater emphasis on acquisition and maintenance of motor skills to the exclusion of other skills, such as functional or wellness skills (Shanck and Lubkin, 1990).

Williams (1987) studied how adolescent girls with disabilities adjust to problems of early adolescence, as a step in assisting with integrating students into mainstream adolescent cultural activities. Nurses are aware that as efforts are made to foster each individual's growth and identity within the community, health care team members will need to acknowledge the individual's desires and needs. Someone will be needed to facilitate knowledge and skill acquisition to meet those needs. Knowledge of sexuality and practice in protective behaviors are also elements in facilitating community membership. Sexual knowledge and sexual behavior assessment and then education in each area can be taught to people of all abilities. Curricula such as the STARS curriculum provide nurses with a basic framework for either one-to-one or group teaching (Heighway, Webster, and Shaw, 1988). Nurses can be the facilitators for the acquisition of these skills.

In the empowerment model, the help giver or facilitator of skills training is directed to create enabling experiences. Nurses have demonstrated their role as "patient educators" and have been creative in initiating enabling experiences. One example in which nurses have readily modified "patient education" instruction is that of teaching parents who have cognitive impairment. Adaptions for such parents include one-on-one instruction, constant reinforcement, incorporating structure into the daily routine, repetitive practice time, keeping instructions identical from one teaching session to the next, anticipating common problems, and coaching the parents in problem solving (Foster, 1988). An important component of the creation of enabling experiences includes an awareness of interactional behaviors between the help giver and the help seeker.

Durst, Trivette, Davis, and Cornwell (1988) summarize eight behaviors necessary during help-giving practices to produce competency for families of children with health impairments. Nurses will benefit by investigating the extent to which these interactional behaviors influence "patient teaching." Indeed, at least one of the behaviors, "allow decision making to rest entirely with the help-seeker," may need to be re-envisioned for some families, but the concept that effective helping needs to incorporate certain help-giver characteristics and practices is an important one in the design of service delivery.

Another approach to improve nursing care is the use of the nursing classification system of nursing diagnosis. Nursing diagnosis, which has been nationally recognized since the 1970s, helps to organize nursing functions and define nursing's practice and scope (Carpenito, 1983). Nursing diagnosis has been presented as one means to help differentiate nursing practice from medical practice, a long-desired differentiation (Patterson and Rowland, 1970). Nurses in residential care facilities have documented common nursing diagnoses and appropriate interventions. Five of the most frequently occurring nursing diagnoses in one facility included ineffective breathing pattern; alteration in bowel elimination, constipation; alteration in nutrition, less than body requirements; fluid volume deficit; and impairment of skin integrity (Miller, Steele, and Boisen, 1987). The challenge for nursing is in transferring the intervention plans to the community setting when persons move from the residential care facility. Nursing diagnosis certainly offers a systematic way to assess and intervene for health care needs that will be commonly encountered in the community.

RAMIFICATIONS OF COMMUNITY-BASED TRENDS

The shift to community membership and meeting the health care support needs of individuals in their own homes presents challenges to the nursing profession. Ramifications of this revolution in service provision to people with disabilities are multiple. Several will be explored in this section.

Nurses in every setting will interact with people who have rehabilitation and habilitation needs. Nurses already draw on their generalist abilities to provide nursing care. With the advent of people living in the community who have complex health care needs, the generalist nurse will need to draw on many new resources to provide quality care. As more technological information unfolds concerning specific health conditions or syndromes, nurses will need to know the implications of these conditions on their nursing assessment, plan, interventions, and evaluations. Although nurses in general cannot be expected to keep up to date on all the latest information, nurses are obliged to at least direct consumers to the most current information.

In the past, nurses in state facilities and in University Affiliated Programs have provided consultation to other nurses and to the community. As a profession, nurses must articulate what professional nurse consultation is needed, decide who can best offer it, and assure that adequate consultation is available. If closing of facilities implies that consultative services will be eliminated, then nurses need to articulate what the loss of that service will mean.

The shortage of nurses in hospitals, in long-term settings, and now in home care places stress on a system in which they are needed to monitor changing health care status or to provide direct nursing care (Buerhaus, 1987; Cairns and Schroeder, 1988; White, 1991). Persons discharged from institutions or who have been cared for at home who have complex health care have needs that must be met. To ensure this objective, innovative models of care are needed. The models should consider the obvious factor of nurse shortage. The principle of using professionals as consultants fits well into the schema of the community framework. However, as indicated previously, there may be few places to train nurses skilled in the needs of persons with complex health care. Creative, efficient suggestions regarding the use of a scarce supply of nurses must also take into consideration the principles of care in the natural setting.

Because large residential facilities have been a primary place in which disabilities nursing practice and specialization has thrived, nursing in small, consumer-based settings is in its infancy. For this nursing practice to grow and mature, it will require nurses' attention and possible new conceptualizations. At this point the scarcity of resources and the commitment to providing care in the least restrictive environment may well come into direct conflict with each other. Mini-institutions may well arise again as people with more intense health care needs are grouped together for most efficient and safe care.

In creating community alternatives, some degree of risk taking may be necessary. As parents can attest, the willingness to risk enhancing a person's dignity is often questioned by health care professionals who are concerned about the risk of safety for the individual. Developing a health care delivery system that is located in the natural setting away from the careful monitoring and supervision of health care professionals will require collaboration between health care professionals who can articulate the challenges and the interventions required to meet the challenges, and the social service providers who can work with the health care challenges.

One conceptualization needed to implement the sharing of health care information is role release (see Rainforth et al., 1995, Chapter 7 in this book). *Role release* is a process in which certain traditional aspects of the nursing role are released to other non-nurse team members, including parents, support persons, or the consumers themselves. Role release is a series of transitions in which specific health care interventions can be carried out by non-nurses according to a personalized program plan. Role release requires continuous team support, consultative backup, and availability of a nurse to provide highly complex interventions that are mandated by law or necessitated by the changing needs of the consumer (Hutchinson, 1978).

Nurses are not the only scarce resource. Financial barriers occur on many levels. First, the health care coverage by Medicaid is not sufficient to provide quality health care for rehabilitation (Shanck and Lubkin, 1990; Steele, 1977). Financial means to pay for equipment and quality services are not fully available under the present Medicaid reimbursement system. Thus, lack of financial means is a barrier. Second, one of the reasons that living in the community was promoted to the public and politicians was that it was less expensive than living in institutions. As persons with more complex health care needs exercise their right to live in the community, it may not be possible to claim that it will be less expensive, because it may well not be. Parents have already had to face this issue when given the choice to either institutionalize their medically fragile infants or to give up parental rights in order that the child live with a foster family. That is, public money could be obtained to provide twenty-four-hour nursing care in foster care, but not for the natural family.

A ramification of empowering consumers to participate fully in decision-making activities implies allowing consumers to prioritize their activities. An important issue in this is whether nurses can optimize health care objectives while respecting consumers' perspectives and preferences. An example of dilemmas resulting from empowering consumers to make their own choices involves a twenty-one-year-old named Becky. Becky was recently able to move into her own apartment after living for fifteen years in foster care. While at the foster home, preventive health care interventions that included X rays of entire body to determine the extent of her congenital anomalies were not done. She and her foster parents prioritized a loving home environment over one disrupted by frequent health care interventions, such as successive stage orthopedic and genito-urinary surgeries—despite these procedures being recommended by her specialty clinic. Although Becky was a vibrant, healthy, young adult when she moved away from home, within six months of her move she was faced with difficult decisions regarding the possible need for life-threatening surgery.

Another complexity that this example illustrates is how nurses can contribute to community support systems for individuals with severe medical disabilities. In Becky's case, by the time she contemplated surgery, her foster parents had retired to another part of the country. Her closest friend was her boyfriend, whom she was planning to marry in the near future. He, however, knew little of the intricacies of the serious medical questions confronting her. Becky also had a community-based social worker/case manager who had a role in coordinating residential services and community health care assistance. As with the boyfriend, he was invested in Becky's welfare, but had incomplete knowledge of her medical dilemmas, and she did not feel comfortable discussing some of these issues with a man.

A nurse was able to provide an assessment of present and potential health care needs and to be supportive of Becky as she made decisions regarding her health care. In addition, Becky's support system, consisting of her boyfriend and her social worker, received written information regarding her congenital anomalies and treatment options. They also consulted frequently with the nurse to discuss ongoing and potential health care concerns. Nurses are challenged to develop competent support systems for persons with disabilities. Members of the support systems will need to be informed so that they can realistically discuss health care interventions.

To implement care in the natural setting, nurses need to be open to people with different and unfamiliar life attitudes and beliefs. A willingness to commit to the resources that the person with disabilities has around him or her and to offer support to those significant others is vital. Time and again, nurses have witnessed how some family members who were originally "written off" as being unfit to provide twenty-four-hour care and management have become well-skilled, self-educated advocates. For many, it was only their determination to stick by their family member that allowed the discharge from the acute care or long-term care facility. For others more fortunate, words of encouragement, efforts to involve them in the care of their loved one, and recognition that they can learn the complex tasks if they wish have empowered family members and significant others to leave with dignity and a sense that they can provide the care. For these individuals, an interaction between the nurse and family members probably occurred in which both sides learned of each other's perceptions about the disabling condition.

In those situations in which care at home seems to have deteriorated and placed the person's health at risk, an organized evaluation process may need to occur. This process could include past and present coping mechanisms, present life stressors on the care provider, and more frequent assessment of the person's physical condition. This evaluation process is to be coordinated with the primary caregiver, and nurses could well be advocates with the primary health care provider.

IMPLICATIONS

The paradigm shift from services in institutional settings to services in one's natural setting has several implications for the education of nurses and the delivery of nursing services. The education of nurses and of community care providers will be explored in this section, along with two aspects of service delivery, continuity of care and case management.

The lack of training that nursing students receive in providing nursing care both for adults with disabilities and for people with rehabilitation needs has implications for nurse educators. Clinical learning sites that are based in the consumers' natural settings and that utilize the consumers' natural liaisons must be sought out or developed by nurse educators. The experience that nursing students will gain in those sites may enable them to develop comprehensive health care plans and to implement nursing interventions that will ensure the adequacy of community-based health care services. In addition, if nursing students apply new knowledge at their clinical sites, such as the natural history of health care changes that occur in adults with disabilities as they age, staff nurses who have not had similar training may learn about community resources, case management, and clinical approaches to primary care that might benefit them in their care for all consumers.

Nursing education that teaches and helps refine the interdisciplinary team process and that provides training in ways to work as coordinated teams will enhance the nurse's role in enabling persons to live in the community. The health care team concept in rehabilitation has evolved for the purpose of ensuring coordinated, nonfragmented care from a number of specialists. However, a danger exists in that teams may fail to meet their expectations and the health care consumer may be even more fragmented after a team conference. To improve the effectiveness of health care teams, education in team functioning, education in describing one's role on the team, and practice as a team member in clearly communicating goal-directed information are all needed (Rothberg, 1981). This implies that whether nurses participate as members of a health care rehabilitation team, an individual service plan (ISP), or a part of a personal futures plan (PFP), they take time to analyze their own performance on that team.

Nursing education that supports the shift of practice from one based on a helping model to one based on an empowerment model will assist in involving consumers in their own health management (Durst et al., 1988). Nurses will benefit from examining their practice for elements that induce or perpetuate dependence on the part of the help seekers. Modifying nursing practices to enable help seekers to assume responsibility for their health status requires training and practice.

Nursing education has a role in helping to change professional attitudes that impede the delivery of health care to all persons in order that they may live in their natural settings. Attitudinal change is difficult until professionals have an opportunity to interact directly with an unfamiliar person. Thus, students will benefit from clinical assignments in which they work directly with people with disabilities and their families. Hospitalizations are times when both students and nurses have an opportunity to learn from persons with disabilities about their care needs and about themselves as persons with unique strengths and perspectives (Durfee and Durfee, 1990).

Nursing research is needed in many areas to ensure service delivery that is consumer focused. One area is the need to generate information on the health care changes that occur in adults with disabilities as they age. Nurses can assist in sorting out what is unique and what is shared with people who are aging and nondisabled. Information is needed on a wide variety of topics—side effects from long-term use of neuroleptics, injury prevention, prevention and treatment of psychiatric disorders, effective patient teaching, and the development of models of community-based health care systems that allow persons with disabilities to age in place.

In addition to reviewing the education of nurses to ensure that they incorporate a commitment to community care for all individuals with disabilities, education of the community care providers that will enable them to advocate with the health care system is needed. Training a staff unskilled in areas concerning health decision making is complicated by high turnover, inadequate recordkeeping, lack of experience in making health care decisions, lack of direction in knowing when to prioritize the placement of medical needs over vocational or other psychosocial needs, and by lack of techniques in assessing persons with subtle or not-so-subtle health care changes that can become life threatening.

Sometimes when a person's health condition is changing, the clues are difficult to objectify. Observations such as "He looks pale." "His appetite is poor." "He didn't sleep well." "His bowels are loose." become known as a result of day-to-day familiarity. Persons with fragile health conditions need continuity of care to ensure that these observations are made. However, recruiting and retaining support providers is complicated by the fact that there is little financial or social incentive to remain in the support provider role. In addition, when health care needs do arise, primary health care providers may not be available, and instead a practitioner unfamiliar with the person may be consulted. This may result in delay of treatment.

The challenge to provide continuity of care can be met by innovative teaching and support strategies. Detailed records describing a person's health status and indicators of a declining health status can be maintained. Videotaping persons during various times of their changing health status might be useful in training support providers and community nurses. The use of a standard plan of care developed between the health care practitioner and the support provider or consumer has been successful in initiating prompt medical treatment for people with complex health care needs who are unable to articulate their health changes. When consistent behavioral indicators of illness are reported, the health care provider can direct treatment before objective medical tests confirm the diagnosis. For some individuals who become quite ill very quickly, this prompt treatment prevents hospitalizations. Developing creative in-service material, such as handouts on the management and monitoring of common health care concerns and phone line telecommunications that allow the support providers to "talk" with the educator, are activities needed to ensure quality of care for persons with multiple needs.

Attention to the definition of case management and the assumed expectations of that role is important. Health care workers are familiar with the primary health care provider as the identified medical case manager.

In the area of rehabilitation or disabilities, case management is a more comprehensive term. Keeping current with terminology allows nurses to dialogue with consumers. For instance, familiarity with the proposed case management models as required in P.L. 99-457 keeps nurses informed of what parents and families seek in their expectation of a case manager. Because many children with disabilities have increased health problems resulting in increased need for health services, nurses would be valuable members of the interdisciplinary teams called for in this legislation (Davis and Steele, 1991).

One outstanding implication for nurses who are committed to providing consumer-directed care in the natural setting will be using resources that enable them to keep informed. Appendix A lists professional resources that will provide updated information especially for adults with developmental disabilities.

CONCLUSION

This chapter reviews the history of nursing care to people with disabilities and contemporary approaches as described in the American nursing literature. The current model for delivering services to people with disabilities has far-reaching ramifications for present-day and future nursing practice. Although historically nurses have been associated with caring for persons with disabilities, and specific nurse leaders have advocated impressively to enhance service delivery, nursing today is not as visible as the other disciplines in promoting and designing health care services for people with disabilities who are living in or planning to return to their home settings. The planning and developing of service delivery models in which health care needs are met in an integrated manner along with other community living needs is a necessity at this time. With the current governmental mandates to downsize or close large institutions where nursing has been consistently active in supporting people, the importance of nursing's involvement in the creative problem-solving process that ensures quality care for people with complex health care needs cannot be underestimated.

REFERENCES

Aggen, R., and Moore, N. (1984). *Standards of nursing practice in mental retardation/developmental disabilities.* Albany, NY: Office of Mental Retardation and Developmental Disabilities.

Andrews, M., and Nielson, D. (1988). Technology dependent children in the home. *Pediatric Nursing, 14,* 111–114.

Avey, M. (1973). Primary care for handicapped children. *American Journal of Nursing, 73,* 658–661.

Barnard, K. (1975). Trends in the care and prevention of developmental disabilities. *American Journal of Nursing, 75,* 1700–1704.

Barnard, K., and Powell, M. (1972). *Teaching the mentally retarded.* St. Louis: Mosby.

Benchot, R. (1984). The mentally retarded adult: A nursing perspective. *Journal of Community Health Nursing, 4,* 235–246.

Benchot, R. (1986). Mentally retarded patients. *Association of Operating Room Nurses Journal, 44,* 768–780.

Bowar-Ferres, S. (1975). Loeb Center and its philosophy of nursing. *American Journal of Nursing, 75,* 810–815.

Brandt, P., and Magyary, D. (1989). Preparation of clinical nurse specialists for family-centered early intervention. *Infants and Young Children, 1,* 51–62.

Buerhaus, P. (1987). Not just another nursing shortage. *Nursing Economics, 5,* 267–279.

Burns, K., and Snyder, M. (1991). Neurological assessment: Adaptations for special populations with mental retardation. *Journal of Neuroscience Nursing, 23,* 107–110.

Caddell, D., and Donaldson, J. (1990). The Hug Center caring for special children. *Caring, 9*(12), 22–25.

Cairns, A., and Schroeder, A. (1988). Editorial. *Journal of Community and Health Nursing, 5,* 85.

Carpenito, L. (1983). *Nursing diagnosis application to clinical practice.* St. Louis: Lippincott.

Chapman, J. (1977). On becoming a helper. In M. Krajicek and A. Tierney (Eds.), *Detection of developmental problems in children* (pp. 193–198). Baltimore: University Park Press.

Crocker, A., Yankauer, A., and the Conference Steering Committee (1987). *Mental Retardation, 25,* 227–232.

Curry, J. (1978). The transition from institution to community living. In J. Curry and K. Peppe (Eds.), *Mental retardation: Nursing approaches to care* (pp. 239–246). St. Louis: Mosby.

Curtis, S., Begin, B., and Blinkhorn, P. (1989). Delivery of nursing services in an Intermediate Care Facility for the mentally retarded. In I. Rubin and A. Crocker (Eds.), *Developmental disabilities: Delivery of medical care for children and adults* (pp. 418–424). Philadelphia: Lea and Febiger.

Davis, B., and Steele, S. (1991). Case management for young children with special health care needs. *Pediatric Nursing, 17,* 15–19.

Diehl, D. (1986). Private practice out on a limb and loving it. *American Journal of Nursing, 86,* 907–909.

Dilorio, C. (1990). An analysis of trends in neuroscience nursing research: 1960–1980. *Journal of Neuroscience of Nursing, 22,* 139.

Durfee, S., and Durfee, M. (1990). Preparing Camille for surgery. *Exceptional Parent, 20,* 28–30.

Durst, C., Trivette, C., Davis, M., and Cornwell, J. (1988). Enabling and empowering families of children with health impairments. *Children's Health Care, 17,* 71–81.

Feeg, V. (1987). Developmental disability services and territorial imperative. *Pediatric Nursing, 13,* 78.

Foster, S. (1988). Approaching the developmentally delayed parent. *Maternal Child Nursing, 13,* 19.

Fraley, A. (1990). Chronic sorrow: a parental response. *Journal of Pediatric Nursing, 5,* 268–273.

Glassman-Feibusch, B. (1984). The nurse's role with mentally retarded clients: Teacher, advocate, listener, doer. *Journal of Community Health Nursing, 1,* 225, 226.

Gleeson, S. (1987). Public sector perspective: Potential nursing services in mental retardation. *Pediatric Nursing, 13,* 81–83.

Granger, C., Seltzer, G., and Fishbein, C. (1987). *Primary care of the functionally disabled.* Philadelphia: Lippincott.

Heighway, S., Webster, S., and Shaw, M. (1988). *STARS—Skills Training for Assertiveness, Relationship Building and Sexual Awareness.* Madison: University of Wisconsin.

Hodgkins, P., and Monfils, M. (1985). Nursing care and treatment of the retarded mentally ill. *Journal of Psychosocial Nursing, 23,* 31–33.

Hulsman, B., and Chubon, S. (1989). A comparison of disabled adults' perceived quality of life in nursing facility and home settings. *Public Health Nursing, 6,* 141–146.

Hutchinson, D. (1978). The transdisciplinary approach. In J. Curry and K. Peppe (Eds.). *Mental retardation: Nursing approaches to care.* St. Louis: Mosby.

Kaufman, J., Lichtenstein, K., and Rosenblatt, A. (1986). A service coordination: A systems approach to medically fragile children. *Caring, 5,* 42–49.

Kimball, K. (1983). Caring for a special patient. *Nursing, 13,* 74–75.

Kirkhart, K., Steele, N., Pomeroy, M., Anguzza, R., French, W., and Gates, A. (1988). Louisiana's ventilator assisted care program: Case management services to link tertiary with community-based care. *Children's Health Care, 17,* 106–111.

Lannon, S. (1990). Assessing seizure activity in mentally disabled adults. *Journal of Neuroscience Nursing, 22,* 294–301.

Lenihan, S. (1985). The young child and the home health care nurse: Problems, challenges and intervention strategies. *Home Healthcare Nurse, 3*, 6–9.

Macedo, A., and Posel, F. (1987). Nursing the family after the birth of a child with spina bifida. *Issues in Comprehensive Pediatric Nursing, 10*, 55–65.

McCoy, P., and Votroubek, W. (1986). Tusson's first homebound ventilator-dependent child, Kim Nichols. *Caring, 5*, 52–57.

McDonald, E. (1985). Medical needs of severely developmentally disabled persons residing in the community. *American Journal of Mental Deficiency, 90*, 171–176.

Meyers, A., Cupples, A., Lederman, K., Branch, L., Feltin, M., Master, R., Nicastro, D., Glover, M., and Kress, D. (1987). Carrying nursing services into the community. *Medical Care, 25*, 1057–1068.

Miller, J., Steele, K., and Boisen, A. (1987). The impact of nursing diagnoses in a long-term care setting. *Nursing Clinics of North America, 22*, 905–915.

Minihan, P. (1986). Planning for community physician services prior to deinstitutionalization of mentally retarded persons. *American Journal of Public Health, 76*, 1202–1206.

Minihan, P., and Dean, D. (1990). Meeting the needs for health services of persons with mental retardation living in the community. *American Journal of Public Health, 80*, 1043–1048.

Murphy, A., and Pueschel, S. (1975). Early intervention with families of newborns with Down Syndrome. *Maternal Child Nursing Journal, 4*, 1–7.

Nehring, W. (1991). Historical look at nursing in the field of mental retardation in the United States. *Mental Retardation, 29*, 259–267.

O'Pray, M. (1987). Working with families with infants with respiratory equipment in the home. *Basics in Comprehensive Pediatric Nursing, 10*, 113–121.

Patterson, E., and Rowland, G. (1970). Toward a theory of mental retardation nursing: An educational model. *American Journal of Nursing, 70*, 651–655.

Peppe, K. (1987). Nursing services. In H. Wallace, R. Biehl, L. Taft, and A. Oalesby, (Eds.), *Handicapped children and youth* (pp. 195–202). New York: Human Sciences Press.

Peppe, K., and Sherman, R. (1978). Nursing in mental retardation: Historical perspective. In J. Curry and K. Peppe (Eds.), *Mental retardation: Nursing approaches to care* (pp. 3–18). St. Louis: Mosby.

The Pepper Report (1991). *Caring, 10*, 15–30.

Rainforth, B., Giangreco, M.F., Smith, P.D., and York, J. (1995). Collaborative teamwork in training and technical assistance: Enhancing community support for persons with disabilites. In O.C. Karan & S. Greenspan (Eds.), *Community rehabilitation services for people with disabilities*. Boston: Butterworth–Heinemann.

Raven, J. (1988). Application of Orem's self-care model to nursing practice in developmental disability. *Australian Journal of Advanced Nursing, 6*, 16–23.

Rothberg, J. (1981). The rehabilitation team: Future direction. *Archives of Physical Medicine and Rehabilitation, 62*, 407–410.

Selekman, J. (1991). Pediatric rehabilitation: From concepts to practice. *Pediatric Nursing, 17*, 11–14.

Shanck, A., and Lubkin, I. (1990). Rehabilitation. In I. Lubkin (Ed.), *Chronic illness: Impact and interventions* (pp. 403–423). Boston: Jones and Bartlett.

Steele, S. (1977). General ideas in relation to long-term illness in childhood. In S. Steele (Ed.), *Nursing care of the child with long-term illness* (pp. 107–152). New York: Appleton-Century-Crofts.

Steele, S. (1986). Assessment of functional wellness behaviors in adolescents who are mentally retarded. *Issues in Comprehensive Pediatric Nursing, 9*, 331–340.

Steele, S. (1987). Deinstitutionalization of persons with mental retardation/ developmental disabilities. *Issues in Comprehensive Pediatric Nursing, 10*, 235–250.

Steele, S., Russell, F., Hansen, B., and Mills, B. (1989). Home management of URI in children with Down Syndrome. *Pediatric Nursing, 15*, 484–488.

Tasch, V. (1988). Parenting the mentally retarded adolescent: A framework for helping families. *Journal of Community Health Nursing, 5*, 97–108.

Tudor, M. (1978). Nursing intervention with developmentally disabled children. *Maternal Child Nursing, 3*, 25–31.

White, J. (1991). The home care nursing shortage. *Caring, 10*, 4–11.

Whitney, A. (1966). Behavioral approaches to the nursing of the mentally retarded. *Nursing Clinics of North America, 1*, 641–647.

Williams, B. (1967). *Lillian Wald.* New York: Julian Messner.

Williams, D. (1987). Becoming a woman: The girl who is mentally retarded. *Pediatric Nursing, 13*, 89–93.

Wilson, D. (1975). *Stranger and traveler.* Boston: Little, Brown.

Yoos, L. (1985). Assessment and management of the developmentally delayed infant in primary care. *Nurse Practitioner, 10*, 24–35.

Ziring, P., Kastner, T., Friedman, D., Pond, W., Barnett, M., Sonneberg, E., and Strassburger, K. (1988). Provision of health care for persons with developmental disabilities living in the community. *Journal of the American Medical Association, 260*, 1439–1444.

Appendix A

Reference List for Information on Health Care Needs of Adults with Developmental Disabilities

American Association of Neuroscience Nurses
224 N. Des Plaines, Suite 601
Chicago, IL 60661
(312) 993-0043

American Association of University
 Affiliated Programs
Nursing Group
8630 Fenton St., Suite 410
Silver Spring, MD 20910
(301) 588-8252

> Nurses at the master's and doctoral levels who are employed at University Affiliated Programs (UAPs) have the mandate to provide exemplary service, training, dissemination, and research in the field of developmental disabilities. The national contact person can direct your questions regarding health care needs to nurses at specific UAPs. Standards for the Clinical Nurse Specialist in Developmental Disabilities/Handicapping Conditions were developed by the nursing group of AAUAP. These standards are available to measure quality care and to guide nursing action.

American Association on Mental Retardation
Nursing Division and Medical Division
1719 Kalorama Rd., N.W.
Washington, DC 20009
(800) 424-3688

> Oldest interdisciplinary professional association that promotes the well-being of individuals with mental retardation and supports those who work in the field. This organization reviews and shapes public policy, encourages research and education, and fosters communication and excellence in service, training, and research. The Nursing Division and the Special Interest Group on Aging have periodic newsletters. A special interdisciplinary group on health care has also been recently organized.

Association of Rehabilitation Nurses
5700 Old Orchard Rd.
Skokie, IL 60077
(708) 966-3433

The Habilitative Mental Healthcare Newsletter
P.O. Box 57
Bear Creek, NC 27207
(919) 742-5686

Monthly newsletter to disseminate up-to-date information on psychiatric aspects of mental retardation.

Janicki, M., and Wisniewski, H.
Aging and Developmental Disabilities
Baltimore: Paul H. Brookes, 1985

This book provides a summary of epidemiological, sociological, and legal issues as well as clinical and service approaches that will assist practitioners in meeting the needs of the elderly who are developmentally disabled. Specific chapters provide information on Alzheimer's disease, musculoskeletal aging, nutrition, dementia, and medications.

National Association of Developmental Disability Councils
1234 Massachusetts Ave., N.W.
Suite 103
Washington, DC 20005
(202) 347-1234

This agency will provide the name and location of each state's Developmental Disability (DD) Council. This council is a mandated agency to assist each state in public policy development. In some states, the DD Council may have pilot funds and models for innovative approaches for community integration. Although a particular DD Council may not have focused on health care issues, they are willing to learn of health care needs and suggestions for service delivery.

National Rehabilitation Information Center
8455 Colesville Rd., Suite 935
Silver Spring, MD 20910-3319
(800) 346-2742

This center offers the most complete collection of research and historical information on rehabilitation issues available in the United States. High-quality reference, research, and referral services are offered in response to site visits, telephoned requests, and electronic mails.

National Society of Genetics Counselors
233 Canterbury Dr.
Wallingford, PA 19086
(215) 872-7608

Provides locations of genetics clinics throughout the United States. A clinical geneticist from one of these clinics may provide up-to-date information regarding specific health needs of adults with genetic conditions.

Rehabilitation Research and Training Center
Consortium on Aging and Developmental Disabilities
3300 Elland Ave.
Cincinnati, OH 45229
Attn: Dr. Ruth Roberts
(216) 375-7956

This clearinghouse provides information and referral for inquiries concerning older persons with developmental disabilities.

15 ⬜⬜⬜
⬜⬜⬜
⬜⬜⬜

Assistive Technology

Gregory Bazinet

INTRODUCTION

In order to serve individuals with special needs, technology often must be applied so that consumers can realize their goals. Just as a pair of glasses helps many people to see better, assistive technology helps others to accomplish, on their own, tasks that previously required the service of others. Assistive technology enables individuals to be more self-supportive in reaching their own personal, social, and professional goals. Services received by individuals with special needs often cause the recipients to become reliant on those services; in the case of assistive technologies, these same individuals often become more self-reliant, building on their own abilities. This chapter will address the role of assistive technology, its evolution, and its contribution to the enablement of individuals with disabilities.

To understand assistive technology, one should understand the definition of *technology*. Simply put, it is a process—the application of scientific knowledge to a practical purpose. This definition implies that the outcome of the application of technology is a facilitation or enhancement of performance.

A good example of assistive technology is the modern running shoe. The technology of today's running shoe helps to absorb surface impacts, decreasing the shock transferred to the bone and muscle structure of the runner. The shoe also supports the foot and provides good traction so that the runner may make greater use of his or her effort.

Likewise, assistive technology might support the efforts of individuals with disabilities. Technology can increase personal mobility, through assisted doorways, ramps, or high-tech wheelchairs or through surgical implants to support neurological stimulation of muscles or prosthetic manipulation through muscular control. Technology can also aid communication, through computer applications to enhance employment opportunities or to support and augment the abilities of those individuals with sight, speech, or hearing impairments (Brown, 1992).

THE PLACE OF ASSISTIVE TECHNOLOGY

Assistive technology is unique in that it provides an interface between an individual's disability and a potential opportunity that most people take for granted. For example, the telephone enables us to communicate over great distances. In the past, an individual who was speech or hearing impaired would not have been able to use the telephone, a device most of us take for granted. With the invention of TDD (telecommunication devices for individuals who cannot hear), an entire segment of the population was provided access to telephone service. This is the purpose of assistive technology: to bridge an individual's disability and that person's inherent ability to succeed on his or her own. Assistive technology connects the consumer to the world and his or her opportunities.

CATEGORIES OF ASSISTIVE TECHNOLOGY

Depending on its functional impact on an individual's life, assistive technology can be classified into three basic categories or environments: living skills, access to environment, and job/work and education. These categories were created through an analysis of the ABLEDATA database system (McCarty and Bazinet, 1990). Each individual with a disability operates from a different and unique level across the categories. A brief overview of the three categories will provide the reader with a better appreciation for the levels and application of technology to meet each individual's needs.

Living Skills

Living skills includes an individual's immediate needs, such as personal care, home management, mobility within the home, communication inside and outside the living environment, and sensory disabilities, as well as the use of orthotics, prosthetics, and therapeutic aids.

Access to Environment

Access to environment encompasses the attempts to support an individual's physical movement from the living skills segment of his or her life toward the larger community. The primary foci in this area of enablement are transportation, available services, opportunities to join in recreation (Colston, 1991) within the community, and surmounting the architectural elements of the community. These areas are of paramount interest as individuals develop self-esteem and confidence in their ability to be members of the community.

Job/Work and Education

Job/work and education focuses on supporting the individual in accessing available educational and vocational opportunities that are appropriate to his or her needs and abilities. To function in the work environment, an individual should have developed a good deal of living skills and established dependable access to the environment, steps that not everyone will achieve to the same degree.

APPLICATION OF ASSISTIVE TECHNOLOGY

When applying assistive technology, the consumer and his or her support team must have information from the three categories mentioned earlier. This input is vital to providing the appropriate technology for each individual's unique needs (Stromberg, 1992).

The appropriate use of technology should also be considered: If the technology is provided, can the individual otherwise (without further intervention or assistance) perform the task or duty? If we can answer with an unqualified yes, we are preparing a true interface.

For example, individuals with severe cerebral palsy may be unable to write with a pencil or pen, but with the use of a computer or word processor, many such individuals are quite capable of communicating and realizing new opportunities. In such situations, assistive technology fulfills an individual's ability to function that for one reason or another has been lost or impaired.

THE "TRAINING WHEEL" APPROACH

The training wheel approach identifies the basic structures required to support an individual in the use of assistive technologies.

Simple and efficient, this method is somewhat as effective as using training wheels to support a child who *wants* to learn to ride a bicycle. "Wanting to learn" is a significant requirement in the use of assistive technology. There must be some degree of desire, regardless of magnitude, to enable an individual to *try*. As with training wheels, a degree of balance must be mastered, and a degree of risk is implied. In the training wheel approach, constant assessment and encouragement, along with input from the consumer, are needed to assess progress and to make modifications as needed.

THE EVOLUTION OF ASSISTIVE TECHNOLOGY

Assistive technology stems from three roots: (1) the parallel to the medical model, (2) the impact of federal legislation, and (3) the growth of improved technology. The medical model, simply stated, starts with identification, follows with diagnosis, and concludes with a prescription that will become the remedy. In the case of assistive technology, a three-step model is also evident; it differs only in that it begins after the initial prescription in the medical model. In the process of providing assistive technology to individuals with special needs, the individual is often first identified in either a hospital, home, school, or work setting. Upon identification, an evaluation is performed to discover the specific needs of the individual; a diagnosis and prescription follow (Parette and Van Bienvliet, 1991).

Rehabilitation efforts have often been prescribed to enable the individual to initiate or reinitiate personal or professional tasks and duties. As a result of the preceding model, rehabilitation engineering was born. Rehabilitation engineering came about as a way to more fully integrate an individual with his or her community through the means of assistive technology.

The combined impact of the Education for All Handicapped Children Act of 1975 (P.L. 94-142) and Section 504 of the Rehabilitation Act of 1973 (P.L. 93-112) has significantly enhanced the growth of technology applications on behalf of people with special needs. This growth is expected to continue because of the Americans with Disabilities Act of 1990 (P.L. 101-136). (See Fifield and Fifield, Chapter 3 in this book, for an elaboration of the impact of these laws on services to people with disabilities.)

As a parallel to the development and implementation of these laws, technology and the population requiring rehabilitation have been growing significantly. In 1973 the first operational microcomputer was displayed. This device would provide new insight into "high tech." Two years later, the Vietnam war ended, in 1975. One of the not-so-obvious results of this contemporary war was the survival of more severely injured men, women, and children than in any previous war. As a result of these parallel developments, coupled with the century's tremendous medical advances, more people were surviving serious trauma and requiring rehabilitation than at any other time in American history. These events, combined with the federal legislation of this era, provided the catalyst to truly apply developing and refined technologies to the direct needs of a new population of individuals with special needs.

CATEGORIES OF ASSISTIVE TECHNOLOGY

Assistive technology has two different, but not mutually exclusive, categories: high tech and low tech. *Low tech* refers to "off-the-shelf" technology (Holt, 1991), which uses readily available materials in both ordinary and unique applications. For example, for an individual who has a problem gripping an eating utensil due to lack of fine motor coordination, one simple solution would be to wrap the handle of the utensil with grip tape to increase its diameter and its "gripability"; of course, this solution is not always effective for every need. Another example of low tech is the remote operation of a television. Off-the-shelf low-tech solutions can cost as little as thirty dollars, plus the time of an able and understanding technician. Low tech implies low cost, as well as local availability of simple technology.

High tech refers to areas of greater complexity, often involving unique application of information, personal requirements, and the customization of technology to meet specific needs. An example of high-tech adaptation is the artificial hand or the Boston Arm. The current hand designs are affixed to the limb of an individual and manipulated by *reading* the neuromuscular commands of the individual. These hands and arms have been in refinement since the 1970s and are coming into more frequent use due to the technical enhancements of computer support and battery technology, as well as refinement of surgical techniques to relocate neuromuscular sensors. In many areas of high-tech adaptation, sensor technology of the 1980s has made possible what yesterday was only a dream. High tech implies more sophisticated technology focused more narrowly on the needs of small groups of individuals. High tech also implies a higher cost of more complex technologies.

High technology, however, can suddenly "spin off" to serve many individuals at reasonable cost. For example, digital speech, which was pioneered for public use by Texas Instruments in its original "Speak and Spell" format, has changed the world of individuals who are sight impaired. Today there are several excellent digitized voice programs that can both read back to an individual from a personal computer as well as speak each letter or word as an individual enters them into the computer.

THE EMPOWERMENT OF ASSISTIVE TECHNOLOGY

The use of assistive technology is unique for each individual. Each person may use a similar technology in a slightly different way. The specific selection and application of technology determines whether it meets the specific needs of an individual.

Several routes to the use of appropriate technology can be developed. For example, those involved in creating the technology must work closely with the individual to try to understand the process and opportunities that the person hopes to realize. Through such person-centered planning, focused on fulfilling the needs of the individual, appropriate interfaces are more likely to be developed. Obviously there are no universal prescriptions, and the individual with the disability must be an active participant (Guzzo and Guzzo, 1991). This ensures mutual understanding as well as a common focus on the direction, application, and use of technology to meet specific needs.

The preceding process assumes that those involved in technology development must try to understand what the technology means for the person in terms of his or her needs and expectations. The process should try to refine the answers to needs that can be well defined. Some of these needs may be quantifiable using dimensions such as colors, textures, weights, and so on. In essence, the developers must attempt to ascertain the degree of freedom required or desired. Also, it is important to clarify what the technology can and cannot do. Clearly, whatever interface is developed cannot do everything and solve all the person's needs. Often it is helpful to work on one area at a time to better focus both energy and resources.

Another aspect of the empowerment of assistive technology is getting to know the person and learning about his or her capabilities and limitations (Frey and Godfrey, 1991). Medical information may also be appropriate so as to better ensure technology decisions that will be both safe and appropriate for the specific needs of each individual. Each situation will be different and require a different set of evaluations. These will become a benchmark on which to develop parameters for use of the appropriate technology (McCarty and Bazinet, 1990).

IDENTIFYING OPPORTUNITIES FOR THE USE OF ASSISTIVE TECHNOLOGY

The California Department of Rehabilitation has developed some excellent guidelines to aid in the development and use of assistive technology.

First is the identification of general objectives: What are the goals of the individual? What functional problem(s) keep the person from realizing the objective(s)? Often a simple interview strategy is not effective in collecting enough information. A visit to the person's home, school, or job site may be required to observe the environment (Konig and Schalock, 1991) and the individual in that environment.

Second, determine the order in which the problems will be solved. This is best dealt with in a collaborative effort with the input of the consumer, peers, and others involved in the environment of application.

Third, identify the *specific* tasks the individual has difficulty performing. This step requires an analysis of the physical and mental requirements of the task and any environmental conditions that may limit function. As part of this analysis, developers must explore the individual's capability to do the task (Rusch and Hughes, 1988); support personnel often help with this exploration. Multiple observations are often required, and input from the individual being assessed should be gathered; after all, who knows better the specific problems than the person who is trying to surmount them? The use of a video camera and VCR are highly encouraged to support the documentation and collection of these data.

Examining and discussing the data with the consumer will generate several suggestions, which should be viewed in three distinct ways. First, is there another way to perform the task? (In a recent situation in which an individual had a difficult time reaching food products in the back of a refrigerator from his wheelchair, a decision was made to "erect a fence" to prevent the food from being pushed to the rear of the refrigerator shelf. Initially the person was not happy with this low-tech solution, but it worked well and the accommodation was installed within twenty-four hours.) Second, if assistive technology is required, what is commercially available with or without modification that will enable the individual to accomplish the desired task? There are several databases available to select possible technological options; however, creative new solutions should not be ruled out. What is locally available and can be put to the task? If steps one and two are not successful in overcoming the obstacles preventing accomplishment of the task, design and fabrication of a "custom device" should be considered. Whenever possible, the consumer should have the opportunity to test and critique the prototypes before the final design is selected.

At this point, a note of caution is required. The individual to be accommodated will have definite expectations. In the design of prototypes, the information collected in the assessment must be constantly reflected upon to allow the most *conservative* design development. Why? Is the assistive technology to become an autopilot for a human being or simply a device to provide personal accommodation? Upon final development and employment of the assistive technology, individual fitting and adjustment of the device and training in its proper and safe use must be stressed. Upon acceptance and employment of the device, the team should follow up to ensure that the solution meets fully the individual's needs (McCarty and Bazinet, 1990).

The development, acceptance, and use of assistive technology also implies liability for the design team and the individual user. All parties involved should constantly observe best-practice roles to ensure that no one has been inattentive or unconcerned in regard to OSHA and ADA mandates, as addressed in both local and federal mandates. For example, if a computer-assisted device failed to operate, would the user face personal harm or injury? The design and use of assistive technologies should in no way put any person or facility in the position of unforeseen harm or injury (McCarty and Bazinet, 1990).

REASONABLE ACCOMMODATION

Many possible solutions regarding assistive technology can arise from the answers to a few basic questions. For example, is accommodation required for performance of the task or learning situation? What effect will the accommodation(s) have on the individual, peers, or the facility and its operations? What improvements will the assistive technologies achieve? How will they be measured? Will the accommodated individual be on a more equal basis with his or her peers? How will the accommodation affect others? Finally, what are the alternatives to the proposed accommodations? Development of clear and reasonable answers to the preceding questions can assure more efficient and effective accommodation for each individual with disabilities.

MODIFICATION OF SCHEDULES

Restructuring living, learning, or working procedures can help eliminate factors found to be incompatible with an individual's capabilities. Restructuring should be planned in concert with past participants, when available, to determine the most agreeable course of modification. As always, provisions must be made for special accommodations, such as readers/interpreters, and instructions for changes in routine operations must be simple, logical, and clearly presented.

FINAL RULES OF THUMB

Each individual is unique. Whether possessing three disabilities or none, each person has different points of view, desires, and ways to solve problems. When employing assistive technology, the focus must always be on how the technology will enable an individual in a specific task. In accommodating an individual to become empowered, remember that if the individual has a dislike or personal reason for not applying himself or herself or the technology, *any* modification may be useless. The purpose of any assistive technology is to enhance the capabilities of an individual, not to eliminate his or her working responsibilities.

Those who assist in the development or matching of assistive technology should not prescribe solutions for the individual with disabilities but plan in a collaborative environment with the individual's unique and focused input. Too often the knowledge and experience of the consumer is neglected, resulting in needlessly complicated or even useless devices. As always, time, budget constraints, and medical factors must be integrated into the formula for success.

Assistive technology continues to grow and develop along with the capabilities of technology, the efforts of concerned professionals, and the desires of people with disabilities. Whether the goal is near or far, each journey of assistive technology must begin with simple steps, with hope that it may allow the person with a disability to experience the wonder of human potential.

REFERENCES

Brown, C. (1992). Assistive technology, computers and persons with disabilities. *Communications of the ACM, 35, 36.*

Colston, L. (1991). The expanding role of assistive technology in therapeutic recreation. *Journal of Physical Education, Recreation and Dance, 4,* 39.

Compton, C. (1989). Assistive technology: Up close and personal. *Seminars in Hearing, 10,* 104.

ED issues final rules on assistive technology (1990). *Education of the Handicapped, 16,* 5.

Farley, R.C., Bolton, B., and Parkerson, S. (1992). Effects of client involvement in assessment on vocational development. *Rehabilitation Counseling Bulletin, 35,* 146.

Fifield, B. and Fifield, M. (1995). The influence of legislation on services to people with disabilities. In O.C. Karan and S. Greenspan (Eds.). *Community rehabilitation services for people with disabilities.* Boston: Butterworth–Heinemann.

Frey, J.L., and Godfrey, M. (1991). A comprehensive clinical vocational assessment: The PACT approach. *Journal of Applied Rehabilitation Counseling, 22,* 25.

Guzzo, P., and Guzzo, B. (1991). Scott's IEP includes technology: One family's journey to obtain assistive technology for their son. *The Exceptional Parent, 302,* 105.

Holt, K.S. (1991). Everyday aids and appliances: Mobility aids and appliances for disabled children. *British Medical Journal, 302,* 105.

Johnson, W.F. (1991). Using local resources in providing assistive technology, or What to do until the rehabilitation engineer arrives. *Vocational Evaluation and Work Adjustment Bulletin, 24,* 125.

Kearly, P. (1988). Historical and philosophical issues in normalization of handicapped individuals. *Child and Youth Services, 10,* 3.

Konig, A., and Schalock, R. (1991). Supported employment: Equal opportunities for severely disabled men and women. *International Labour Review, 130,* 21.

McCarty, T., and Bazinet, G. (1990). *How to recognize opportunities and interfaces for people with disabilities.* University of Maine.

Mosley, C.C. (1988). Job satisfaction research: Implications for supported employment. *Journal of the Association for Persons with Disabilities, 13,* 211.

Parette, H., Jr., and Van Bienvliet, A. (1991). Rehabilitation assistive technology issues for infants and young children with disabilities: A preliminary examination. *Journal of Rehabilitation, 57,* 27.

Parker, S., Buckley, H., and Truesdell, A. (1990). Barriers to the use of assistive technology with children. *Journal of Visual Impairment, 84,* 532.

Peterson, C., and Foley, B. (1992). If you can move your head, you can move your world: Accessing the arts through assistive technology. *Arts and Activities, 4,* 28.

Position paper: Occupational therapy and assistive technology (1991). *The American Journal of Occupational Therapy, 45,* 1076.

Rogers, J., and Hold, M. (1992). Assistive technology device use in patients with rheumatic disease: A literature review. *The American Journal of Occupational Therapy, 46,* 20.

Rusch, F., and Hughes, C. (1988). Supported employment: Promoting employee independence. *Mental Retardation, 26,* 351.

Simmons, T., and Fleier, R. (1992). Development of Supportive Employment Programs for Adults with Developmental Disabilities. *Journal of Rehabilitation, 58,* 35.

Stromberg, E. (1992). ADA-inspired revolution is focusing attention on assistive technology. *The Hearing Journal,* June, 23.

Supported employment: An alternative model for vocational rehabilitation of persons with severe neurologic, psychiatric, or physical disability (1991). *Archives of Physical Medicine and Rehabilitation, 72,* 101.

APPENDIX A

Assistive Technology Resources—Nationwide Organizations

ABLEDATA, Adoptive Equipment Center
Newington Children's Hospital
181 East Cedar Street
Newington, CT 06111

> ABLEDATA is the largest single source of information on disability-related consumer products, with more than 15,000 commercially available products. Products are organized in fifteen categories of assistive technology. A custom search of the database enables you to locate and compare assistive products. For more information about ABLEDATA, or to request an ABLEDATA search, call 1-800-344-5405 or, in Connecticut, (203) 667-5405 (voice or TDD).

Accent on Information (AOI)
P.O. Box 700
Bloomington, IL 61701
(309) 378-2961

> AOI is a computerized system of information on products and devices that assist persons with disabilities in such areas as grooming, furniture, home management, mobility, and written and oral communication. Two types of information are available: references to publications, including sources; and brief descriptions of equipment, with addresses of manufacturers and distributors. For a fee, searches of the AOI system are made on specific topics. AOI also produces publications providing information on new products.

Alexander Graham Bell Association for the Deaf, Inc.
1537 35th Street, N.W.
Washington, DC 20007
(202) 337-5220

American Association for the Advancement
  of Science (AAAS)
Project on the Handicapped in Science
1776 Massachusetts Avenue, N.W.
Washington, DC 20036
(202) 467-4400

> AAAS Project on the Handicapped in Science (PHS) promotes opportunities in science for people who are physically challenged. PHS is an advocacy and information resource service for professionals and students of science who are handicapped.

American Foundation for the Blind (AFB)

15 West 16th Street	500 North Michigan Ave.	1860 Lincoln Street
New York, NY 10011	Chicago, IL 60611	Denver, CO 80203
(212) 620-2000	(312) 321-1880	(303) 861-9355
1660 L Street, N.W.	100 Peachtree Street	760 Market Street
Washington, DC 20036	Atlanta, GA 30303	San Francisco, CA 94102
(202) 467-5996	(404) 525-2303	(415) 392-4845

> AFB has consultant staff who work in the areas of children and youth; rehabilitation, orientation, and mobility; employment; low vision; aging; radio information services; special population groups; and recreation. Their headquarters are in New York and Washington, D.C., in addition to the four regional offices listed above.

American Parkinson Disease Association
147 East 50th Street
New York, NY 10022
(212) 421-5890

American Speech and Hearing Association
10801 Rockville Pike
Rockville, MD 20852
(301) 897-5700

Amyotrophic Lateral Sclerosis Society of America
15300 Ventura Boulevard
Suite 315
Sherman Oaks, CA 91403
(213) 990-2151

Arthritis Foundation
211 Park Avenue South
New York, NY 10003
(212) 677-5790

Association for Children with Learning Disabilities
 (ACLD)
4156 Library Road
Pittsburgh, PA 15234
(412) 341-1515

> A national organization of parents and professionals. ACLD's vocational committee studies and promotes vocational needs of people who are learning disabled.

Association for the Education of the Visually Handicapped
919 Walnut Street
Philadelphia, PA 19107
(215) 923-7555

Provides materials and information for people who are visually handicapped.

The Association for the Severely Handicapped (TASH)
Information Department
1600 West Armory Way
Seattle, WA 98119
(206) 283-5055

Information and materials requests on all aspects of education and services for people who are severely handicapped are answered by TASH's Information Department. TASH maintains a library of resource materials. The Information Department also conducts surveys of integrated schools and parent needs.

Center for Labor Research and Studies
Job-Related Physical Capacities Research Project (JRPC)
Florida International University—Tamiami Campus
Miami, FL 33199
(305) 552-2768

JRPC comparison system is an interactive computer system used in conjunction with already existing computerized career information. A person uses the system to explore interest areas and, in addition, is evaluated by a physician using a JRPC format to analyze the individual's physical capacities for ninety-eight different activities, such as walking, lifting, and reaching. Ratings on these capacities are then fed into the computer. Jobs in which the individual has expressed an interest (or all jobs meeting the person's physical specifications) are displayed on the screen or printout. The jobs are described in the same terms as the physical capacities that the physician rated. The kind of information a person receives includes a listing of the physical capacities necessary for the performance of the job, the percentage of people working at that job (from JRPC field sample) who say that his or her capacities would be sufficient, number of hours per day one might expect to use that capacity, and aids that are easily available to help overcome a specific functional handicap at the work site.

Council for Exceptional Children (CEC)
1920 Association Drive
Reston, VA 22091
1-800-336-3728
(703) 620-3660

CEC is a professional association interested in the educational needs of all exceptional children. CEC operates the Educational Resources Information

Center (ERIC) Clearinghouse on Handicapped and Gifted Children. The clearinghouse has bibliographies and abstracts in such areas as program accessibility for handicapped students. Brochures are available describing the association's services and publications.

Electronic Industries Foundation (EIF)
Project with Industry
2001 Eye Street, N.W.
Washington, DC 20006
(202) 457-4913

EIF has developed a program to train people who are handicapped to work in the electronic industries. Rehabilitation resources and industries work together to identify, train, and place potential employees. Currently, area EIF offices are located in Los Angeles, San Francisco, and Massachusetts.

Epilepsy Foundation of America
1828 L Street, N.W.
Washington, DC 20036
(202) 293-2930

Handy-Cap Horizons, Inc.
3250 East Loretta Drive
Indianapolis, IN 46227
(317) 784-5777

A travel club that arranges group tours around the world for people who are handicapped and elderly.

Helen Keller National Center for Deaf–Blind
  Youths and Adults
111 Middle Neck Road
Sands Point, NY 11050
(516) 944-8900

Innovative Matching of Problems to Available
  Rehabilitation Technology (IMPART)
IMPART Demonstration Center
Bexar County Easter Seal Center
2203 Babcock Road
San Antonio, TX 78229
(512) 699-8988

Industrial Home for the Blind operates the center to provide evaluative and rehabilitative services to deaf-blind youths and adults in a residential setting. Reprints of articles of research on sensory aids conducted by the center are available to inquirers.

International Association of Laryngectomies
American Cancer Society
777 Third Avenue
New York, NY 10017
(212) 371-2900

International Association of Parents
 of the Deaf
814 Thayer Avenue
Silver Spring, MD 20910
(301) 585-5400

Just One Break (J.O.B.)
373 Park Avenue South
New York, NY 10026
(212) 725-2500

> J.O.B. is a job placement agency for people who are physically disabled. Free of charge, J.O.B. applicants receive skill testing, vocational evaluation, and a ninety-day follow-up after placement. These services are available to potential employees and employers in the New York City metropolitan area. In addition, J.O.B. conducts research and demonstration projects, provides training seminars, and distributes printed material.

Library of Congress
Division for the Blind and Physically
 Handicapped (DBPH)
Washington, DC 20542
(202) 287-5100

> The Library maintains a collection of reading matter in braille and recorded form that is loaned free of charge to individuals unable to hold, handle, or read conventional printed matter. Listening equipment, including attachments such as speed controls, are also loaned to eligible individuals. The library's DBPH produces two publications that announce new book releases, have feature articles, and give information on library programs. The publications are *The Talking Book Topics*, available in print and on floppy disk, and *Braille Book Review*, available in print and braille. Reference circulars, available from DBPH, provide information on subjects relevant to blindness and physical handicaps.
>
> The Library of Congress works with a network of cooperating local libraries to distribute reading material equipment. Many local libraries maintain their own special materials collection. Contact your local library for more information and details.

Mainstream, Inc.
1200 15th Street, N.W.
Washington, DC 20005
1-800-424-8089 (also for TTY)
(202) 833-1136

> This organization provides information on federal laws and regulations concerning employment and education of handicapped people. Their hotline, equipped with a TTY, is answered by people who will answer questions on compliance with affirmative action regulations. If unable to answer questions, a confidential referral is made to the appropriate federal office. Mainstream produces a series of publications and sponsors conferences on issues regarding the rights of handicapped persons.

Muscular Dystrophy Associations of America, Inc.
810 Seventh Avenue
New York, NY 10019
(212) 586-0808

Myasthenia Gravis Foundation, Inc.
15 East 26th Street
New York, NY 10010
(212) 889-8157

National Amputation Foundation
12-45 150th Street
Whitestone, Long Island, NY 11357
(212) 767-8400

National Association for Retarded Citizens
2709 Avenue "E" East
Arlington, TX 76011
(817) 261-4961

National Association for Visually Handicapped (NAVH)

305 East 24th Street   3201 Balboa Street
New York, NY 10010   San Francisco, CA 94121
(212) 889-3141   (415) 221-3201

> AVH provides publications; adult and youth services including group programs; counseling to families and programs for the elderly; parent discussion groups; professional and public education; field testing of optical aids in cooperation with manufacturers; and information on and referral to community services.

National Association of the Deaf
814 Thayer Avenue
Silver Spring, MD 20910
(301) 587-1788

National Braille Association
85 Godwin Avenue
Midland Park, NJ 08432
(201) 447-1484

    Recorded, large-print, and braille materials are available through this association.

National Easter Seal Society for Crippled Children and Adults
2023 West Ogden Avenue
Chicago, IL 60612
(312) 243-8400

National Federation of the Blind
1800 Johnson Street
Baltimore, MD 21230
(301) 659-9314

National Labour Market Board
Sundbybergsvagen 9
S-171 99 Solna
Sweden

    In connection with the International Year for Disabled Persons, the National Labour Market Board is planning to compile a catalog of solutions to various vocational problems. For further information, write to the above address.

National Library of Medicine
National Institutes of Health
8600 Rockville Pike
Bethesda, MD 20209

National Library Service for the Blind and Physically Handicapped
Library of Congress
1291 Taylor Street, N.W.
Washington, DC 20502

National Multiple Sclerosis Society
205 East 42nd Street
New York, NY 10017
(212) 986-3240

The National Rehabilitation Information Center (NARIC)
4407 Eighth Street, N.E.
The Catholic University of America
Washington, DC 20017
Main office: (202) 635-5826
Information specialist: (202) 635-5822
TTY: (202) 635-5884

> NARIC is funded by Rehabilitation Services Administration (RSA) to improve information delivery to the rehabilitation community by (1) supplying copies of research reports and audiovisual materials prepared with RSA funding, as well as journal articles, conference proceedings, and other types of publications; (2) preparing bibliographies tailored to specific requests; (3) helping you locate the answers to factual questions, such as dates, places, names, addresses, or statistics. *Pathfinder* is published by NARIC six times a year.

National Society to Prevent Blindness
79 Madison Avenue
New York, NY 10016
(212) 684-3505

National Spina Bifida Association of America
343 South Dearborn
Chicago, IL 60604
(312) 663-1562

National Spinal Cord Injury Foundation
369 Elliot Street
Newton Upper Falls, MA 02164
(617) 964-0521

National Technical Information Service
U.S. Department of Commerce
5285 Port Royal Road
Springfield, VA 22161

Office of Special Education and Rehabilitative Services
Department of Education
400 Maryland Avenue, S.W.
Washington, DC 20202
(202) 471-3740

> The function of this office is to develop and implement educational policy to fulfill mandates of Part B, Education of the Handicapped Act (P.L. 91-230) as amended by P.L. 43-380 and P.L. 94-142, Education of All Handicapped Children Act of 1975.

Office of Technology Transfer (OTT), Veterans Administration
252 Seventh Avenue
New York, NY 10001
(212) 620-6659

> OTT operates under the Rehabilitation Engineering Research and Develop-
> ment Service to transfer research results into clinical practice. Their publica-
> tions disseminate information on new devices and techniques developed in
> the rehabilitation engineering program. OTT maintains a reference collection
> on rehabilitative engineering available to anyone, but helpful primarily to
> those in medical, allied health, and engineering fields.

Smithsonian Science Information Exchange
1730 M Street, N.W.
Washington, DC 20036

Technology Utilization Program
National Aeronautics and Space Administration
600 Independence Avenue, S.W.
Washington, DC 20545

Texas Rehabilitation Commission
118 East Riverside Drive
Austin, TX 78704
(512) 447-0100

> IMPART has engineers who help handicapped individuals make use of ad-
> vanced technology. Engineers are located at the Texas Rehabilitation Com-
> mission and the Southwest Research Institute Applied Rehabilitation En-
> gineering Center in San Antonio. IMPART helps people overcome difficulties
> encountered at work and at home by locating existing adapted technology or
> creating new items. This service is available to any person who is vocationally
> challenged and to individuals and agencies working with handicapped people.

Tools, Equipment, and Machinery Adapted for the Vocational Education
  and Employment of Handicapped People
Wisconsin Vocational Studies Center, University of Wisconsin–Madison
Madison, WI 53706-1796
(608) 263-3696

TRACE Research and Development Center for the Severely
  Communicatively Handicapped
314 Waisman Center, 1500 Highland Avenue
Madison, WI 53706

Source: Compiled by Timothy L. McCarty and Gregory Bazinet for the E-Team Educational
Module: "How to Recognize Opportunities and Interfaces for People with Disabilities,"
School of Applied Science, University of Southern Maine, Gorham, ME 04038 (207-780-5440).

APPENDIX B

Assistive Technology Resources—Rehabilitation Engineering Centers, by State and Country

Rancho Los Amigos Hospital
7601 East Imperial Highway
Downey, CA 90242
(213) 922-7167

Rehabilitation Engineering Center
Children's Hospital at Stanford
520 Willow Road
Palo Alto, CA 94034
(415) 327-4800

Rehabilitation Engineering Center
Smith-Kettlewell Institute of Visual Sciences
2232 Western Street
San Francisco, CA 94115
(415) 563-2323

> In addition to rehabilitation engineering research, the center produces publications.

San Francisco Lighthouse for the Blind
1155 Mission Street
San Francisco, CA 94103
(415) 431-1481

The George Washington University
Medical Rehabilitation R and T Center
2300 Eye Street, N.W.
Washington, DC 20037
(202) 676-3801

People to People Committee for the Handicapped
Directory of Organizations Interested in the Handicapped
1522 K Street, N.W., Room 1130
Washington, DC 20005
(202) 638-2487

> This directory lists the names, addresses, phone numbers, and officers of 118 organizations of or for persons with handicaps. Each listing also describes the structure and purpose of the organization, its principal programs, major publications, newsletters, and journals.

Rehabilitation Engineering Center
Northwestern University
345 East Superior Street, Room 1441
Chicago, IL 60611
(312) 649-8649

Rehabilitation Engineering Society
 of North America
1701 South First Avenue, Suite 504
Maywood, IL 60153

> The society is made up of consumers, therapists, manufacturers, providers, and engineers who develop technology for people with disabilities.

Schwab Rehabilitation Hospital
Departments of Vocational Services and
 Occupational Therapy
Technical Aids Evaluation, Training, and Demonstration
 Laboratory for the Physically Disabled
1401 South California Boulevard
Chicago, IL 60608
(312) 522-2010

> The technical aids laboratory is designed to give individuals with disabilities and social service specialists easy access to and information about technical aids for people who are handicapped. Evaluation of equipment and training in the use of aids are among the services offered.

Rehabilitation Engineering Center
University of Iowa
Orthopedics Department
Dill Children's Hospital
Iowa City, IA 52242
(319) 356-1616

Cerebral Palsy Research Foundation of Kansas, Inc.
4320 East Kellogg Street
Wichita, KS 67128
(316) 683-5627

> The foundation produces a publication describing its research, *Tech Brief.*

Rehabilitation Engineering Center
Children's Hospital Medical Center
300 Longwood Avenue
Boston, MA 02115
(617) 734-6000

Tufts University
Medical Rehabilitation R and T Center
171 Harrison Avenue
Boston, MA 02111
(617) 956-5625

Rehabilitation Engineering Center
University of Michigan
225 West Engineering
Ann Arbor, MI 48109
(313) 764-1817

University of Minnesota
Medical Rehabilitation R and T Center
860 Mayo Building
Minneapolis, MN 55455
(612) 373-8990

National Institute for Rehabilitation Engineering
97 Decker Road
Butler, NJ 07405
(201) 838-2500

New York University
Medical Rehabilitation R and T Center
400 East 34th Street
New York, NY 10016
(212) 679-3200

Telephone Pioneers of America
30-C 1847
195 Broadway
New York, NY 10017

> The Telephone Pioneers of America is the world's largest voluntary association of industrial employees. It is composed of men and women in the United States and Canada who have served eighteen or more years in the Bell System companies, certain Canadian telephone industry companies, and Rochester Telephone Corporation. Working through ninety-four chapters in forty-eight states and Canada, Pioneers devote their free time to a wide range of community service activities. Pioneers' basements become workshops for the repair of recording machines for individuals who are blind and the manufacture and design of "talking toys" for children with autism. Special preschool programs have tested thousands of children for vision and hearing problems; older Americans have been screened for glaucoma and hypertension. To contact the Pioneer chapter in your area, consult your local telephone directory.

United Cerebral Palsy Association, Inc.
66 East 34th Street
New York, NY 10016
(212) 481-6300

Case Western Reserve University
2219 Adelbert Road
Cleveland, OH 44106
(216) 368-2000

Rehabilitation Engineering Center
Krusen Research Center
Moss Rehabilitation Hospital
12th Street and Tabor Road
Philadelphia, PA 19141
(215) 329-5715

The University of Tennessee
Department of Orthopedic Surgery
1248 La Paloma Street
Memphis, TN 38114

Applied Rehabilitation Center
Southwest Research Institute
2203 Babcock Road
San Antonio, TX 78229
(512) 699-0386

Texas Institute for Rehabilitation and Research
1333 Mousund Avenue
Houston, TX 77025
(713) 979-1440

Rehabilitation Engineering Center
University of Virginia
P.O. Box 3368
University Station
Charlottesville, VA 22903
(804) 924-0311

University of Washington
Medical Rehabilitation R and T Center
Seattle, WA 98195
(206) 543-3600

Science for the Handicapped Association (SFHA)
SSS 201
University of Wisconsin–Eau Claire
Eau Claire, WI 54701
(715) 836-4164

> Association members include science educators of students who are emotionally, mentally, physically, or socially handicapped. The association was formed to promote science for all students with disabilities in the schools. This is done through information dissemination at national conferences, publications, and a bibliography on science for students with disabilities. SFHA recently became an Associated Group of the National Science Teachers Association.

TRACE Research and Development Center for the Severely
Communicatively Handicapped
314 Waisman Center
1500 Highland Avenue
Madison, WI 53706
(608) 262-6966

> The TRACE Center works in cooperation with the Communication Aids and Systems Clinic of the University of Wisconsin–Madison to study and develop techniques and aids that augment existing vocal skills of the clinic patient. Information on communication aids and techniques is collected, documented, and disseminated by the Center through publications and is also available on computer database.

Rehabilitation Engineering Center
Undersecretary of State of Rehabilitation
Ministry of Social Affairs
Mugamaa Building, Tahrir Square
Cairo
Egypt

Rehabilitation International
Information Service
Stiftung Rehabilitation
P.O. Box 101 409
D-6900
Heidelberg 1
Germany

> Stiftung Rehabilitation maintains a computerized system of available modified products.

Rehabilitation Engineering Center
Institute of Orthopedic Surgery and Rehabilitation
Academy of Medicine
Dzierzynskiego 135, 61 545 Poznan
Poland

Swedish Engineering Employment Association
Box 5510
S-114 85 Stockholm
Sweden
468 631750
Telex 170 45

> This association has formed a computer-based central information system
> called "Miljobanken," which contains solutions to various work environment
> problems. Members of the Swedish Engineering Employment Association can
> join the "Miljobanken" system free of charge; nonmember firms and institu-
> tions can join for a fee.

Rehabilitation Engineering Center
University of Ljubljana
Department of Electrical Engineering
61001 Ljubljana, Trzaska 25
Yugoslavia

Source: Taken from Tools, Equipment, and Machinery Adapted for the Vocational Education and Employment of Handicapped People (ERIC #ED198272) by John Gugerty, Arona
Faye Roshal, Mary D.J. Tradewell, and Linda Anthony. Originally published in 1981 by
the Wisconsin Vocational Studies Center, University of Wisconsin–Madison; now the Center on Education & Work, School of Education, University of Wisconsin, Madison, WI
53706-1796.

16

Shifting Paradigms in School Environments: Special Education and the Role of the Educator

Kay A. Norlander

The greater integration of special and general education is an educational development long overdue. Effecting it stirs and rearranges an extraordinary political, economic, and educational network of agencies, institutions, and individuals. . . . Significant change affects entire ecosystems, arousing passions, changing human behaviors, and exposing reefs not marked on any charts.

— Goodlad (1993, p. 3)

Special education within the school community is undergoing dramatic changes. For these changes to be both successful and farsighted, educators must share common values about the education of all children in least restrictive environments. Currently, values and attitudes about what a teacher's job is, are not always ones that allow for the full integration of students with disabilities into the educational community. Rather, we continue to find many students with disabilities, including those with mild handicaps to learning, placed in special education settings for large portions of their school day. We justify these pull-out or resource-room programs as beneficial to the learner, when in fact there is little evidence to support the effectiveness of this model of service delivery. Similarly, many students with more severe disabilities are still educated, albeit in public schools, in self-contained arrangements.

If the community is to be effective in changing this paradigm toward the belief that individuals with disabilities can and should be fully integrated into our society, then the place called school is the logical place to start. In fact, most people spend their first formative years in this environment. The configuration of this community shapes attitudes and values and has a lasting effect on each individual's ability to understand and be responsive to diversity.

Historically, persons, in this case children, with disabilities, were largely undereducated in or excluded from public schools. Litigation ending "separate but equal" schools and Brown v. Board of Education (1954) signaled the movement away from school exclusionary practices. This landmark case, about desegregation, formed a base for court cases and legislation in special education. These court cases and laws were also about "desegregation," but this time focused on children with disabilities.

It was almost twenty years after the Brown case that the Pennsylvania Association for Retarded Citizens (PARC), a group led largely by parents, challenged the Commonwealth of Pennsylvania to provide special education services to children with mental retardation. The PARC case, in 1972, was immediately followed by Mills v. Board of Education in the District of Columbia (1972), a case that extended the rights gained in the PARC case to all children with disabilities. Yet it took formal, federal legislation to nationalize equal educational opportunities for children and adults with disabilities. (See Fifield and Fifield, Chapter 3 in this book, for their discussion of legislative influences on services to people with disabilities.)

Ensuring equal access to agencies receiving public funding, including educational, was guaranteed to all persons with disabilities in 1973 by Section 504 of the Rehabilitation Act. This legislation was followed in 1975 by the Education of All Handicapped Children Act (EHA), Public Law 94-142—now called the Individuals with Disabilities Act (IDEA). This law set forth the right of all children, regardless of disability, to be afforded a free, appropriate, public education in the least restrictive environment. Components of this legislation ensured parental participation, individualized educational planning, nondiscriminatory testing, the provision of necessary related services, and the principle of zero reject. This law has been amended a number of times to now include infants and toddlers and has suggested that individual planning also include transition plans.

Most recently, guarantees for persons with disabilities have been extended and reconfirmed with the passage of the Americans with Disabilities Act (ADA) in 1990. "This act guarantees equal access to all aspects of life—not just those that are federally funded—to people with disabilities and implements the concept of normalization" (Smith and Luckasson, 1992, p. 27).

Since the 1950s we have witnessed slow but steady progress; we have become deliberate in our efforts to educate children and adults with disabilities in least restrictive environments. Goodlad and Lovitt (1993, p. v) state:

> Although the mission of enculturating all is at the core a moral one, it is now defined in part by legal terms. There are no legitimate arguments for denying access to knowledge. The educational environments provided in schools are to be minimally restrictive and maximally educative.

But legislation alone will not be enough: the teacher must be informed, skilled, and willing to accommodate diversity in his or her classroom. Acts of Congress and of the courts will guarantee access. Yet unless the professionals directly involved in actualizing these rights are prepared, unless schools are organized to ensure equal opportunities for all, these guarantees may in fact be less than adequate. Shifts in our current paradigms of education, its practice, and its organization must take place across grades and teaching disciplines. These shifts must span ethnic, cultural, and socioeconomic differences as well as be responsive to persons with disabilities.

PHASES OF SCHOOL DESEGREGATION

Institutionalization and School Segregation Ending in the Mid-1970s

The year is 1970. Meet Jeffrey, a five-year-old with cerebral palsy and blindness, who has spent his entire young life in a small institution in Philadelphia. For much of this time Jeffrey has been in a crib, receiving little stimulation. While many of the workers in this institution are caring individuals, they are undereducated for the work that needs to be done with children like Jeffrey, and they are overworked. Consequently, children like Jeffrey are often left alone for long periods of time. Jeffrey is also not included in the public school, nor is he receiving any "educational" services in the institution. In 1971, Jeffrey, now six, begins to go to "school" for the first time. The school is a day care center located within the same community as the institution and is in a local church basement. All of the other students in this center are students with disabilities. The children range in age from three to nine years old. None have ever been in public school. Their disabilities are severe, multiple, and often accompanied by behavioral difficulties. These are a group of children who not only are from minority backgrounds, but also have been concomitantly discriminated against because of disability.

Can you imagine Jeffrey's first day in the day care center, his first ride on a bus, and the teacher's trepidation? Jeffrey spent the first several weeks crying (sometimes screaming) in a corner of the basement classroom. As he had not been held by many people, the teacher's attempts to physically comfort him were of little help. Yet, over time, Jeffrey did make his way out of his corner, beginning on hands and knees to explore his new environment.

Jeffrey's teacher had a background in social work. She learned about Jeffrey's community, his home (the institution), and of course, his local public school. Linking with other community agencies, she found out about his physical and medical conditions, his blindness, and his reported "mental retardation." She asked herself about an IQ of "25" found in a file. What does this mean? How could they have tested this young man, given his present circumstance? She joins the Pennsylvania Association for Retarded Citizens and, along with parents and other concerned professionals, begins the fight against exclusive and discriminatory educational practices.

During the years prior to the PARC case (1972) and P.L. 94-142 (1975), there were many children like Jeffrey who had not been included in our communities or our schools. While Jeffrey was finally outside of his crib and the institution, he continued to live in an institutional setting and was not part of the regular (public) school community. The efforts of groups such as PARC and of forward-thinking legislators helped us begin the movement to deinstitutionalize our schools.

DEINSTITUTIONALIZATION OF SCHOOLING: 1976–1986

The year is 1984 (almost ten years after the passage of P.L. 94-142) and Josh, a fourth-grader with severe learning and reading disabilities, is in trouble. Why is this so and what part have teachers and the organization of his school played in causing Josh to refuse to go to school? Let's first examine Josh's educational history.

Josh began kindergarten at age five and was referred for evaluation by his classroom teacher in February of that year due to "slowness" in learning letters and numbers. At that time his level of "intellectual" functioning was evaluated as "above average" and his identified needs were "successful classroom experiences" and "positive reinforcement." By grade four, Josh still needed the same things. Yet, success was hard to come by; for Josh could not read even first-grade text with fluency and his perceived noncompliance with most classroom (academic) tasks allowed for more "punishment" than "reinforcement." Because Josh has an excellent vocabulary and because he is "smart," the teacher often stated that he "just isn't trying, paying attention, or acting his age."

Back to Josh's educational history. At six years of age Josh moved on to grade one and was subsequently retained in this grade for a second year and received remedial reading services during this second year of first grade. At age eight we find that Josh was in grade two. In the fall of that year he is again evaluated as having "above average intelligence" but is found to be below "expected" levels of performance in reading, written language, and mathematics. The psychologist states, "Although Josh can be expected to achieve at grade level, this has not been the case despite having been retained and despite receiving Chapter I remedial reading."

In grade three Josh was labeled or classified as a student with a learning disability. In the beginning of the year he was placed for most of his day in the third grade, with resource room support. As the year progressed, Josh found it more and more difficult to "keep up" with the class, the teacher became frustrated, and so did Josh. By the end of the year, Josh was spending the majority of the day in the resource room.

Fourth grade begins. The Child Study (Planning and Placement) Team meets, along with Josh's parents, and decides, "due to his significant reading difficulties and his inability to keep up academically with the rest of the class," that he should be placed in a self-contained special education classroom. Many of the students in this class have other presenting difficulties, such as emotional problems and mental retardation. By the middle of this year the parents are convinced that they have made a mistake in allowing Josh to be segregated in this classroom. Clearly his learning problems are not improving and he is now refusing to attend school. His parents are told that they need counseling. When asked, "What three wishes would be?" one of Josh's wishes was "to learn everything quickly so I don't have to go to school." Something is wrong, someone is in trouble; but one should ask, "Is it Josh and his parents or is it the educational system and its teachers who are in trouble?"

Josh's teachers have not done a very good job collaborating with each other, with Josh's parents, or with Josh himself. Yet this lack of communication or collaboration may not be their fault alone. In implementing P.L. 94-142, and in an effort to provide a "least restrictive" education for Josh, we the educational community are still plagued with attitudes about curriculum, excellence, and homogeneity in classrooms. It is difficult to integrate Josh because he is different. The laws have helped—he is in school, he has been evaluated, his parents are involved, and an educational plan is in place. But in putting these services in place, the laws have also, with no malice or intent, fostered new layers of segregation: self-contained classrooms, resource rooms, and other pull-out programs designed to provide a continuum or "cascade" of services from least restrictive (the regular classroom with no support) to most restrictive (an institutional setting) (Deno, 1970; Reynolds, 1973).

In the case of Josh, it is important to review the legal meaning of least restrictive environment (LRE). Public Law 94-142 (IDEA) defines LRE as follows:

> . . . to the extent appropriate, handicapped children, including children in public or private institutions or other care facilities, are educated with children who are not handicapped, and that special classes, separate schooling, or other removal of handicapped children from the regular education environment occurs only when the nature or severity of the handicap is such that education in regular classes with the use of supplementary aids and services cannot be achieved satisfactorily. . . . [20 U.S.C., section 1412(5)(B)]

For Josh, the legal issue became one of what was least restrictive. The use of supplemental aids had not been adequately explored, and a state hearing officer ruled that Josh should be educated in the regular classroom with appropriate curricular modifications and support services.

The Era of Community Integration: Effects on School Practice (1986–Present)

Since 1986 and Madeleine Will's controversial stance on mainstreaming, the Regular Education Initiative (REI) (Will, 1986a, 1986b), the educational community and parent advocacy groups have debated the meaning of least restrictive environment and the extent to which children with disabilities should be included in regular classroom settings. Will's position is that our dual system of service delivery is neither efficient nor effective. Many (Lilly, 1986; Reynolds, Wang, and Walberg, 1987; Stainback and Stainback, 1985; Wang, 1987) agreed with Will's position on consolidating services for students with disabilities into regular classroom settings, thus forming "partnership[s] between regular education and special programs and the blending of the intrinsic strengths of both systems" (Will, 1986b, p. 12). This group of authors, along with Will, would "argue that regular education can accommodate 'the full range and types of exceptional children' [Wang, 1987, p. 7]" (in Holcutt, Martin, and McKinney, 1991). Yet others have disagreed with Will, pointing to the lack of involvement by regular educators themselves in the Regular Education Initiative (Lieberman, 1985; Messinger, 1985). Lieberman (1985) argued that Will's proposal had not included regular educators and therefore was flawed from the outset. He likened the REI to a wedding to which the bride (regular education) had not been invited. But thanks to people like Mara Sapon-Shevin (1992a, 1992b), who offers "marriage counseling" to the two partners of the marriage, regular and special educators are beginning to talk to one another and work toward shared responsibility in the education of all children.

More recently there has been a further movement in the cycle of mainstreaming efforts called "Inclusive Education" (see Slee, 1991; Villa, Thousand, Stainback, and Stainback, 1992). This form of mainstreaming or integration would see every child, no matter how severe the disability, educated with appropriate supports, in the regular classroom with age peers. While this is difficult to envision, where implemented with forethought, administrative support, teacher education, parental involvement, and support service, it has been shown to be a successful method of integration.

Regardless of philosophical position, the shift in thinking and practice must be one that stresses maximum inclusion. Consequently, as we approach the twenty-first century, it is the hope of many that our schools will look dramatically different; that students like Norma, a young girl with developmental disabilities, will be able to be educated in her local public school, in a classroom with other children of like age; that the educational environment would be one of accommodation and acceptance; and that diversity in the ways in which children learn and play be seen as a benefit rather than a hindrance. Let's visit Norma, seven years old and in the second grade.

Norma has a number of characteristics that might be considered "different" from those of the "average" second grader. Norma has very limited speech and uses a communication board to express herself. She does this with minimal success, but is getting better at making her needs, learnings, and wishes known. Norma has been classified as a student with mental retardation. Norma loves to listen to music, play with her classmates, and help others. While Norma does not read like other second graders, she does participate in language arts activities while the other students in her class are working on reading, writing, and spelling. Part of the reason for her successful integration is the teacher's reorganization of the classroom using a whole language approach to the teaching of reading (see Fisher and Hiebert, 1990; Goodman, 1990; Palincsar and Klenk, 1993). This approach allows for the integration of reading across subject areas and puts much less emphasis on the homogeneous grouping of students. Norma's teacher is also committed to incorporating the philosophies and techniques of cooperative learning (see Johnson and Johnson, 1989; Slavin, 1991; Slavin and Stevens, 1991) into her classroom. These classroom reorganizations and instructional techniques allow her to be flexible in accommodating the individual differences of her students.

Norma has been fully included in public school classrooms since kindergarten. She is fortunate to have parents who insisted on her total integration from the start of school. At first the school was quite anxious about this parental request, feeling that a self-contained special education classroom within the school building would be the "least restrictive environment" for Norma. Norma's parents cited sections of P.L. 94-142, reminding us that it was possible that Norma could be educated in the regular classroom with supplemental aids and support services. The school and the teachers, both general and special, were convinced, and appropriate support services, including a classroom aide and speech and language assistance, were put in place. The MAPS program was used as a model in formulating services for Norma that included not only the traditional planning team, but also her brothers and other children, "friends," at the school. This "planning process [is] used to facilitate full participation for children with challenging educational needs" (Forest and Lusthaus, 1990, p. 32). (For more information on the MAPS—Map Action Planning System see Forest and Snow, 1987.) Without the careful coordination among school professionals—including the building administrator—and Norma's parents, her siblings, and classmates and friends, her inclusion in second grade might not have been successful; it could have in fact been more restrictive.

Inclusive educational models are becoming more widely advocated and implemented, allowing for students like Norma, Josh, and Jeffrey to be educated in regular education settings. (For three excellent case studies of school systems committed to the philosophy of inclusive education, see Kaskinen-Chapman, 1992; Schattman, 1992; Stainback, Stainback, Moravec and Jackson, 1992; all found in the text *Restructuring for Caring and Effective Education: An Administrative Guide to Creating Heterogeneous Schools*, 1992, edited by Villa, Thousand, Stainback, and Stainback.) But for these models of integration to be widespread and accepted among teachers and other school professionals, significant changes in teacher preparation and school organization must take place.

WHERE EDUCATION NEEDS TO MAKE SIGNIFICANT CHANGES

Teacher Roles and Their Preparation

Clearly there is a need for teachers who can facilitate the integration of students with disabilities into their classrooms and school communities. The examination of traditional teaching roles is essential if integration of all children is to be an effective practice. The role of the "special" educator must be more effectively linked with that of the "regular" educator. New ways of fostering this "shared responsibility" must begin early in the preprofessionals' preparation and carry on into continued professional practice.

> New staff roles must be developed so that teachers may more readily work together to improve instruction and so that experienced and talented teachers can support beginning teachers, plan and develop new curricula, or design and implement staff development (O'Neil, 1990, p. 6).

Unfortunately, most teacher preparation programs separate their students by area of teaching discipline (Goodlad and Field, 1993; Lilly, 1986; Sarason and Doris, 1979; among others). Sarason and Doris analyzed the "gulf" between regular and special educators in 1979, yet not enough has changed in the ensuing years. They remind us that

> . . . school personnel are graduates of our colleges and universities. It is there that they learn there are at least two types of human beings (handicapped and non-handicapped) and if you choose to work with one of them you render yourself legally and conceptually incompetent to work with the other (p. 391).

The separate preparation of teachers who work with children with and without disabilities must end:

> . . . the facts do indicate that special educators and regular educators have jointly participated in a system that has divided and separated teachers in the same way that it has categorized and isolated students (Sapon-Shevin, 1988, p. 106).

Sapon-Shevin suggests that the lack of "parallel discourse" between the two, often distinct, teaching professions is an impediment to educational reform as it impacts the integration of students with disabilities. Others such as Davis (1989) would agree that a lack of discussion among colleagues within both schools and schools of education is a major hindrance to reform. Therefore, there is an obvious need for a more collaborative model of teacher preparation.

It has become quite apparent that special educators must be prepared to accept new responsibilities in a collaborative model of education. Reynolds, Wang, and Walberg (1987) propose that the categorization of students has inadvertently forced the concomitant categorization of teachers, advocacy groups, and funding systems. Consequently, the need is not only for regular educators to become prepared to accept students with handicaps into their classrooms, but also for special educators to be ready, willing, and—most important—able to assist in this effort (Sapon-Shevin, 1988). Too often it is the special educator who hides behind labels or categories (Shepard, 1987; Stainback, Stainback, Courtnage, and Jaben, 1985). Lilly (1987) suggests that special educators must view themselves as integral parts of the "general education community." Our schools of education must foster this attitude through both coursework and practice.

The improvement of student performance and the ability of a school to provide innovative and successful educational experiences are predicated on the quality of the teachers empowered to orchestrate and deliver instruction. The direct interactions between a teacher and his or her pupils is paramount to the success or failure of many students (Trueba, 1989). To fill this critical role, teachers must be afforded professional preparation committed to diversity, individualization, and integration. In examining regular education's readiness to accommodate students with learning problems, the Baker and Zigmond (1990) study cuts to the heart of the matter. Their findings suggest that while many teachers are willing, their instructional techniques are based on traditional practices such as following the sequence of instruction found in the text; routines for all, not for individuals; whole class instruction; undifferentiated assignments; and worksheets, control, and conformity. Baker and Zigmond (1990, pp. 525–526) summarize the problem in the following way:

> Teachers cared about children and were conscientious about their job—but their mind-set was conformity, not accommodation. In these regular education classes, any student who could not conform would likely be unsuccessful. It is not surprising that students who displayed persistent behavior problems or who were noisy or off task during the extended periods of independent seatwork were referred out for special education.

Clearly, teachers must not only learn to work with one another in a coordinated effort to make school more accessible for all, but they must also acquire new techniques for accommodating instructional diversity. But this will also require that school structures allow teachers to be able to take on this challenge.

School Reform and Reorganization

In addition to enabling teachers to work more effectively, together, and for changes in current instructional organizations to occur, there is a need for "special education" to be more fully integrated into the broader context of school reform. Sapon-Shevin (1987) cautions that conflicts are implicit in the "goal of excellence." In an era of continual calls for reform, restructuring, and excellence, we must bear in mind that excellence for all must be sensitive to individuals for whom traditionally conceived measures of excellence may be a form of discrimination (Holcutt, Martin, and McKinney, 1991; Sapon-Shevin, 1987; Shaw et al., 1990; Toch, 1984). We must be conscious of the parallels between discourse on school reform and the restructuring of special education services (Audette and Algozzine, 1992; Sailor, 1991; Skrtic, 1991) and begin to work together in this process of equal access and the reorganization of schooling. Sailor (1991, p. 18) suggests,

> Those special educators associated with, or indeed committed to, the current directions in reform, such as those indicated by LRE mandate for social and academic integration and the retention of special education students in general education classrooms, might well consider forming a strong alliance with the school restructuring process under way in the dominant reform movement within general education. With an increasing likelihood of further progress in special education reform being closely linked with (if not co-opted by) processes of change in the bigger picture of general school organizational reform, an opportunity exists to realign all educational systems to work more effectively and efficiently for all children at the school site.

Efforts to reorganize schools to better accommodate the diverse and changing population found in America's schools are essential. Audette and Algozzine (1992), in an article discussing the "transformation of American public education" as it interfaces with the "free and appropriate education of all students," state,

> School reform is a dominant force in contemporary education. What happens in the next few years as a result of this movement to improve our schools may determine, in fact, what an "appropriate" education is and whether students with disabilities will be "appropriately" educated in the schools of the next century (p. 8).

Thus, as school reform and restructuring efforts reconfigure our buildings and classrooms for all children, we clearly must have teachers who understand the needs of students with disabilities as well as the organization of schools. If not, we will perpetuate the absence of special education concerns in our discussions on educational reform (Ferguson, 1989). In this regard, the restructuring of teacher preparation programs is tightly linked to the success of school change (Carnegie, 1986; Case, Lanier, and Miskel,

1986; Goodlad, 1984; The Holmes Group, 1986; National Commission on Excellence in Education, 1983).

WHAT CAN EDUCATORS DO TO FOSTER INCLUSIVE EDUCATIONAL PRACTICES?

Within the context of restructured schools and changes in the way teachers are prepared for the role of professional educator, there are a number of critical variables that will foster shared decision making, collaboration, and thus more effective methods of integrating students with diversity into the classroom. While these variables are numerous, several are essential.

Foster Positive Attitudes toward Diversity

The attitudes held by each of us about diversity greatly influence the complexion of our communities. As students with disabilities are more likely to be included in general education settings, the attitudes held about these individuals and their right to inclusion must be addressed openly. When teachers view the inclusion of students with differences as a problem rather than a challenge, then efforts to integrate these individuals will be unsuccessful. Similarly, when parents of the general education population view integration as something that takes away from their sons or daughters, we will face another roadblock to the creation of equity in education.

Hilliard (1991) asks the educational community and society at large if "we have the will to educate all children." He relates this discussion to the issues of school restructuring, attitude toward diversity, and excellence for all. He states,

> To restructure we must first look deeply at the goals that we set for our children and the beliefs that we have about them. Once we are on the right track there, then we must turn our attention to the delivery systems, as we have begun to do. Decentralization is right. Cooperative learning is right. Technology access for all is right. Multiculturalism is right. But none of these approaches or strategies will mean anything if the fundamental belief system does not fit the new structures that are being created (p. 36).

Encourage Collaboration among Educators

Collaboration among teachers, parents, administrators, as well as other related services personnel is essential to the successful integration of students with disabilities into school communities (Morsink and Lenk, 1992; see Rainforth et al., Chapter 7, this book). Models of collaboration have ranged from consultation to team teaching. Imbedded in all of these is a philosophy of shared responsibility for the education of all students. Collaborative teams have been suggested as a powerful method for creating restructured schools (Thousand and Villa, 1992). Yet, in many cases, the special educator or other "specialist" is an advice giver rather than a player in the delivery of educational service. This "consultation" model of collaboration does not lend itself to team members working together on a regular basis in the instructional process. Pugach and Johnson (1991) provide an excellent discussion of this problem. They debate the relationship between consultation and collaboration, citing the many problems with our current, hierarchical practice of consultation. They suggest that educators and other related services professions must learn how to "deliberate" together.

> Only in the context of joint deliberation does consultation have the potential to change the way adults interact in schools. In our opinion, consultation will never be successful as long as it represents special education's answers to the problems of general education. We must develop a partnership in which problems and solutions are shared equally. With joint deliberation as the guiding principle toward the development of such a partnership, the goal of collaboration—which places special education as a lateral, not a vertical, source of assistance—is surely within our grasp (pp. 88–89).

Engender Administrative Support

The support of school administration is essential to changing our current school organization, thereby creating not only an atmosphere of acceptance for diversity, but also one that lends itself structurally to integration. Leadership that is based on models of shared decision making (see Gardner, Chapter 6, this book; Hess, 1992; Maeroff, 1993; Provenzo, 1989) will encourage teachers to take responsibility for their classrooms and their students. Further, it makes teachers equal partners in the organization and operation of their school. As medical doctors typically have a significant say in the operation of the hospital they choose to be affiliated with, teachers must have input into the decisions that affect the running of the school in which they work. In a discussion of this form of leadership, Case and Shibles (1990, p. 19) suggest that,

> For restructuring to occur, leadership needs to be built on shared authority and responsibility, not on delegated authority and responsibility. In the broad sense this means investing power in others and increasing their own opportunities

for authority, responsibility, choice, and influence. . . . Leadership in restructured schools involves providing maximum involvement of individuals and groups, encouraging initiative taking, creating a culture of cooperation, cultivating connection, building capacity, and developing a professional problem-solving capacity.

Create Flexibility in Curriculum Demands and Grouping Practices

Homogeneous grouping and standard curricula are two common school practices that are culprits in the segregation of students, one from another. The issues of curriculum and grouping practices are inextricably intertwined. Much of the segregation that has taken place in schools has been "well intentioned." Moving students with handicaps into isolated classrooms with other children with learning problems was an alternative to modifying the curriculum within the regular classroom. Although this model did provide individualized instruction to the student with disabilities, it failed to create an environment for that individual that would allow for normal social development and in many cases disallowed the individual from reaching his or her full potential academically.

There are numerous cases of students with learning disabilities who have not been afforded the necessary high school curriculum to enter college, even though they had the "potential" to succeed in this type of curriculum. Likewise, students with behavior disorders are often segregated due to their "misbehaviors." Yet these grouping practices provide the student with few positive behaviors to model. As stated earlier, while these practices were initially well intentioned,

> It seems, however, that we have been quite guilty of trying to educate those with disabilities by moving them away from the regular curriculum via a separate special education track. In doing so, we have succeeded in isolating the students physically and socially and have severely limited their opportunity for exposure to the established regular education curriculum (White and White, 1993, pp. 91–93).

Institute Alternative Assessment Practices

Student evaluation is an integral part of the teacher's job. Teachers, parents, and, of course, the students themselves need to know what has been learned and what should be taught next. The evaluation of students based upon standard criteria is common practice. Teachers evaluate their students on a daily basis. They also, at given periods of time (e.g., the end of an instructional unit or the end of the marking period), test their students to evaluate progress. School systems and states have similar practices. They will evaluate the "success" of their schools based on the collective test scores of all of the students in a given group. When these evaluations are based solely on standardized tests of achievement, a very narrow picture of productivity or potential is painted. This scenario of "testing" must therefore be expanded to encompass a more comprehensive assessment model. We need not throw away the concept of evaluation; it is an important one. But we must begin to view evaluation in a much broader context. The assessment of individual differences is an important educational practice and, in fact, for persons with disabilities, is a requirement of P.L. 94-142. Yet even in this specific case of assessment, current practice still relies heavily on an evaluation model that is "test" based. Competent diagnosticians would be looking for much more information than just a test score. They would be searching for clues to a problem. Similarly, they might be attempting to determine why a particular line to treatment has been successful.

It is clear that the identification of a student's strengths and weaknesses within the school environment is a necessary and important practice, yet many current assessment or evaluation procedures have not changed along with other curriculum and organizational reforms. The educational system is making strides in accommodating diversity in the classroom. If this is to continue, assessment practices must do more than simply group, label, or classify students; they must shift toward the use of varied assessment techniques that search for a student's learning capabilities as well as areas that may require additional, different, or modified instruction. Alternative forms of assessment include situational assessment, observational procedures, curriculum-based assessment, authentic assessment (such as portfolios), and outcome-based assessments.

No matter which form of assessment is chosen, care must be taken to ensure that test procedures are not affected by the individual's disability. If they are, they would be biased and discriminatory. Overton (1992, p. 31) states,

> Assessment can be discriminatory . . . The laws mandate that the instruments used to assess one skill or area do not discriminate or unduly penalize a student because of an existing handicap[ping] condition. For example, a student who is referred for reading difficulties should not be penalized on a test that requires the student to pronounce nonsense syllables because a speech articulation problem is present.

In our efforts to ensure the right to an evaluation, the evaluation team must always remember that the goal is not simply classification, but also the "diagnosis" of the particulars such that a student can be better educated.

CONCLUSION

For the paradigm shifts discussed in this chapter to take place, teachers will need to be empowered to make choices about the learning that occurs in their classrooms. Teachers must find their own voice in the change process and must be allowed to "take control." "Taking control of one's justifications involves reflection on practices, that is, on activities and their theoretical frameworks, and an ability to articulate them to others in a meaningful way" (Richardson, 1990, p. 16).

In the final analysis, ensuring equal access to education for all students may be as much a matter of values as of preparation. Fundamental beliefs and assumptions about persons with "disabilities" must shift from those that foster segregated service delivery systems to ones that ensure equity in education. And, given the challenge of educating an increasingly diverse population of students, new foundations of thinking and practice must be built. We must find in our schools, including postsecondary educational settings, teachers who are willing and able to make appropriate curricular adaptations and who understand the diversity of learners in their classrooms.

We must break barriers among teachers, redesign curricula that will allow access to learning for a larger range of students, make strong commitments to preparing teachers differently, and recruit a teaching force from diverse backgrounds who possess both analytical skills and compassion for people. If the current educational culture, influenced by personal attitude and school organization, has fostered much of what continues to segregate and isolate students from educational opportunities, then we must begin to challenge these attitudes and organizations. We must take bold new looks at the needs of the school and the individual. We will need to conduct business very differently. We will need to work together; this will be hard work—changing basic beliefs and habits always is. Valuing diversity will not be easy; yet it is our moral obligation to try.

REFERENCES

Americans with Disabilities Act of 1990. P.L. 101-336.

Audette, B., and Algozzine, B. (1992). Free and appropriate education for all students: Total quality and the transformation of American public education. *Remedial and Special Education, 13*(6), 8–18.

Baker, J., and Zigmond, N. (1990). Are regular education classes equipped to accommodate students with learning disabilities? *Exceptional Children, 56*(6), 515–527.

Brown v. Board of Education, 347 U.S. 483 (1954).

Carnegie Forum on Education and the Economy (1986). *A nation prepared: Teachers for the 21st century.* Washington, DC: Author.

Case, C.W., Lanier, J.E., and Miskel, C.G. (1986). The Holmes Group report: Impetus for gaining professional status for teachers. *Journal of Teacher Education, 37*(4), July–August, 36–43.

Case, C.W., and Shibles, M. (1990). Restructuring schools: A review. Occasional Paper I, Connecticut Leadership Academy.

Davis, E.W. (1989). The Regular Education Initiative debate: Its promises and problems. *Exceptional Children, 55*(4), 440–446.

Deno, E. (1970). Special education as developmental capital. *Exceptional Children, 37,* 229–237.

Education of All Handicapped Children Act (1975). 20 U.S.C. sections 1400 et seq. and amendments.

Ferguson, D.L. (1989). Severity of need and educational excellence: Public school reform and students with disabilities. In D. Biklen, D. Ferguson, and A. Ford (Eds.), *Schooling and disability: Eighty-eighth yearbook of the National Society for the Study of Education* (pp. 25–58). Chicago: University of Chicago Press.

Fifield, B. and Fifield, M. (1995). The influence of legislation on services to people with disabilities. In O.C. Karan and S. Greenspan (Eds). *Community rehabilitation services for people with disabilities.* Boston: Butterworth–Heinemann.

Fisher, C.W., and Hiebert, E.H. (1990). Characteristics of tasks in two teaching approaches to literacy instruction. *Elementary School Journal, 91*(1), 3–18.

Forest, M., and Lusthaus, E. (1990). Everyone belongs with the MAPS action planning system. *Teaching Exceptional Children,* Winter, 32–35.

Forest, M., and Snow, J. (1987). *More educational integration.* Toronto: G. Allan Rocher Institute.

Gardner, J.F. (1995). Maintaining quality and managing change: Administration in transition. In O.C. Karan and S. Greenspan (Eds.). *Community rehabilitation services for people with disabilities.* Boston: Butterworth–Heinemann.

Goodlad, J.I. (1984). *A place called school.* New York: McGraw-Hill.

Goodlad, J.I. (1993). Access to knowledge. In J.I. Goodlad and T.C. Lovitt (Eds.), *Integrating general and special education* (pp. 1–22). New York: Macmillan.

Goodlad, J.I., and Field, S. (1993). Teachers for renewing schools. In J.I. Goodlad and T.C. Lovitt (Eds.), *Integrating general and special education* (pp. 229–252). New York: Macmillan.

Goodlad, J.I., and Lovitt, T.C. (Eds.) (1993). *Integrating general and special education.* New York: Macmillan.

Goodman, K. (1990). Whole-language research: Foundations and developments. *Elementary School Journal, 90,* 207–221.

Hess, G.A. (Ed.) (1992). *Empowering teachers and parents: School restructuring through the eyes of anthropologists.* Westport, CT: Bergen and Garvey.

Hilliard, A., III (1991). Do we have the will to educate all children? *Educational Leadership,* September, 31–36.

Holcutt, A.M., Martin, E.W., and McKinney, J.D. (1991). Historical and legal context of mainstreaming. In J.W. Lloyd, N.N. Singh, and A.C. Repp (Eds.), *The Regular Education Initiative: Alternative perspectives on concepts, issues, and models.* Sycamore, IL: Sycamore Publishing.

The Holmes Group (1986). *Tomorrow's teachers.* East Lansing, MI: Author.

Johnson, D.W., and Johnson, R.T. (1989). *Leading the cooperative school.* Edina, MN: Interaction Book Co.

Kaskinen-Chapman, A. (1992). Saline Area Schools and inclusive community CONCEPTS [Collaborative Organization of Networks: Community Educators, Parents, The Workplace, and Students]. In R.A. Villa, J.S. Thousand, W. Stainback, and S. Stainback (Eds.), *Restructuring for caring and effective education: An administrative guide to creating heterogeneous schools* (pp. 169–185). Baltimore: Paul H. Brookes.

Lieberman, L.M. (1985). Special education and regular education: A merger made in heaven? *Exceptional Children, 51*(6), 513–516.

Lilly, M.S. (1986). The relationship between general and special education: A new face on an old issue. *Counterpoint, 6,* 10.

Lilly, M.S. (1987). Lack of focus on special education in literature on educational reform. *Exceptional Children, 53*(4), 325–326.

Maeroff, G.I. (1993). *Team building for school change: Equipping teachers for new roles.* New York: Teachers College Press.

Messinger, J.F. (1985). Commentary on a rationale for the merger of regular and special education or, Is it now time for the lamb to lie down with the lion? *Exceptional Children, 51*(6), 510–512.

Mills v. Board of Education of the District of Columbia, 348 F. Supp. 866 (1972).

Morsink, C.V., and Lenk, L.L. (1992). The delivery of special education programs and services. *Remedial and Special Education, 13*(6), 33–43.

National Commission on Excellence in Education (1983). *A nation at risk: The imperative for educational reform.* Washington, DC: U.S. Government Printing Office.

O'Neil, J.W. (1990). Piecing together the restructuring puzzle. *Educational Leadership, 47*(7), 4–10.

Overton, T. (1992). *Assessment in special education: An applied approach.* New York: Merrill.

Palincsar, A.S., and Klenk, L. (1993). Third invited response: Broader visions encompassing literacy, learners, and contexts. *Remedial and Special Education,* 14(4), 19–25.

Pennsylvania Association for Retarded Children v. Commonwealth of Pennsylvania, 343 F. Supp. 279 (E.D. Pa., 1972).

Provenzo, E.F., Jr. (1989). School based management and shared-decisionmaking in the Dade County Public School. In J.M. Rosow and R. Zager (Eds.), *Allies in educational reform.* San Francisco: Jossey Bass.

Pugach, M. (1987). The national education reports and special education: Implications for teacher preparation. *Exceptional Children,* 53(4), 308–314.

Pugach, M.C., and Johnson, L.J. (1991). Rethinking the relationship between consultation and collaborative problem solving. In E. Meyen, G.A. Vergason, and R.J. Whelan (Eds.), *Challenges facing special education* (pp. 79–90). Denver: Love Publishing.

Rainforth, B., Giangreco, M.F., Smith, P.D. and York, J. (1995). Collaborative teamwork in training and technical assistance: Enhancing community support for persons with disabilities. In O.C. Karan and S. Greenspan (Eds.) *Community rehabilitation services for people with disabilities.* Boston: Butterworth–Heinemann.

Rehabilitation Act of 1973, Section 504, 19 U.S.C. section 794.

Reynolds, M. (1973). Two policy statements approved by CEC delegate assembly. *Exceptional Children, 40,* 71.

Reynolds, M., Wang, M., and Walberg, H. (1987). The necessary restructuring of special and regular education. *Exceptional Children, 53*(5), 391–398.

Richardson, V. (1990). Significant and worthwhile change in teaching practice. *Educational Researcher, 19*(7), 10–18.

Sailor, W. (1991). Special education and the restructured school. *Remedial and Special Education, 12*(6), 8–22.

Sapon-Shevin, M. (1987). The national reports and special education: Implications for students. *Exceptional Children, 53*(4), 300–307.

Sapon-Shevin, M. (1988). Working towards merger together: Seeing beyond distrust and fear. *Teacher Education and Special Education, 11,* 103–110.

Sapon-Shevin, M. (1992a). Introduction. In R.A. Villa, J.S. Thousand, W. Stainback, and S. Stainback (Eds.), *Restructuring for caring and effective education: An administrative guide to creating heterogeneous schools* (pp. xvii–xx). Baltimore: Paul H. Brookes.

Sapon-Shevin, M. (1992b). Marriage advice. In R.A. Villa, J.S. Thousand, W. Stainback, and S. Stainback (Eds.), *Restructuring for caring and effective education: An administrative guide to creating heterogeneous schools* (pp. 3–5). Baltimore: Paul H. Brookes.

Sarason, S.B., and Doris, J. (1979). *Educational handicap, public policy, and social history.* New York: Free Press.

Schattman, R. (1992). The Franklin Northwest Supervisory Union: A case study of an inclusive school system. In R.A. Villa, J.S. Thousand, W. Stainback, and S. Stainback (Eds.), *Restructuring for caring and effective education: An administrative guide to creating heterogeneous schools* (pp. 143–159). Baltimore: Paul H. Brookes.

Shaw, S.F., Biklen, D., Conlon, S., Dunn, J., Kramer, J., and DeRoma-Wagner, V. (1990). Special education and school reform. In L.M. Bullock and R.I. Simpson (Eds.), *Critical issues in special education: Implications for personnel preparation* (pp. 12–25). Denton, TX: University of North Texas.

Shepard, L.A. (1987). The new push for excellence: Widening the schism between regular and special education. *Exceptional Children, 53*(4), 327–329.

Skrtic, T.M. (1991). The special education paradox: Equity as the way to excellence. *Harvard Educational Review, 61*(2), 148–206.

Slavin, R.E. (1991). Synthesis of research on cooperative learning. *Educational Leadership, 48*(5), 71–82.

Slavin, R.E., and Stevens, R.J. (1991). Cooperative learning and mainstreaming. In J.W. Lloyd, N.N. Singh, and A.C. Repp (Eds.), *The Regular Education Initiative: Alternative perspectives on concepts, issues, and models.* Sycamore, IL: Sycamore Publishing.

Slee, R. (1991). Learning initiatives to include all students in regular schools. In M. Ainscow (Ed.), *Effective schools for all* (pp. 43–67). London: David Fulton Publishers.

Smith, D.D., and Luckasson, R. (1992). *Introduction to special education: Teaching in an age of challenge.* Boston: Allyn and Bacon.

Stainback, S., and Stainback, W. (1985). The merger of special and regular education: Can it be done? A response to Lieberman and Messinger. *Exceptional Children, 51*(6), 517–521.

Stainback, W., Stainback, S., Courtnage, L., and Jaben, T. (1985). Facilitating mainstreaming by modifying the mainstream. *Exceptional Children, 52*(2), 144–152.

Stainback, W., Stainback, S., Moravec, J., and Jackson, H.J. (1992). Concerns about full inclusion: An ethnographic investigation. In R.A. Villa, J.S. Thousand, W. Stainback, and S. Stainback (Eds.), *Restructuring for caring and effective education: An administrative guide to creating heterogeneous schools* (pp. 305–324). Baltimore: Paul H. Brookes.

Thousand, J.S., and Villa, R.S. (1992). Collaborative teams: A powerful tool in school restructuring. In R.A. Villa, J.S. Thousand, W. Stainback, and S. Stainback (Eds.), *Restructuring for caring and effective education: An administrative guide to creating heterogeneous schools* (pp. 73–108). Baltimore: Paul H. Brookes.

Toch, T. (1984). The dark side of the excellence movement. *Phi Delta Kappan,* November, 173–176.

Trueba, H. (1989). Culture, selfhood, and standardization. *The Holmes Group Forum, 2*(3). East Lansing, MI: Author.

Villa, R.A., Thousand, J.S., Stainback, W., and Stainback, S. (Eds.) (1992). *Restructuring for caring and effective education: An administrative guide to creating heterogeneous schools.* Baltimore: Paul H. Brookes.

Wang, M. (1987). *Implementing the integration mandate of the Education of All Handicapped Children Act of 1975.* Paper presented at the Bush colloquium on policy implementation. Chapel Hill, NC.

White, A.E., and White, L.L. (1993). A collaborative model for students with mild disabilities in middle schools. In E. Meyen, G.A. Vergason, and R.J. Whelan (Eds.), *Challenges facing special education* (pp. 91–104). Denver: Love Publishing.

Will, M.C. (1986a). Educating children with learning problems: A shared responsibility. *Exceptional Children, 52*(5), 411–416.

Will, M.C. (1986b). *Educating children with learning problems: A shared responsibility. A report to the Secretary.* Washington, DC: U.S. Department of Education, Office of Special Education and Rehabilitation Services.

17

The Psychiatrist's Role in the Care and Treatment of Individuals with Disabilities: Changing Paradigms

Frank J. Menolascino

INTRODUCTION

Since the time of Itard's work with the Wild Boy of Aveyron, psychiatry has had many opportunities to more fully understand human existence and its fundamental concerns. Yet the history of the care and treatment of individuals with disabilities has had cycles of hope and despair. Psychiatry has been a major influence in this history. At times, new light has been shed on human vulnerabilities and ways to bring human fulfillment, joy, and interdependence. At other times, oppression and dehumanization has ruled.

In the hopeful cycles, there has been probing into the meaning and purpose of life, the hunger for feelings of companionship, the impact of aloneness and emotional loss, and the dynamic role of the family and community in the lives of vulnerable individuals. In the darker cycles, individuals with disabilities passed through periods wherein isolation, segregation, and dehumanization vanquished integration, respect, and dignity.

This chapter reviews the history of psychiatry from the time of Itard's work with Victor, "The Wild Boy of Aveyron," to the present day. This analysis also points out the underlying value systems that were prevalent in various periods as well as the major clinical and programmatic structures that resulted from such belief systems. Finally, this chapter examines in depth the current ideological and subsequent clinical and programmatic shifts that are guiding psychiatry in its care and treatment of individuals with disabilities.

AN ERA OF HOPE

Psychiatrists as Educators

In the early part of the nineteenth century, Itard (1832), a pupil of the Parisian psychiatrist Pinel, published a report on his five-year project of "educating the mind" of Victor, the "Wild Boy of Aveyron" (Itard, 1832). Victor was, in all probability, a child with severe mental retardation who had been abandoned by his family. Itard took the child under his care, and his subsequent report sparked the beginning of scientific concern with disabilities as a challenge in biology, sociology, education, and psychiatry.

Prior to his work with Victor, Itard had dedicated his career to the education of individuals who were deaf based on philosophical commitment to the Cartesian theory of the mind as a *tabula rasa*. Itard was convinced that Victor could be educated by a system of sensory input and habit training. His report revealed his recognition of the significance of motivation, needs, and transference in his work with the child. This report is the first detailed published monograph on dynamic psychotherapy in an individual with mental retardation.

After Itard's pioneering work, Seguin (1846), a Parisian neuropsychiatrist, opened the world's first school for children with disabilities. This was soon followed by similar schools across the continent and England. Seguin based his pedagogy on Itard's work and described his approach as a program of physical, intellectual, and moral training (Seguin, 1846).

Meanwhile, in the United States Dorothea Dix and others were describing institutional conditions in which individuals were destitute of appropriate care and protection, bound with chains, tied by ropes, and beaten with rods. Howe, a Boston neuropsychiatrist inspired by Seguin's work, set out to establish special schools and asylums with Seguin's guidance. Once psychiatrists and others perceived the needs of individuals with disabilities and were able to implement a hopeful training approach, schools and institutions began to spring up.

The early part of the nineteenth century opened an era of hope for "educating the minds of idiots." Wolfensberger (1969) termed the early period (1850–1880) one of "making the deviant undeviant." This period emphasized increasing adaptive skills and strengthening the individual's will: substituting capacities for incapacities and substituting burdens of society with contributors. Wilbur (1852) pointed out that these early institutions were designed to help the person become "more capable of self-assistance, of self-support, of self-respect, and of obtaining the greatest degree or comfort and happiness with their small means." Hope prevailed. Yet a differentiation had begun to creep into this hopeful outlook. Howe (1849) warned against making his Massachusetts institution an establishment for incurables; instead, he defined it as a temporary boarding school solely for children able to return to the community. Howe (1849) urged public policy that excluded "the epileptic or insane children."

A PARADIGM OF DESPAIR

Psychiatrists as Protectors

The rationale for institutional care slowly began to change in the last part of the nineteenth century. It became increasingly difficult for institutions to live up to the promise of making each individual a productive member of society. Fernald (1892) commented: "We find the superintendents regretting that it was not expedient to return to the community a certain number of cases who had received all the instruction the school had to offer." Pity slowly replaced benevolence and protection substituted for training. Fernald (1912) described the rationale for psychiatry to take a preeminent role in the care of individuals with disabilities since the rationale of institutions was changing from training to custodial care: "The biological, economic, and sociological bearings of feeble-mindedness have overshadowed the fact that it is fundamentally and essentially a medical question."

The rationale for long-term care came about slowly. Although the early hospital–schools had a record of successfully reintegrating individuals into the community, there were some who could not become productive members of society, plus, as Wolfensberger (1976) pointed out, many residents had no home to return to and thus had to remain in the institution. Thus, a rationale evolved for long-term care. Fernald (1892) stated, "It gradually became evident that a certain number of these higher grade cases needed life-long care and supervision, and that there was no suitable provision for this permanent custody outside these special institutions." Pity and paternalistic charity began to replace the earlier developmental model that had evolved between 1870 and 1880.

Psychiatrists became key leaders in a growing national system of state hospitals and gave little objection to the change from a psycho-pedagogical service model to a medical one. Each hospital-school had a superintendent, always a physician, and generally a psychiatrist. Living units were supervised by nurses. Residents were kept under the controlling watch of nursing stations. Residents were viewed as patients. Butler (1883) described the new ideology as: "Give them an asylum, with good and kind treatment; but not a school. A well-fed, well-cared idiot, is a happy idiot." Johnson (1897) posited the rationale for the asylum: "They must be kept quietly, safely away from the world, living like angels in heaven, neither marrying, nor given in marriage."

By the beginning of the twentieth century, the institution had evolved into a permanent residential placement. The physician–psychiatrist provided oversight and shaped the institution into a place to protect vulnerable individuals from the complexities of community living. Johnson (1897) summarized this social policy: "A belief in the necessity of the permanent care of all this defective class is professed by every superintendent of every state school for the feeble-minded in the United States." Institutions became safe havens, and psychiatry had succumbed to a custodial role.

Psychiatrists as Jail Keepers

At the time that Europe and the United States were establishing institutions as training centers and later as protective havens, another fateful trend was developing. Bourneville (1880) and his colleagues were emphasizing their "defect theory," which assumed that there was always a relationship between disabilities and fixed central nervous system pathology. This theory opened the door to a dark period in care and treatment. Those with more severe disabilities were seen as beyond the reach of education and those with mild disabilities were treated as social misfits tainted by blighted genes. Individuals gradually became viewed as burdens and threats to the well-being of society. Not only were they seen as a "tremendous burden to the thrifty taxpayer" (Kerlin, 1886), but also as "useless . . . and mischievous" (Wilmarth, 1906).

The late nineteenth and early twentieth centuries ushered in an indictment. Individuals with disabilities became viewed as a menace to society. Wilmarth (1906) quoted the position of the National Conference on Charities and Correction: "My child, your life has been one succession of failures. You cannot feed and clothe yourself honestly. You cannot control your appetites and passions." What had initially been seen as a noble undertaking soon became a process of protecting society from dangerous individuals.

Fernald (1912) summarized this emerging trend as due to (1) the widespread use of intelligence tests; (2) the eugenics alarm, that is, the perception that individuals with disabilities were the causes of delinquency, crime, and sexual immorality, and other forms of social evil and disease; and (3) the perception that such disabilities were spreading like wildfire.

These trends gathered a force in the development of social policy. Protection began to turn into incarceration. Butler (1915) described the rationale for this trend: "While there are many anti-social forces, I believe that none demands more earnest thought, more immediate action than this. Feeble-mindedness produces more pauperism, degeneracy, and crime than any other force. It touches every form of charitable activity. It is felt in every part of our land." Butler (1915) later increased the scare: "When we view the number of feeble-minded, their fecundity, their lack of control, the menace they are, the degradation they cause, the degeneracy they perpetuate, the suffering and misery, and crime they spread—these are the burden we must bear."

Women, in particular, were singled out as a danger to society. Bullard (1909) indicted women with disabilities as "a plague-spot" on society who posed a greater danger to society than "even the violently insane." Fernald (1912) emphasized, "The feeble-minded are a parasitic, predatory class, never capable of self-support . . . they cause incredible sorrow at home and are a menace and danger to the community. . . . It has been truly said that feeble-mindedness is the mother of crime, pauperism, and degeneracy."

As institutions turned into jail-like settings, one of the primary rationales put forth was the eugenics alarm. Individuals with disabilities were seen as "the defilement of the race" (Fernald, 1912). Sterilization became a major goal of care. Barr (1902) urged: "One cannot fail to recognize the necessity for the enforcement of measures which experience has demonstrated as absolutely needful steps toward prevention, viz: the separation, sequestration, and asexualization of degenerates."

Individuals with special needs underwent a six-decade period in which segregation via commitment and often compulsory sterilization were the essential treatment "goals" for a large percentage of them. These goals also coincided with a public desire to save money. Education, care, and treatment became a thing of the past. Institutions were no more than large labor camps.

The Psychiatrist as Gatekeeper

By 1920 psychiatrists and other professionals began to recognize that some individuals with disabilities were not the menace they had been made out to be. Taft (1918) pointed out that perhaps "the high grade types" might be able to adjust to community living, and he proposed a new social policy as a partial alternative to institutionalization based on the registration, supervision, and control of individuals with disabilities in the community. This could have signaled the beginning of a new role for psychiatry, that is, the provision of support to individuals with disabilities in the confluences of family and community life. But the call was not heeded. The states failed to provide any alternatives to custodial care, and the vast majority of psychiatrists, except for those few who supervised institutions, drifted away from the care and treatment of individuals with disabilities.

Wolfensberger (1976) indicated,

> By 1925, however, a curious situation had developed. . . . The only major rationale left was relief for hard pressed families of retarded individuals. . . . Community services did not develop fast enough, and this is probably one of the major reasons institutions did not change. . . . Any institution . . . that has much momentum but no viable rationale is likely to strive for self-perpetuation on the basis of its previous rationales and practices. And I believe that this is what happened. . . .

Psychiatrists, as the principal leaders of institutional control, became the overseers of these vast places. What Focault (1965) described as the rationale of the asylums of eighteenth-century France matched those of North American institutions in the first half of the twentieth century:

> *Homo medicus* was not called into the world of confinement as an *arbiter*, but rather as a guardian, to protect others from the vague danger that exuded through the walls of confinement. . . . The atmosphere was not one of benevolent neutrality. If a doctor was summoned, it was because people were afraid—afraid of the strange chemistry that seethed behind the walls of confinement, afraid of the powers forming there that threatened to propagate.

The psychiatrist, with the power to segregate, sterilize, and commit, did not any longer wish to deal with the care and treatment of individuals in the spirit of Itard. Pinel (1806) analyzed the duties and roles of the psychiatrist–superintendent: "He must be endowed with a firm character, and on occasion display an imposing strength. He must threaten little but carry out his threats, and if he is disobeyed, punishment must immediately ensue." Focault (1965) further stated that the psychiatrist had to be " . . . Father and Judge, Family and Law—his medical practice being for a long time no more than a complement to the old rites of Order, Authority, and Punishment."

The first phase of the care and treatment of individuals with disabilities placed psychiatrists as preeminent leaders in the care and treatment of individuals with mental retardation. The psychiatrist as "enlightened educator" was transformed to the behavioral pathologist responsible for the identification, segregation, and isolation of "deviants." The "defect position" ushered in a tragic interlude (1900–1920) that left a long-lasting imprint on the role of psychiatry. Institutions changed from training centers to low-budget warehouses that placed a premium on forced labor as a means of institutional support. Institutions became like prisons. Psychiatrists played the role of warden. Education was replaced by incarceration. Psychiatry, which had initially played a dynamic and hope-giving role, became the leading profession in the warehousing of individuals with disabilities.

A CHANGING PARADIGM

Parents as Victims

From the dawn of time, most families have cared for their children with special needs at home in spite of the lack of almost any societal supports. Families received some hope with the work of the early French and American neuropsychiatrists. But they soon suffered from the "scientific" study of disabilities through the eugenics movement. Barr (1902) had accused parents of being the cause of the problem: "Heredity is herein proven law, as inexorable in the descending as it is beneficent in the ascending scale." This destructive posture persisted in full strength until recently.

If not seen as the direct causes of the disability, parents generally felt accused by psychiatrists. Avis (1985) pointed out: "Practices in institutions seemed to separate parents from their children." Parents were ridiculed for being "neurotic" and having poor child-rearing practices. They were viewed as the source of the child's problems. Psychiatrists and other professionals described them as rigid, perfectionistic, emotionally impoverished, and depressed (Marcus, 1977). Bettleheim advocated "parentectomy," institutionalizing the child to replace parents with institutional staff and professionals considered more competent.

In the 1950s, psychiatry did not know what its role should be in relation to individuals with special needs. Wolfensberger (1972) noted that during this time period, "The mental health field, and especially psychiatry, appears to be in a state of ferment and uncertainty that amounts to a crisis." Institutions had long ago lost their therapeutic meaning and were simply adrift. The majority of psychiatrists were still clinging to the medical model.

Parents as Catalysts of Change

Because psychiatrists and other professionals were not responding to the needs of individuals with disabilities or their families, parents began to organize on a local level in the 1930s. The National Association for Retarded Children was formed in 1950 with the expressed purpose of "creating opportunities for children and providing hope and support to families." This heralded a new era of hope once again, in which the nation would undergo a slow, but irrevocable, change in the care and treatment of individuals with disabilities.

Psychiatrists in Turmoil

Primarily due to parental advocacy, the 1950s and 1960s witnessed a gradual change in the role of psychiatrists. Those involved in institutional care seemed locked into a medical model that was equal to human warehousing. Parents bypassed these recalcitrant professionals and started to establish alternatives to institutions. Turnbull and Turnbull (1986, p. 11) commented that parents recognized that they had to set out on their own if the institutional model were to disappear:

> Local parent groups organized classes in community buildings or church basements and solicited financial support from charitable organizations. Over the years, parent organizations initiated services in education, recreation, residential living (group homes), and vocational alternatives.

This social change process slowly began to attract some psychiatrists back to a more hopeful and helpful posture.

Families had to navigate through negative psychiatric views. Beddle and Osmond (1955) equated parental response to the birth of a child with a disability as equivalent to "child loss" and that institutionalization was seen as death without the proper ties. For example, Aldrich (1947) commented that the prognosis for the child with Down syndrome was bleak: "I have often remarked that the better they were, the worse off they were.... There is only one adequate way to lessen all this grief, ... immediate commitment to an institution at the time of diagnosis. This is preventive medicine."

Although institutions still held a strong grasp on the attitudes and recommendation of physicians, psychiatrists, and other health care professionals, other professionals were slowly inculcating a new model. Wein-gold and Hormuth (1953) advocated for the rights of the child: "Home care of the mongoloid child cannot be undertaken unless and until the professional persons with whom the child and family come in contact are ready and willing to afford him the rights of childhood."

As parents were organizing as advocates, psychiatry was torn between the "grief model" that held that (1) the parent was a patient, (2) psychiatric help consisted of therapy that delved into the parent's parent, and (3) resolution involved the dissipation of guilt. By throwing the focus on the parent-as-the-problem, psychiatry continued to adopt a nihilistic view of the individual with a disability.

But countervailing forces also began to take shape. Olshansky (1962) disputed the grief model and urged a more therapeutic approach that involved the entire family as well as the community. He pointed to the social factors surrounding the birth of a child with a disability and held that "chronic sorrow" was not neurotic but "an understandable nonneurotic response to a tragic fact." He saw the resolution of this as the need for parents to have an opportunity to ventilate their feelings and, equally important, the need for society to provide concrete, community-based services such as day care centers, special classes, and sheltered workshops.

Farber (1960) postulated that most family structures were not demolished by the birth of a child with special needs, but underwent "a role organization crisis." He theorized that, for children to remain with their families, three sources of conflict had to be resolved: novelty shock, value conflicts, and situational stress.

Subtle changes began to take place in how psychiatrists and other mental health professionals approached families. Hastings (1948) remarked, "The correct handling of the child usually lies in the correct management of the parent." But parental management was still generally tainted by prejudice against the child and the subsequent recommendation of removal from the family, since the child is a "mental cripple" and will remain so throughout life (Murray, 1969).

The fledgling parental advocacy movement began to formulate new management approaches based on their self-defined needs. In an informal study of parents of individuals with disabilities, Zwerling (1954) found that parents wanted guidance from psychiatrists and other medical personnel based on realistic, but hopeful, attitudes instead of the common dehumanizing values so often expressed in "negative aspects of the child to the total exclusion of any assets in the child." He also found that the parents' most bitter memory "concerned their being advised to institutionalize their retarded child . . . to put the child away."

Psychiatrists in Change

The scandalous conditions of state institutions slowly began to be recognized. The 1962 Report of the President's Panel on Mental Retardation (President's Panel, 1962) described institutional conditions as poor and later as "plainly a disgrace to the nation and to the states that operate them" (President's Committee on Mental Retardation, 1968). Psychiatry had to undergo a substantial transformation if it was to play any positive role in this individual and social change process. Blatt (1970) warned that psychiatry itself must change: "You will come to save us, bringing your science and your prestige and your power, yet knowing so pitifully little of either whom you will help now or the conditions that gave rise to this problem." This plea brought no quick response.

Dybwad (1970) pointed out that the medical model continued to prevail and grow:

> Both the American Medical Association and the American Psychiatric Association have expressed themselves strongly that institutions serving the mentally retarded should be directed by physicians and, insofar as the latter association is concerned, specifically by psychiatrists. . . . [Yet] a realistic index of the medical professions, including the field of psychiatry, is to be found in the articles published in the professional journals and the papers submitted to large scientific meetings. The number of papers written by psychiatrists over the past ten years on aspects of psychiatric treatment in institutions for the mentally retarded is indeed minimal.

Psychiatry was often more of a roadblock to constructive change than a help. Dybwad (1970, p. 555) pointed out that in those institutions under the direction of a psychiatrist,

> the lack of application of the principles of dynamic psychiatry in the administrative organization, in interstaff relationships, in the day to day care of the residents, and in the relationships with the families is astounding. . . . The use of restraint and isolation, with children and adults alike, over prolonged periods is to be noted in this context.

He went on to define a role for psychiatry: ". . . first in the specific therapeutic interventions with those residents who give evidence of distinct emotional disturbance and, indeed, psychosis, and, second, in promoting a climate of mental hygiene throughout the institution. . . ."

Potter (1970) reminded Dybwad that only a minority of institutions were administered by psychiatrists and that psychiatry's tradition was based on the orientation of the neuropsychiatrists of the nineteenth century that made those early institutions "... hives of patient activity, with vigorously pursued programs of training and education." He went on to state that most psychiatrists avoided the care and treatment of individuals with disabilities due to "the unhappy and uninspiring image of the mentally retarded."

Menolascino (1970) recognized the need to redefine psychiatry's role:

> We have to remind ourselves that diagnosis and treatment are the core specialty of psychiatry—not research and administration. . . . I believe that we must broaden our discussion to include other human management personnel, rather than persevering in the 'psychiatrist alone' posture of the past.

He not only urged psychiatrists and other professionals to reenter the field of care and treatment, but also advocated for a much broader professional and change-oriented approach. He asked psychiatrists to assume new roles, especially coordinating and motivating other disciplines and encouraging enlightened training, leadership, and a commitment to optimizing human fulfillment.

At the same time, Menolascino (1970) delineated the major barriers presented by psychiatrists: the mental age myth, a disproportionate preoccupation with severe disabilities and ignoring of individuals with mild disabilities, treatment nihilism, and the lack of trained and sensitive psychiatrists. The last barrier was recognized as a major systemic roadblock. Ironically, psychiatry, which had inspired the humane education of individuals with special needs, had become apathetic to their needs. As late as 1970, Menolascino (1970) reported,

> The United States has only a handful of psychiatrists, clinical psychologists, and psychiatric social workers prepared to respond to the demands and opportunities of implementing the mental health aspects of a national program of action for the mentally retarded.

At best, psychiatrists had become institutional "gatekeepers." Clinical "skills," most notably, the administration of institutional settings, had eclipsed skills in psychiatry.

Specifically, Menolascino recommended:

1. The psychiatrist should serve as a "generalist," correlating and interpreting diagnostic findings of a multidisciplinary team into meaningful therapeutic prescriptions.

2. Psychiatrists should specialize in special-interest areas such as family support, psychopharmacology, and the diagnosis and treatment of specific mental disorders.
3. Psychiatrists need to embrace community psychiatry by integrating individuals with disabilities of all ages into the burgeoning community psychiatry movement.

Cytryn (1970) urged the training of psychiatric residents in the diagnostic and treatment process of individuals with special needs. He pointed out the benefits and opportunities of such training: (1) the use of methods among individuals with mild disabilities that had been applied to the prevention of emotional difficulties in normal children; (2) the increased knowledge related to the reciprocal interaction of affective and cognitive factors in learning, and of the biochemical and neurophysiological corollaries to the adaptation of the human organism to stress; (3) the differentiation of innate developmental forces and environmental influences; (4) the experience of interpreting emotional affective needs in nonverbal individuals; (5) the ability to study the evolution of personality defenses in their primitive forms; and (6) the appreciation of the dynamic interplay of organic and dynamic factors in human behavior.

Wolfensberger (1970) added a research dimension to psychiatry in terms of its possible contribution to individuals with disabilities and their families. He advocated for research by psychiatrists and other disciplines in areas such as the diagnosis of etiological syndromes, assessment of infant development and personality, and, especially, psychopharmacology. Freeman (1970) pointed out that research possibilities were at a very primitive level, since so little systematic information was available in institutions.

Menolascino (1965) emphasized that research should begin in the delineation of psychiatric syndromes in individuals with special needs. At that point in time, the major recognized psychiatric disorders were described as chronic brain syndromes, functional psychoses, adjustment reactions of childhood, and psychiatric disturbances not-otherwise-specified. This basic diagnostic approach had much more than a theoretical rationale.

The 1960s witnessed a flirtation with the diagnostic and treatment roles of the psychiatrist, but much remained to be done. Psychiatry had to formulate specific diagnostic and treatment modalities designed for individuals with disabilities. Menolascino (1970) emphasized that appropriate diagnosis was a prelude to a multimodal treatment approach:

It is my opinion that the most important aspect of a successful treatment approach to these particular children and their families is the use of multiple treatment modalities such as supportive play therapy (with focus on nonverbal aspects), psychotropic medications, family counseling, aid in seeking community resources, and last, sequential follow-through visits to assure the continuity of needed community services.

Psychiatry was set to embark on a journey back to its origins based on hope, education, and community integration.

Normalization as the Defining Value

Nirje (1969) introduced the principle of normalization as the guiding value in the care and treatment of individuals with disabilities. This helped to shape not only future services, but also the role of the psychiatrist as well. Nirje defined normalization as "making available to all mentally retarded people patterns of life and conditions of everyday living which are as close as possible to the regular circumstances and ways of life of society." This principle redefined the entire field of services to individuals with special needs, including psychiatry.

Nirje pointed out, "The normalization principle does not just affect the lives of retarded people, it has a deep effect on those who work with them, their parents, and society itself." Bank-Mikkelsen (1969), commenting on similar changes in Denmark, reminded his North American colleagues that, although psychiatrists had begun to show interest in diagnosis and treatment, they were still ensconced in the hospital model and that, for normalization to occur, psychiatrists had to look toward community care.

Grunewald (1969) called for an array of community-based residential, educational, and vocational services. Institutions had decreased from nearly 200,000 residents in the late 1960s to slightly more than 100,000 in the late 1980s (White, Lakin, and Brunininks, 1989). It was within this community model that psychiatrists would have to learn to work.

For psychiatrists, it meant new responsibilities and a changing locus of service delivery. No longer would institutions be seen as the place for individuals with special needs, including those with allied psychiatric disorders. Individuals with disabilities remained in the community, and increasing numbers began to return home from institutions. With a multidisciplinary approach, psychiatrists began to play a more specialized role appropriate to their discipline. They often gravitated toward university clinical and training programs, especially the newly formed University Affiliated Facilities designed to provide clinical training, demonstrate new techniques, and provide inpatient and outpatient services.

A major contribution of psychiatry at this time was a slow, deepening return to the recognition of the full sentient nature of individuals with special needs. Menolascino (1965) observed that "the majority of high level retarded children, if their family environment is reasonably healthy, do not have evidence of emotional disturbances in their earlier years." Chess (1970) analyzed their highly vulnerable nature in an environment organized primarily for youngsters of average intelligence and compared the impact of each level of mental retardation to the child's capacity to cope with environmental pressures.

Psychiatrists had been reluctant to apply psychotherapy to individuals with special needs because, as Albini and Dinitz (1965) reported, there was no benefit to its use due to the lack of insight and sufficient verbal communication skills. But some psychiatrists creatively ventured into psychotherapy in spite of these caveats. Sternlicht (1966) listed nonverbal communication techniques such as play therapy, finger painting, and music therapy as mechanisms for psychotherapy. Astrachan (1955) successfully used group therapy by constantly structuring and individualizing goals. Clarke and Clarke (1958) began to emphasize the need for allied supports such as language and communication therapy, remedial education, and social rehabilitation. Goodman and Rothman (1961) concluded that group therapy and group play helped individuals learn to control their impulses, observe routine rules, and accept their handicapping condition.

Behavioral Therapy

At a time when psychiatrists were essentially ignoring individuals with disabilities, behavioral therapists began to enter into institutions and implement applied behavior analysis with marked and surprising success. Fuller (1949) reported the first institutional study of "a vegetative organism." This opened the door to the widespread use of behavior modification in the United States. Gardner (1970) pointed out: "This is of special significance in view of the limited number of trained psychiatric personnel who are presently available to provide service to the mentally retarded," since "behavior modification procedures can be applied by caretaker personnel."

Although behaviorists provided direly needed attention and help, a corollary effect was the diminution of the perception of the sentient nature of individuals with disabilities. Residents became viewed as sets of observable behaviors rather than individuals with an emotional dimension.

The maladaptive behaviors most often selected for treatment included aggression, self-injury, noncompliance, hyperactivity, destructive and disruptive behavior, and stereotypy (Matson and Barrett, 1982). Therapy began to consist of a system of reward and punishment that often disregarded the fullness of the human condition. The most common intervention strategies consisted of positive and negative reinforcement to enhance desired behaviors and punishment to suppress undesired behavior. Positive effects were found with a variety of procedures; however, punishment techniques fell under sharp national scrutiny and were restricted or banned by some states and professional organizations.

Psychiatrists as Druggists

When behavior modification failed in its use of positive reinforcement, a twofold trend crept into institutional settings and community settings. Punishment-based interventions were often instituted, ranging from time-out to mist sprayed in the face to the use of electric shock. When these failed, psychiatrists were called in to prescribe psychoactive drugs. Gualtieri (1991), looking at the previous three decades, commented:

> The psychiatric community has become largely disaffected from the developmentally disabled. . . . Learning theorists and educators have assumed the responsibility of constructing programs and planning treatments for this group of patients.

Yet the question of dealing with individuals who failed to respond to behavior modification remained. With the introduction of chlorpromazine in the mid-1950s, psychiatrists had an answer.

The prevalence of pharmacotherapy increased dramatically with the availability of neuroleptic medication. Lipman (1970) surveyed institutions to determine the extent of the use of psychotropic drugs and found that 39 percent of the residents received thioridazine or chlorpromazine. Sprague (1977) also reported widespread use (approximately 50 percent). Hill et al. (1984) found 30 percent were receiving neuroleptic medications. Hill et al. also reported that approximately 20 percent of individuals living in the community were receiving neuroleptic medications. Reasons for drug use were almost always linked to "behavior control," such as hyperactivity, aggression, and self-injury, and not the treatment of diagnosed psychiatric conditions.

Gualtieri (1991) reviewed this trend from the mid-1950s to the end of the 1980s and concluded:

> The epidemic of neuroleptic overuse among mentally retarded people is one of those tragic experiments that nature, or history, will sometimes play. For thirty years and as recently as only a few years ago, the simple fact of being mentally retarded and residing in an institution meant that one was treated,

like as not, with neuroleptic drugs. The doses were high, the treatment went on for years, and there was little or no attention given to the side effects that the drugs could have.

Three major trends emerged in the 1960s through the 1970s that had a profound effect on psychiatry's role with individuals with disabilities. First, the psychiatrist-as-gatekeeper was quickly disappearing. Psychiatrists, and other medical personnel, were no longer seen as the heads of institutions—making decisions to admit, to commit, and to release residents. Instead, they became a part of an interdisciplinary team process. Second, their institutional role as distributor of drugs became essential. When all else failed, the psychiatrist was looked on to prescribe a drug to control behaviors. Psychiatric diagnosis was rare and other forms of psychiatric treatment were even rarer. Third, at the same time, a growing number of psychiatrists began to work in the community. At first, these were psychiatrists attached to university centers; but more community psychiatrists began to gradually care for the mental health needs of individuals with special needs. These psychiatrists began to adapt and apply diagnostic and psychotherapeutic approaches with some success.

A RETURN TO HOPE

The New Psychiatrist

The trends of the last three decades converged in the 1980s to establish new roles for psychiatrists. Diagnosis began to take on major importance. Psychiatrists began to view their role as a therapeutic profession. A prelude to care and treatment was an appropriate diagnosis (Eaton and Menolascino, 1982). Earlier studies and commentaries on the vulnerability of individuals with special needs to suffer from a mental illness began to be more fully understood and appreciated. The Piagetian model was proposed as applicable to this understanding (Menolascino, 1979). Beyond this, psychiatrists were challenged to formulate new diagnostic insights as to the presence and nature of mental illness. Menolascino, Gilson and Levitas (1986) described this thus:

In general, psychiatric diagnoses in the retarded follow traditional diagnoses. But we must be aware that these diagnoses are often modified by atypical features which are seen as unique behaviors in retarded individuals and not as signs and symptoms of mental illness. . . . When diagnosing a mental illness, the clinician must rely on the signs (observed behaviors) and less on the symptoms (verbally reported stress or dysfunction) that characterize the various psychiatric disorders, especially in those individuals with severe degrees of mental retardation.

Diagnosis also began to include formal measures used in general psychiatry and adaptations of these. Focus was given to interview techniques to evaluate the individual. Van Ornum and Mordock (1984) emphasized the need to interview caregivers, along with personal interviewing of the individual often through indirect questioning, with an understanding of expressive and receptive language characteristics, along with direct interactions and observations.

Clinicians began to rely more on adaptive behavior scales rather than formal intelligence quotients. Similarly, a number of scales to identify psychiatric symptoms began to be used, including the *Rotter A2 and B2 Behavioral Scales*, the *Child Behavior Checklist*, the *Beck Depression Inventory*, the *Child Depression Inventory*, and the *Standardized Assessment of Personality* (Gath and Gumley, 1984; Matson et al., 1984; Reid, Ballinger, Heather, and Melvin, 1984). In addition, scales designed specifically for individuals with special needs were developed, including the *Psychopathology Instrument for Mentally Retarded Adults* (Senatore et al., 1985) and the *Aberrant Behavior Checklist* (Aman et al., 1983).

Menolascino, Gilson, and Levitas (1986) defined these initial understandings as critical because of the need (1) to establish communication with a person whose capacity for formal or abstract thought may be limited; (2) to recognize psychosocial needs and strengths regardless of the level of disability; (3) to gather a complete personal-developmental history; (4) to correlate presenting symptoms with predictable crises such as the birth of siblings, starting school or changing teachers, puberty and adolescence, sexual development, dating and socialization, emancipation of siblings, transition to the world of work, moving from home, changing residences or residential support staff, relationships with staff, inappropriate expectations, and aging, illness, and the death of parents.

Psychotherapy began to take on an increased role, although Szymanski (1980) noted: "Paradoxically, there seem to have been more studies on psychotherapy with retarded persons published in earlier years than recent years." Nevertheless, psychotherapy began to be adapted to individuals with special needs. Szymanski (1980) urged psychotherapists to " . . . be (and feel comfortable in this role) a 'real person' and not only a neutral therapeutic mirror . . . [but] a direct role model." Therapists were encouraged to share their own life experiences in order to overcome the probable lack of abstract thinking and to form a strong, personal therapeutic alliance. It began to be recognized that sometimes behavioral problems were actually symptoms of underlying emotional stress and that the behavior problems were age-inappropriate expressions of these deeper feelings. Therapists focused on the recognition of these feelings and the appropriate ways to express them. Menolascino, Gilson, and Levitas (1986) pointed out that " . . . the therapist will want to help the retarded person to begin to experience anxiety, sadness, anger, and guilt as signals and clues to the person's inner life and as reactions to the world around them."

Bergman (1976) summarized the goals of psychotherapy among individuals with special needs:

> (1) the expression and resolution of dysphoria, anger, and resentment related to realistic cognitive limitations and experiences of social stigmatization and rejection; (2) the enhancement of self-esteem and personal competence within reasonable boundaries; (3) the development of greater capacity to recognize, process, and resolve internalized conflict adaptively; (4) the ability to assume greater personal independence and emancipation from family and others; and (5) the broadening of social skills and competencies necessary for successful social group acceptance and participation.

For the first time in years, many psychiatrists and other mental health professionals had started to recognize the full sentient nature of individuals with disabilities and apply psychodynamic techniques to meet their needs.

Group psychotherapy increased in use. Fletcher (1984) reported a recognition of its usefulness and an acceptance of it as an integral part of the therapeutic process. Various group techniques were utilized. Schramski (1984) emphasized role playing, encompassing allied activities such as role reversal, scene setting, and group sociometric exercises. Monfils (1985) cited the use of theme-centered group therapy, involving a central theme or idea around which group interaction could revolve. Monfils (1985) listed several other techniques: sharing information and experiences, peer and therapist modeling, confrontation, group support and encouragement, problem solving, and group cohesion.

Behavior modification had reached its peak in the 1980s and had started to encounter marked opposition due to its avoidance of the inner person and its increasing use of punishment procedures. Meyer and Evans (1989) postulated a "non-aversive" behavioral approach that was designed to enable individuals with disabilities "to have access to family-scale community living, supported work, normalized leisure life styles, meaningful social interactions with family and friends, and to take advantage fully in the variety of community experiences. . . ." McGee, Menolascino, Hobbs, and Menousek (1987) developed a "gentle teaching" approach that precluded the use of restraint and punishment and focused on the development of bonded relationships between individuals and their caregivers. A trend was initiated to ensure individuals with behavior problems the benefits of applied behavioral analysis without the use of punishment and restraint.

Likewise, the use of neuroleptics came under serious question. Gualtieri (1989) noted: "Psychiatrists became wedded to a deceptively simple and reductionist framework: one behavior, one drug . . . a single disorder, a single treatment. . . ." Psychopharmacological treatment goals most often focused on one symptom, behavioral control. Little attention was given to the effects of medications on patients' cognitive and social abilities, nor to their long-term neurological effects, as seen in tardive dyskinesia.

This concern, coupled with more sensitive diagnostic and therapeutic intervention strategies, led to a decrease in the use of neuroleptics and "behavior control" drugs. It also resulted in the more targeted use of a variety of new drugs based on more precise psychiatric diagnoses. Ratey and Gualtieri (1991) pointed out that "with the advent of new drugs (especially serotonergic agents) . . . neuropsychiatry is experiencing a dramatic philosophical reorganization." Menolascino, Ruedrich, and Kang (1991) attributed much of this to improvements "in the measurement and recording of atypical and abnormal behaviors via descriptive scales . . . [that] are increasingly replacing the hypothesized presence of signs or symptoms of mental illness." With such refinements, the use of medications began to take an adjunct role aimed at specific underlying mental disorders, and medications were used along with a multitude of other therapeutic and programmatic interventions.

By the 1980s, psychiatry had started to more comprehensively focus on the needs of individuals with special needs. The foundations had been established for the formulation of appropriate diagnostic processes with sufficient specificity to validate the presence of the entire range of mental illnesses. Attention had begun to be given to previously unidentified psychiatric diagnoses, especially the affective disorders and the presence of mental illness in those with severe disabilities, along with the possibility of heretofore unidentified neuropsychiatric disorders. A range of therapeutic and programmatic intervention models had been adapted or created to indicate that psychiatric needs could be met.

Diagnostic, therapeutic, and programmatic attention was given to specific groups of individuals with disabilities. It had been established that a primary role of general psychiatry was to include those with mild disabilities and allied psychiatric needs. Special attention had not yet generally been provided to issues surrounding those with antipersonality disorders. It was recognized that, for those with moderate disabilities, psychiatrists needed a deeper understanding of relevant cognitive and communication factors as well as the environmental stressors that contributed to emotional vulnerability. Psychiatry had only just touched on the psychosocial needs of those with severe disabilities, especially challenges presented by the lack of verbal communication, preoperational cognitive abilities, and allied medical and sensorial needs.

The foundation of community psychiatry had been established. Once again, psychiatrists were beginning to play a central role in helping, through (1) providing psychotherapy and counseling to parents in accepting and understanding the meaning of special needs, especially in relation to children with severe medical needs, and guiding them in finding in-home supports and other community alternatives; (2) offering therapeutic support to individuals with behaviors potentially harmful to the community and, at the same time, protecting the community from harm; (3) using nonaversive intervention strategies, especially for those individuals most at risk to emotional disorders; (4) mobilizing parental advocacy and legislative change for the creation of community alternatives; and (5) preventing or alleviating specific mental disorders.

The evolving role of psychiatry gained force with the establishment of the National Association for the Dually Diagnosed (NADD), in 1983. This voluntary association of professionals and parents dedicated itself to " . . . the well-being of persons with mental retardation and mental illness . . . through cross boundary research, training, and developmental services" (Fletcher and Menolascino, 1989). This organization posited several rationales for the involvement of psychiatry (Fletcher and Menolascino, 1989):

1. Deinstitutionalization had focused increasing attention on mental health needs.
2. The negative emotional effects of institutionalization had become evident once individuals returned to their communities.
3. Diagnosis of mental illness along the entire spectrum of psychiatric disorders was possible.
4. The establishment of integrated programs and services for these individuals was preferable to segregated ones.
5. Individuals with mental retardation and mental illness had the same rights as any other citizen.
6. To ensure community integration and human rights, the future required new and improved services, more innovative basic and applied research, and more relevant and in-depth training.

A PARADIGM OF INTERDEPENDENCE

Overview

The paradigm that psychiatrists inherited at the turn of the twentieth century and that endured for more than five decades was one of hopelessness designed to control individuals through segregation, isolation, and asexualization. From the 1950s through the 1970s, psychiatry entered into a new paradigm that was given much impetus by parent-advocates. Most psychiatrists were hard pressed to join in the national deinstitutionalization movement. The field was at a crossroads. Many psychiatrists chose to remain in institutions and maintain an ideology based on control with the modern form of restraint, drugs. However, a handful of psychiatrists resolved to advocate for substantive change and practice creative psychiatry in the community.

The introduction of normalization brought the seedlings of a new paradigm, one constructed on individual and social change. A few psychiatrists actively participated in the clinical and social dimensions of this revolution. Now, in the last decade of the twentieth century, psychiatry has returned to the origins articulated by Itard more than a century and a half ago:

> When we consider the full extent of this development [i.e., Victor's progress], we find among other real improvements, that he has a knowledge of the conventional value of symbols of thought and the power of applying this knowledge. . . . This has led to an extension of the pupil's relations with the people around him, his ability to express his wants to them, to receive orders from them, and to effect a free and continual exchange of thoughts with them. . . . Victor is aware of the care taken of him, susceptible to fondling and affection, sensitive to the pleasure of doing things well, ashamed of his mistakes, and repentant of his outbursts. . . .

If Itard had lived in the middle part of the twentieth century, he surely would have been astonished and chagrined at the state of affairs. By then, nearly 200,000 children and adults were warehoused in institutions. Buildings built for one thousand individuals were crammed with two thousand. He would have seen magic-like pills being given to almost every resident and then watched them stumble away in a state of oblivion. He would have been perplexed at psychiatry's role, wondering how the majority of psychiatrists simply ignored this state of affairs while a few actually perpetuated it. Itard would have been one of the first to call for substantive change, the return to the developmental model, and the adoption of the principle of normalization.

The New Paradigm

Psychiatry has begun to enter into an era of hope for all individuals with disabilities, including those with the most challenging problems. The therapeutic goal of psychiatry is changing from control and compliance through the use of reward and punishment to human inter-dependence through mutual change. Not only has the locus of services changed from the institution to the community, but also the purpose of service has changed. Menolascino and McGee (1982) described interde-pendence as a different way of looking at persons with severe behavioral difficulties. Each person is seen as an equal, as a person who experiences pain, hungers for justice, and longs for joy and companionship.

This leads psychiatrists and others not only to see individuals with special needs in another light (i.e., not as sick, hopeless, useless, repugnant, or defective, but as full human beings with respect and dignity) and to make a commitment to clinically help the individual, but also to effectuate programs, services, and supports that ensure community integration. This involves putting aside aversive practices that revolve around the elimina-tion of so-called behavioral problems and creating new caregiving models based on warmth, affection, tolerance, and interventions that start with unconditional valuing instead of behaviorism's sterile giving of "reward" for deeds done. It signals the need for the marked decrease in the use of "behavior-control" drugs and the use of drugs as a short-term adjunct to other treatment modalities. It requires creative clinical interventions and the disposition to provide care across the life span.

Psychiatrists as Advocates

The new paradigm also calls on psychiatrists to assume an active role in the development of an array of community-based residential, vocational, and recreational options to meet the needs of all individuals with disabilities. For individuals with mental illness, this does not mean "special" residences, classrooms, or work sites, but rather small, inte-grated, family-scale settings in the community. Clinical interventions are for naught if individuals with these needs have no place to live in the community, attend school, work, or recreate. Indeed, the lack of such services would return psychiatry to the dark ages of long-term institutional care.

Psychiatrists need to take a leadership role in the development of community alternatives. Just as community-based programs evolved in the 1970s and 1980s for individuals with mental retardation in general, so too will they evolve for those with mental illness and behavioral challenges in particular in the 1990s.

The new paradigm requires an evolving array of services: ongoing use of generic specialized services such as outpatient psychiatric services; avail-ability of acute psychiatric care services; an array of in-the-community residential alternatives such as small, family-like homes or supervised apartments; and well-supervised and supportive foster care, adoptive homes, respite care, case advocacy, supported work, work enclaves, integrated classrooms, and leisure time activities.

Psychiatrists as Specialists

Special attention will have to be given to individuals with more unique needs: those who are in the criminal justice system, the elderly, those with more severe levels of mental retardation and allied behavioral problems, and those with acute psychiatric needs. The applicable guiding criteria remain the same: nonaversive interventions, the minimal use of psychoactive drugs, the avoidance of segregation, family-scale interventions, ongoing support, the use of a multimodal approach, and community integration.

The psychiatrist of the 1990s will be expected to diagnose and treat the most complex individuals, indeed, individuals who will be on the brink of expulsion from community programs. A key role will involve caring for and treating individuals with extremely disruptive behaviors, some even violent and destructive, but always finding ways to maintain them in the community. The psychiatrist will have to counsel and guide staff and parents, teach direct caregivers how to help, oversee long-term community placements, and serve as an advocate for the individual.

The new psychiatrist will become much more attuned to the individual's interactions with the environment as well as his or her personal and present history, in terms of not only observed behaviors, but also the interpretation of inner states and personal vulnerabilities. Sovner (1990) has pointed out that dysfunction often occurs because of a misrepresentation of information and subsequent exaggeration of maladaptive behavior. Such difficulties may promote problems in interactions and behaviors. Internal stimulus control dysfunctions can produce internal chaos, personal distortions, impulsivity, hypervigilance, increased physiological stress, and aggression (Glass and Singer, 1973). This understanding leads to greater empathy and warmth toward the afflicted person and, thus, enhances the therapeutic process.

As the use of medications to control behaviors decreases and as diagnosis becomes sharper, lessened and more refined medication use will be employed. Biology and behaviors will be seen as complementary and not antagonistic . . . to minimize side-effects and maximize desired effect (Ratey and Gualtieri, 1991). In an increasing multimodal approach, psychopharmacology will continue to be used, but in conjunction with nonaversive behavior change processes and psychotherapy.

Psychiatrists as Researchers

Research will also play a significant role in psychiatry's future (Stark and Menolascino, 1992). It will continue to probe into the nature and causes of disabilities. Issues such as early screening and identification will be focused on to prevent or diminish the impact of mental illness, much as the early screening and treatment of PKU helped prevent mental retardation and the dramatic reduction of its related psychosis and seizure activity. Bregman and Hodapp (1991) have pointed out,

> An important task for the future will be the development of more sophisticated procedures for judging the relative importance of biological and psycho-social vulnerabilities that underlie cognitive impairment. It will be critical to identify the psycho-social variables that serve a protective function among biologically predisposed individuals.

Current research in genetics and the use of neuroimaging technology such as positron–emission tomography (PET) offer hope for the future.

The use of PET has tremendous research and treatment implications for psychiatry—the identification of neurophysiological variables related to mental illness, brain areas involved, and those areas affected by psychopharmacological and psychotherapeutic interventions. PET will be used increasingly to investigate a number of mental disorders, including autism, attention deficit disorder, affective disorders, schizophrenia, panic disorders, dementia, the psychiatric dimensions of Huntington's disease and Parkinson's disease, and obsessive–compulsive disorders.

PET applications include clinical neuroimaging and psychiatric interpretation of the instances of mental illness, which both enhances and confirms the diagnostic and treatment process, as in the case of Alzheimer's disease or a schizophrenic psychosis in nonverbal individuals. Positron–emission tomography is also an excellent tool for evaluating the "adaptive" effects of allied disabilities, such as seizure activity, on mental disorders. Additional applications involve the long-term evaluation of the effects of psychotropic drugs, as well as the compilation of normative PET databases. Finally, PET should help give great understanding to the molecular-genetic basis of a wide number of the major mental illnesses.

Research in psychopharmacology will focus on more efficacious and less toxic medication regimens. Peripheral Beta-blockers, anticonvulsants, opioid receptor antagonists, amantadine, and other medications will be further examined as to their effect on underlying psychiatric disorders without conveying severe side effects and inhibiting cognitive ability (Herman, 1991; Chandler, Barnhill, and Gualtieri, 1991). The immediate and long-term treatment goals of such chemicals will be community integration and the ability of the individual to function as fully as possible.

The psychiatrist will play a central role—a role that goes beyond diagnosis and treatment and involves substantive social change. It demands political mobilization and the inclusion of parents as primary change agents. All individuals, regardless of the level or type of disability, including those with the most severe behavioral challenges, will be served in the mainstream of community life.

The psychiatrist will no longer participate in throwing these individuals into the deep wells of institutions nor leave them abandoned in the valleys of chemical restraint. Nor will the psychiatrist allow them to rust away in the cold environment of human warehouses, as they have in the recent past and still do even today. The challenge is to keep them within the mainstreams of our communities, to support them, and fully help them.

In so doing, the psychiatrist of today will give rebirth to the posture of the French psychiatrist Jean-Marc Itard in his care of the Wild Boy of Aveyron. Like Itard, the psychiatrists of today will look for "windows into the soul" and thus greatly embellish the lives of individuals with disabilities, as well as their own.

REFERENCES

Albini, J.L., and Dinitz, S. (1965). Psychotherapy in disturbed and defective children: An evaluation of changes in behavior and attitudes. *American Journal of Mental Deficiency, 69*(4), 560–567.

Aldrich, C.A. (1947). Preventive medicine and mongolism. *American Journal of Mental Deficiency, 52,* 127–129.

Aman, M.G., Vamos, M., and Werry, J.S. (1983). Factor structure and norms for the revised behavior problem checklist in New Zealand. *Australian Journal of Psychiatry, 17*(4), 354–360.

Astrachan, M. (1955). Group psychotherapy with mentally retarded female adolescents and adults. *American Journal of Mental Deficiency, 60,* 152–156.

Avis, J. (1985). Through a different lens: A reply to Alexander, Warburton, Waldron, and Mas. *Journal of Marital and Family Therapy, 11*(2), 145–148.

Bank-Mikkelsen, N. (1969). Metropolitan area in Denmark-Copenhagen. In R.B. Kugel and W. Wolfensberger (Eds.), *Changing patterns in residential services for the mentally retarded* (pp. 227–254). Washington, DC: President's Panel on Mental Retardation.

Barr, M. (1902). The imperative call for our present to our future. *Journal of Psycho-Asthenics, 7,* 5–8.

Beddle, A., and Osmond, H. (1955). Mothers, mongols and mores. *Canadian Medical Association Journal, 73,* 167–170.

Bergman, C.C. (1976). The role of clergy in serving the mentally retarded. *Journal of Religion and Health, 15*(2), 100–107.

Blatt, B. (1970). Empty revolution beyond the mental. In F.J. Menolascino (Ed.), *Psychiatric approaches to mental retardation* (pp. 542–551). New York: Basic Books.

Bourneville, D. (1880). Sciercuse tubercuse des convulsion cerebrales. *Archives of Neurology, 1,* 91, 391.

Bregman, J.D., and Hodapp, R.M. (1991). Current developments in the understanding of mental retardation: Biological and phenomenological perspectives. *Journal of the American Academy of Child and Adolescent Psychiatry, 30,* 707–719.

Bullard, W. (1909). The high-grade mental defectives. *Journal of Psycho-Asthenics, 14,* 14–15.

Butler, A. (1883). Editorial: Does the education of the feebleminded pay? *Proceedings of the Association of Medical Officers of American Institutions for Idiots and Feebleminded Persons,* 152.

Butler, T.H. (1915). A simplified eldrige-green latern. *British Medical Journal, 2819,* 73.

Chandler, M. Barnhill, L.J., and Gualtieri, C.T. (1991). Amantadine: Profile of use in the developmentally disabled. In J.J. Ratey (Ed.), *Mental retardation: Developing pharmacotherapies. Progress in Psychiatry, 32,* 139–162. Washington, DC: American Psychiatric Press.

Chess, S. (1970). The child psychiatrist's role in mental retardation. *Archives of General Psychiatry, 23*(2), 122–130.

Clarke, A.M., and Clarke, A.D.B. (Eds.). (1958). *Mental deficiency: The changing outlook.* Glencoe, IL: The Free Press.

Cytryn, L. (1970). The training of pediatricians and psychiatrists in mental retardation. In F.J. Menolascino (Ed.), *Psychiatric approaches to mental retardation* (pp. 552–574). New York: Basic Books.

Dybwad, G. (1970). Roadblocks to renewal of residential care. In F.J. Menolascino (Ed.), *Psychiatric approaches to mental retardation* (pp. 552–574). New York: Basic Books.

Eaton, L., and Menolascino, F.J. (1982). Psychiatric disorders in the mentally retarded: Types, problems and challenges. *American Journal of Psychiatry, 139,* 1297–1303.

Farber, B. (1960). Perceptions of crisis and related variables and the impact of a retarded child on the mother. *Journal of Health and Human Behavior, 1,* 108–118.

Fernald, W. (1892). Some of the methods employed in the care and training of feeble-minded children of the lower grades. *Proceedings of the Association of Medical Officers of American Institutions for Idiots and Feebleminded Persons*, 450–457.

Fernald, W.E. (1912). The burden of feeble-mindedness. *Journal of Psycho-Asthenics*, *17*, 87–111.

Fletcher, R. (1984). Group therapy with mentally retarded persons with emotional disorders. *Psychiatric Aspects of Mental Retardation Reviews*, 3(6), 21–24.

Fletcher, R.J., and Menolascino, F.J. (Eds.) (1989). *Mental retardation and mental illness: Assessment, treatment, and service for the dually diagnosed*. New York: Lexington Books.

Focault, M. (1965). Madness and civilization in the age of reason. Translated from the French by Richard Howard. New York: Pantheon Books.

Freeman, R.D. (1970). Psychopharmacology and the retarded child. In F.J. Menolascino (Ed.), *Psychiatric approaches to mental retardation* (pp. 294–367). New York: Basic Books.

Fuller, P.R. (1949). Operant conditioning of a vegetative human organism. *American Journal of Psychology*, 62, 587–590.

Gardner, W.I. (1970). Use of behavior therapy with the mentally retarded. In F.J. Menolascino (Ed.), *Psychiatric approaches to mental retardation* (pp. 250–275). New York: Basic Books.

Gath, A., and Gumley, D. (1984). Down's syndrome and the family: Follow-up of children first seen in infancy. *Developmental Medicine and Child Neurology*, 26(4), 500–508.

Glass, D.C., and Singer, J.E. (1973). Experimental studies of uncontrollable and unpredictable noise. *Representative Research in Social Psychology*, 4(1), 165–183.

Goddard, H. (1912). *The Kallikak family*. New York: Macmillan.

Goodman, L., and Rothman, R. (1961). The development of a group counseling program in a clinic for retarded children. *American Journal of Mental Deficiency*, 65, 780–782.

Grunewald, K. (1969). A rural county in Sweden: Malmohus County. In R.B. Kugel and W. Wolfensberger (Eds.), *Changing patterns in residential services for the mentally retarded* (pp. 255–285). Washington, DC: President's Panel on Mental Retardation.

Gualtieri, C.T. (1989). Pharmacotherapy for mentally retarded people. Treatment of psychiatric disorders: A task force report of the American Psychiatric Association. Washington, DC: American Psychiatric Association, Vol 1–3, 67–99.

Gualtieri, C.T. (1991). *Neuropsychiatry and behavioral pharmacology*. New York: Springer-Verlag.

Hastings, D. (1948). Some psychiatric problems of mental deficiency. *American Journal of Mental Deficiency, 52,* 260–262.

Herman, B.H. (1991). Effects of opioid receptor antagonists in the treatment of autism and self-injurious behavior. In J.J. Ratey (Ed.), *Mental retardation: Developing pharmacotherapies. Progress in Psychiatry, 32,* 107–137. Washington, DC: American Psychiatric Press.

Hill, B.K., Rotegard, L., and Bruininks, R.H. (1984). The quality of life of mentally retarded people in residential care. *Social Work, 29*(3), 275–281.

Howe, S. (1849). The condition and capacities of the idiots in Massachusetts. *American Journal of Insanity, 5,* 374–375.

Itard, J.M.G. (1832). *The Wild Boy of Aveyron.* New York: Appleton-Century-Crofts.

Johnson, G.E. (1897). What we do, and how we do it. *Journal of Psycho-Asthenics, 2,* 98–105.

Kerlin, I. (1886). Provisions for imbeciles. *Proceedings of the Association of Medical Officers of American Institutions for Idiots and Feebleminded Persons,* 1–17.

Lipman, R.S. (1970). The use of psychopharmacological agents in residential facilities for the retarded. In F. Menolascino (Ed.), *Psychiatric approaches to mental retardation.* New York: Basic Books.

Marcus, L. (1977). Patterns of coping in families of psychotic children. *American Journal of Orthopsychiatry, 47*(3), 388–399.

Matson, J.L., and Barrett, R.P. (1982). *Psychopathology in the mentally retarded.* New York: Grune and Stratton.

Matson, J.L., Kazdin, A.E., and Senatore, V. (1984). Diagnosis and drug use in mentally retarded, emotionally disturbed adults. *Applied Research in Mental Retardation, 5*(4), 513–519.

McGee, J., Menolascino, F.J., Hobbs, D.C., and Menousek, P.E. (1987). *Gentle teaching: A non-aversive approach to helping persons with mental retardation.* New York: Human Sciences Press.

Menolascino, F.J. (1965). Emotional disturbance and mental retardation. *American Journal of Mental Deficiency, 70,* 248–256.

Menolascino, F.J. (1970). Psychiatry's past, current and future role in mental retardation. In F.J. Menolascino (Ed.), *Psychiatric approaches to mental retardation* (pp. 709–744). New York: Basic Books.

Menolascino, F.J. (1979). Handicapped children and youth: Current–future international perspectives and challenges. *Exceptional Children, 46*(3), 168–173.

Menolascino, F., Gilson, S.F., and Levitas, A.S. (1986). Issues in the treatment of mentally retarded patients in the community mental health system. *Community Health Journal, 22,* 314–327.

Menolascino, F., and McGee, J.J. (1982). Persons with severe mental retardation and behavioral challenges: From disconnectedness to human engagement. *Journal of Psychiatric Treatment and Evaluation, 5*(2–3), 197–193.

Menolascino, F.J., Ruedrich, S.L., and Kang, J.S. (1991). Mental illness in the mentally retarded: Diagnostic clarity as a prelude to psychopharmacological interventions. In J.J. Ratey (Ed.)., *Mental retardation: Developing pharmacotherapies. Progress in Psychiatry, 32,* 19–33. Washington, DC: American Psychiatric Press.

Meyer, L., and Evans, I.M. (1989). Chapter 17 in *Nonaversive intervention for behavior problems: A manual for home and community.* Baltimore: Paul H. Brookes.

Monfils, M.J. (1985). Theme-centered group work with the mentally retarded. *Social Casework, 66*(3), 177–184.

Murray, F.B. (1969). Conservation in self and object. *Psychological Reports, 25*(3), 941–942.

Nirje, B. (1969). A Scandinavian visitor looks at U.S. institutions. In R.B. Kugel and W. Wolfensberger (Eds.), *Changing patterns in residential services for the mentally retarded.* Washington, DC: President's Panel on Mental Retardation.

Olshansky, S. (1962). Chronic sorrow: A response to having a mentally defective child. *Social Casework, 43,* 190–193.

Pinel, P. (1806). *A treatise on insanity.* London: Hafner.

Potter, H.W. (1970). Human values as guides to the administration of residential facilities for the mentally retarded. In F.J. Menolascino (Ed.), *Psychiatric approaches to mental retardation* (pp. 575–584). New York: Basic Books.

President's Committee on Mental Retardation (1968). *The edge of change.* Washington, DC: Government Printing Office.

President's Panel on Mental Retardation (1962). *Report to the President: A proposed program for national action to combat mental retardation.* Washington, DC: Government Printing Office.

Ratey, J.J., and Gualtieri, C.T. (1991). Neuropsychiatry and mental retardation. In J.J. Ratey (Ed.), *Mental retardation: Developing pharmacotherapies. Progress in Psychiatry, 32,* 1–17. Washington, DC: American Psychiatric Press.

Reid, A.H., Ballinger, B.R., Heather, B.B., and Melvin, S.J. (1984). The natural history of behavioral symptoms among severely and profoundly mentally retarded patients. *British Journal of Psychiatry, 145,* 289–293.

Schramski, T.G. (1984). Role playing as a therapeutic approach with the mentally retarded. *Psychiatric Aspects of Mental Retardation Reviews, 3*(7–8), 25–31.

Seguin, E. (1846). *Treatment moral, hygiene et education des idiots et des autre enfants arrieres.* Paris: Bailliere.

Seguin, E. (1866). *Idiocy and its treatment by the physiological method.* New York: William Wood.

Senatore, V., Matson, J.L., and Kazdin, A.E. (1985). An inventory to assess psychopathology of mentally retarded adults. *American Journal of Mental Deficiency, 89*(5), 459–466.

Sovner, R. (1990). Treating mentally retarded adults with psychotropic drugs: A clinical perspective. In R.J. Fletcher and F.J. Menolascino (Eds.) (1989), *Mental retardation and mental illness: Assessment, treatment, and service for the dually diagnosed* (pp. 158–183). New York: Lexington Books.

Sprague, R.L. (1977). Methylphenidate in hyperkinetic children: Differences in dose effects on learning and social behavior. *Science, 198*(4323), 1274–1276.

Stark, J.A., and Menolascino, F.J. (1992). Mental retardation and mental illness in the year 2000: Issues and trends. In L. Rowitz (Ed.), *Mental retardation in the year 2000* (pp. 149–162). New York: Springer-Verlag.

Sternlicht, M. (1966). The clinical psychology internship. *Mental Retardation, 4*(6), 39–42.

Szymanski, L.S. (1980). Psychiatric diagnosis of retarded persons. In L.S. Szymanski and P.E. Tanguay (Eds.), *Emotional disorders of mentally retarded persons.* Baltimore: University Park Press.

Taft, J. (1918). Supervision of the feeble-minded in the community. *Mental Hygiene, 2*, 434–442.

Turnbull, A.P., and Turnbull, H. (1986). *Families, professionals and exceptionality: A special partnership.* Columbus, OH: Charles E. Merrill.

Van Ornum, W., and Mordock, J.B. (1984). Crisis counseling with children and adolescents: A guide for nonprofessional counselors. *Children Today, 13*(3), 336–361.

Weingold, J.T., and Hormuth, R.P. (1953). Group guidance of parents of mentally retarded children. *Journal of Clinical Psychology, 9*, 118–124.

White, C.C., Lakin, K.C., and Bruininks, R.H. (1989). Persons with mental retardation and related conditions in state-operated residential facilities: Year ending June 30, 1988 with longitudinal trends from 1950 to 1988 (Report #30). Minneapolis: University of Minnesota, Institute on Community Integration.

Wilbur, H. (1852). *First annual report of the trustees of the New York State Asylum for Idiots to the legislature of state.* Albany, NY: State Printers.

Wilmarth, A. (1906). To whom may the term feeble-minded be applied? *Journal of Psycho-Asthenics, 10*, 203–205.

Wolfensberger, W. (1969). The origin and nature of our institutional models. In R.B. Kugel and W. Wolfensberger (Eds.), *Changing patterns in residential services for the mentally retarded.* Washington, DC: President's Committee on Mental Retardation.

Wolfensberger, W. (1970). Facilitation of psychiatric research in mental retardation. In F.J. Menolascino (Ed.), *Psychiatric approaches to mental retardation* (pp. 663–689). New York: Basic Books.

Wolfensberger, W. (1972). *The principle of normalization in human services.* Toronto: National Institute on Mental Retardation.

Wolfensberger, W. (1976). On the origin of our institutional models. In R. Kugel and A. Shearer (Eds.), *Changing patterns in residential services for the mentally retarded* (pp. 35–82). Washington, DC: President's Committee on Mental Retardation.

Zwerling, I. (1954). Initial counseling of parents with mentally retarded children. *Journal of Pediatrics, 44,* 469–479.

18 ⬚⬚⬚ ⬚⬚⬚ ⬚⬚⬚

The Changing Roles of Psychologists: The Influence of Paradigm Shifts

Harvey N. Switzky

INTRODUCTION

The paradigm shift as regards thinking about persons with disabilities and providing services to them and their families happened during my professional life as a psychologist. I was an eyewitness to the changes that occurred during this period, and this chapter will reflect my own firsthand experiences. In a sense, this chapter will be a qualitative retrospective case history of the phenomena (Denzin and Lincoln, 1994; Yin, 1989). As such, it will also be idiosyncratic and personal, and reflect my own interpretations and biases. I will try to document the evolutionary process of the shifting paradigms in services to persons with disabilities as regards the changing role of psychologists. Bradley and Knoll (Chapter 1, this book) break the paradigm change process into three distinct phases: (a) the era of institutionalization, dependence, and segregation; (b) the era of deinstitutionalization and community development; and (c) the era of community membership.

SHIFTING PARADIGMS: PHASE ONE

First Job: Psychologist/Educator (1966–1968)

As an educational psychologist specializing in mental retardation and developmental disabilities, I was totally unaware that I was a true pioneering psychologist, combining the roles of educator and psychologist. A throwback to Binet (1911), who viewed himself as both a psychologist and an educator, my role deviated from the standard role of psychologists in the mid-1960s, which was one primarily concerned with IQ testing, assessment, and diagnosis.

I was the "child development supervisor" at the Trudeau Memorial Center for Mentally Retarded Children in Warwick, Rhode Island, a suburb of Providence. In 1966, the year I began this job, there was no P.L. 94-142, the Education of All Handicapped Children Act (1975), and many "subtrainable" children and youths were not receiving any organized educational services or any services at all from the state. Any services they received were provided by organized groups of parents whose children were handicapped—for example, United Cerebral Palsy and The Association for Retarded Children.

The Trudeau Center came about as the result of an innovative experiment between the State of Rhode Island and the Kent County Chapter of The Association for Retarded Children. The State of Rhode Island would provide the seed money to establish a "full-year day care center/school" and "community center" for those children and youth with disabilities not served by the public schools. We hired three "teachers," all of them parents of children with disabilities with extensive experiences that only life can provide. Our curriculum was fully developmental and we served about forty-five to fifty children. We began serving our children in the church basement across the street from the site where the Trudeau Center was being built.

There were no Individual Educational Plans nor Interdisciplinary or Transdisciplinary Staffings. There were only the students, the teachers, the families, and me—a psychologist/educator running the program by the seat of my pants, drawing from my experiences as a developmental psychologist and my experiences with learning theories, especially the work of B.F. Skinner (Bower and Hilgard, 1981; Holland and Skinner, 1961; Skinner, 1953). During my two years at the Trudeau Memorial Center, I set up and administered an innovative full-day, full-year educationally oriented day care center (it wasn't officially a school), with close community involvement for children with severe disabilities based on the principles of behavior modification.

There were two innovations concerning my experiences at the Trudeau Center: I spent a great deal of my time (a) visiting children and their families in their real-world settings, usually their homes, performing what would be called now "family systems analysis" (Turnbull and Turnbull, 1986) and "ecobehavioral analysis" (Schroeder, 1990) and (b) providing real-world experiences for my students in the community, such as going on field trips to the supermarket or eating lunch at fast food restaurants.

At least in Rhode Island at that time, it was rare that professionals in the disability field spent any time visiting families on their home turf and "actually listening" to them and observing what was really happening among members of the family and their relative (whether sibling, cousin, nephew, niece, or grandchild) with a disability. I learned that I was one of the few professionals who supported the family in maintaining their child at home. Most professionals strongly advised institutionalizing children with severe disabilities because the situation was "hopeless." I also learned that families were not given any real information regarding the true nature of the child's handicap. The families were treated as ignorant and stupid and not worth the bother, with the end result that families felt guilty, ambivalent about their child, out of control, and powerless. I also witnessed a lot of marital discord during my home visits, with the burden of caring for the child falling primarily on the mother. This was true for families who were very well-to-do and were pillars of the community, as well as for families who were very poor.

It was very rare during this period to see children with severe disabilities in the real world of the community. Just using my common sense, I came to the conclusion that if my students were really going to learn anything about the real world, they had to participate in it, so I organized field trips all around the community. We did not go to anywhere fancy, just ordinary places that any child would have access to. I organized wagon trains consisting of children in wheelchairs, children on foot, and teachers and parents. We were well received by the citizens of Warwick, Rhode Island, in our trips to the supermarket, the park, the restaurants, the library, and the small shops of the town.

Our children were "learning by doing" by actively participating in learning tasks—another pedagogical idea viewed by the psychologist/educator Binet (1908a, 1908b) as the veritable heart of special education methods of instruction—inadvertently, and serendipitously, applied by me in our programs at Trudeau. Here was another example of a pedagogical practice pioneered by a psychologist/educator from the early twentieth century, and even one earlier (Seguin, 1866) that had been forgotten in the United States by the mid-1960s. It is my thesis that the paradigms which dominate Bradley and Knoll's phase two (the era of deinstitutionalization and community development) and phase three (the era of community membership) are rediscoveries, reworkings, and extensions of Continental European models regarding mental retardation and mental retardation service systems that evolved during the late nineteenth and early twentieth centuries.

Looking back on my experiences at Trudeau, I guess we were the vanguard of a movement to provide more dignity, more responsibility, and more self-worth both to children with disabilities and their families and to teachers. We were trying to create active students, active teachers, and active parents who could really function as active "self-regulated" problem solvers (Bandura, 1993). I knew that other programs in Providence and surrounding communities were just getting started, but the programs at Trudeau were the first. We had a constant stream of visitors: other "educators," people from the State of Rhode Island, and students and professors from neighboring colleges. We even were interviewed by a reporter from *The Providence Journal*. Rhode Island was a very progressive state at that time as far as setting up community models of educational service for children with severe disabilities and their families. (Unfortunately such children were still being excluded from the schools during this period.)

Visiting a Large State Institution for Mentally Retarded Persons (1968–1969)

I conducted my dissertation research on institutionalized subjects residing at the Ladd School. It was there that the State of Rhode Island had set up in cooperation with Brown University a psychology laboratory devoted to doing basic research in mental retardation, another innovation for the State of Rhode Island. To collect data, it was necessary to get as large a sample of subjects as possible, which forced me to visit every living unit that existed at the Ladd School, as well as the School Department and the Department of Psychology.

Psychologists in the Department of Psychology, like most others in the mid-1960s in large state institutions, were totally dominated by the medical-custodial model (Fernald, 1915; Goddard, 1910; Sarason and Doris, 1969). They spent their time testing, assessing, and diagnosing the "degenerate, sick, incurable" armies of individuals of all ages who were maintained in the custodial, medically oriented institution, where for the sake of society's safety, these persons could be kept under total twenty-four-hour control (Switzky, 1988; Switzky et al., 1988). As far as I could tell, the psychologists were running an individual intelligence testing factory. When I was given access to the IQ test scores of the subjects who were to be in my dissertation research sample, I found to my horror that the files were very incomplete. The newest information on the majority of the residents was more than two years old. I was going to have to do my own IQ testing. (I wondered how the psychologists spent their day.)

My trip to the School Department was quite disappointing as well. The school was in utter disorder. I could not tell what the curriculum was or what the teaching goals were. I also found that the teachers were held in very low regard by all the members of the organization and they knew it. I never saw such sad, morose, and unmotivated teachers. They knew they were trapped in an organization that had lost its way and in jobs that had no meaning.

I visited every living unit and program at the institution to get my subjects and test them in the laboratory. One thing that I immediately found out was that each unit or program rarely socialized with the others. People went to their jobs and interacted only with people in their unit or program, though everybody was very pleased to visit with and assist me. They must have been profoundly bored with their work, because they went to extensive lengths to maintain social contact with me to such an extent that I was afraid I wasn't going to collect enough data for that day to complete my dissertation research on time.

I rarely witnessed any kind of "active programming" in the living units. The living units shocked me because they really did remind one of the films of Nazi concentration camps in Eastern Europe. I even went into the locked wards, where the most violent residents were maintained. It was very strange when they locked the door behind me and I was left with a caretaker (often a small woman) surrounded by fifty to sixty very large, naked residents. I was so desperate to find enough subjects to finish my dissertation that I could not afford to neglect any subject population. However, I found that I could not use any subjects in the locked wards because their functioning level was just too low.

Another thing that confused me during my visits to the Ladd School was that often I could not tell who was a resident and who was a caretaker. There were many high functioning people residing at the school who wore ordinary street clothes; many times I thought they were caretakers.

Another shocking set of experiences occurred during my own psychological evaluation of the residents: many of the residents had normal IQ test scores. I could not understand how individuals with normal levels of intelligence could be institutionalized. (How naive I was then.) I really grappled with myself over this problem. Since I was a visitor at the Ladd School, I did not want to "rock any boats," because I wanted to collect my dissertation data and finish up. I finally decided to tell the assistant superintendent, who liked to talk with me at least once a week, about my research. With great trepidation I told him what I had discovered about the

IQ test scores of some of the residents. He smiled and told me not to worry. We never discussed the matter any further; I am not sure that anyone ever did anything to right what I viewed as a grievous wrong. I ended up collecting data at the Ladd School for almost nine months, experiencing firsthand the era of institutionalization, dependence, and segregation.

Over the years I have learned that there often is a great discrepancy between the professional's "ideal role," as espoused by professional societies and trainers of professionals, and the professional's "actual day-to-day working role." This is analogous to the constitutive definition of a construct and the operational definition of a construct. There are also historical distortions of ideas as theories are developed and used, and as ideas travel from Continental Europe to England and the United States (Switzky, 1988, in press; Switzky et al., 1988). Sternlicht and Bialer (1977a, 1977b) divide the ideal role of the psychologist as historically encompassing clinical, consulting, administrative, training, and research functions.

Unquestionably, the most successful research enterprise that psychologists pioneered was the psychology of individual differences (Galton, 1892), especially what Cattell in 1890 called "mental tests" to assess various aspects of human potential and human capacity (Herrnstein and Boring, 1966a). Ebbinghaus, though better known for his work on human memory, in 1895 was involved in discovering methods of measuring the mental capacity of schoolchildren by the use of tests of computation, memory span, and sentence completion (Herrnstein and Boring, 1966b). Ebbinghaus's work apparently deeply influenced Binet, who contended that a psychology of individual differences (Binet and Henri, 1895) should focus mental tests directly on higher mental processes rather than, as proposed by Cattell, primarily on sensory and perceptual processes (Herrnstein and Boring, 1966c).

In Binet's original conception, a psychology of individual differences constituted a natural and scientific home for the psychological study of various disabilities, since intelligence is a major source of differences among individuals. For example, mental retardation could be studied as a set of quantitative variations in behavioral and psychological processes (Haywood and Paour, 1992), and that is exactly what Binet and Simon (1905a, 1905b, 1905c) proposed to invent, a set of scientifically correct criteria for the operational definition and diagnosis of mental retardation. Rather than use an unstandardized clinical interview, Binet and Simon (1905a, 1905b, 1905c) proposed the need for a carefully and precisely defined method of describing the behavioral and psychological manifestations of the various conditions that constitute the overall diagnostic category of mental retardation. They also proposed a standardization in nomenclature and assessment of the levels of intelligence of the condition in measurement operations, so that in a reliable and valid way mental retardation could be distinguished from mental illness.

Binet and Simon (1905a, 1905b, 1905c) constructed the first metric scale of intelligence that recognized the importance of the assessment of adaptive behavior; they field-tested it on 250 residents of an institution at Vaucluse, France (Haywood and Paour, 1992; Pollack and Brenner, 1969). The original Binet–Simon Scale was a questionnaire that measured both "intelligence" and "adaptive" behavior as regards "appearance, language use, identity, family, awareness of age and knowledge of body, body movements, dressing, vocabulary, attention to bodily needs, time and place concepts, and even went up to knowledge of geography, the military, reading, writing, calculating, occupations, and elementary geometry" (Haywood and Paour, 1992, pp. 2-3).

If psychologists in the United States had maintained the original model of "intelligence" proposed by Binet and Simon (1905), as well as their ideas concerning the role of the psychologist as an educational psychologist —Binet believed that only individuals who had great experience with the science of pedagogy and the scientific method were qualified to use the Binet–Simon Scales—much of the current feuding and confusion regarding the relationship of "intelligence" and "adaptive behavior" would have been avoided (Greenspan, Switzky, and Granfield, in press). In addition, if psychologists in the United States had not forgotten the challenge of Itard (1801/1932), Seguin (1846, 1866), and Binet (1911)—that it was possible to train the intellect of individuals who were mentally retarded by teaching them to use what would be called today active educational cognitive and metacognitive strategies (Borkowski et al., 1990; Borkowski et al., 1992)—a lot of needless suffering by students and their families, teachers, and society in general would have been avoided.

Goddard (1910) translated and adapted the intelligence tests developed by Binet and Simon for the United States as an efficient tool to identify children with mental retardation. But the psychosocial, historical *Zeitgeist* concerning persons with mental retardation during the late nineteenth and early twentieth centuries was quite different in England and the United States than in Continental Europe. Attitudes toward persons with cognitive disabilities in the United States had always been ambivalent (Sarason and Doris, 1969; Switzky, 1988; Switzky et al., 1988). Strong, latent, negative attitudes toward persons with mental retardation and other developmental disabilities burst forth with ferocity and viciousness during this period, with a resulting hysteria over the possible harmful effects of allowing such persons to remain in the community. Three trends were responsible for this change in attitude: (a) the rise of the philosophy of social Darwinism, (b) the rediscovery of Mendel's Laws in combination with the rise of the eugenics movement, and (c) the development, Americanization, and subsequent widespread use of intelligence tests (Fernald, 1915; Sarason and Doris, 1969; Switzky et al., 1988).

Darwin's theory implied that the evolution of a species was due to variations in traits among the members of the species, hereditary transmission of traits, and the natural selection of those traits most fit to survive the struggle of existence. The philosophers of social Darwinism of the 1880s considered persons with disabilities to be members of an inferior race that, in accordance with natural law, should be allowed to die out as quickly as possible.

Galton (1883), during this same period, disseminated the idea that society should improve the human race by checking the birthrate of the unfit while increasing the birthrate of the fit, which evolved into the science of eugenics. Eugenics was concerned with using the techniques of selective breeding to improve the inborn qualities of the human race. The rediscovered Mendel's Laws of Inheritance were applied to the inheritance of human characteristics by those in the eugenics movement.

Researchers of that period presented numerous studies to prove not only that certain disabilities were inherited as Mendelian characteristics (Davenport, 1911; Fernald, 1912; Goddard, 1915), but also that they were related to all forms of social degeneracy, criminality, pauperism, and immoral behavior (Fernald, 1912; Goddard, 1912; Jefferis and Nichols, 1921; *Man and Abnormal Man*, 1905; *Report of the Royal Commission on the Care and Control of the Feebleminded*, 1908; Shannon, 1917). Eugenicists also produced evidence that persons with mental retardation and other developmental disabilities had a higher birthrate than did the rest of society, and if these trends continued, they argued, society would become more enfeebled, the general level of intelligence would decrease, and social degeneracy, crime, and immorality would increase substantially (Stoddard, 1922). These frightening prospects caused the social Darwinists and the eugenicists to join forces to order many persons with disabilities to submit to ever-increasing amounts of restrictive "social control."

Goddard's translations and "misuse" of the intelligence tests invented by Binet and Simon indicated that mental retardation was much more widespread than had been previously expected. The "morons," a new class of higher functioning persons with mental retardation discovered by Goddard (1915), were thought to be extremely numerous throughout the population at large. The supposed discovery that "morons" existed in greater numbers than had been previously believed aggravated the superheated hysterical and fearful atmosphere of the times.

As a result of trends that began in the late nineteenth century, many persons with disabilities came to be viewed as a menace to society and were held responsible for all types of social evils, sexual disease, corruption, crime, sexual immorality, prostitution, and moral and physical degeneracy. The offered solution was to protect society from the "contagion" of such persons by isolating them through compulsory commitment to and permanent detention in large state institutions, and by the imposition of rigid social controls. The result of this movement was the creation of an institutional environment where "degenerate, sick, subhuman" individuals of all ages were maintained in custodial, medically oriented institutions and, for the sake of society's safety, kept under total twenty-four-hour control.

Ironically, during this period public school classes for children with disabilities increased dramatically. This was a manifestation of the doctrine of social control imposed by a frightened society. Because there was a chronic shortage of custodial institutions—only 10 percent of the population of individuals with disabilities was ever institutionalized, other arrangements had to be invented to socially control the "degenerate" population of children with disabilities. One such arrangement was the establishment of special education classes in the public education system as a kind of "holding tank" system, where children with disabilities could be socially controlled and monitored until their ultimate placement in a custodial institution.

What I had witnessed at the Ladd School were the vestiges of a treatment model that had been frozen in time. In spite of a large mass of evidence that accumulated from the 1920s to the 1950s, which strongly suggested that persons with cognitive and other developmental disabilities were not a menace to society and could be successfully habilitated and integrated into the community (Anderson, 1922; Fernald, 1919, 1924; Kuhlmann, 1940; Wallace, 1929; Wallin, 1924), residential institutions and public school programs fell into a kind of drift, perhaps because of lack of public interest and lack of money for backup social services.

Psychologists have a strong clinical function as well. Lightner Witmer, who was trained at the University of Leipzig, Germany, and is viewed as the father of both school and clinical psychology in the United States, established the first psychological clinic for children in 1892 at the University of Pennsylvania (Irvine, 1969). Witmer viewed the role of the clinical psychologist in very broad terms: to discover the relationships between cause and effect in applying various pedagogical remedies to children who are suffering from general or special retardation. One might say he was the first clinical psychologist/school psychologist concerned with the problems of exceptional children in the United States (Gardner, 1968). (I expect that he, Binet, and Simon would have been fast friends.)

In 1896 in an address before the American Psychological Association, Witmer defined what he believed should be the role of a clinical psychologist. There were four component dimensions: (a) the investigation and assessment of mental development using clinical methods and statistical techniques in exceptional children; (b) the provision of diagnostic and clinical services to teachers of exceptional children on a consultative basis; (c) the training of teachers, social workers, and physicians concerning the psychological aspects of exceptionality so that these allied professionals could provide service delivery to exceptional populations; and (d) the training of psychologists for the evaluation and treatment of exceptional children so that they could work in an interdisciplinary fashion within the school system. Unfortunately, Witmer's ideas (which I believe flowed from the same Continental European sources as those of Binet and Simon) were ignored by the psychologists in the United States for the same reasons that Binet and Simon's ideas were ignored: the time and place were not right, and the Zeitgeist in the late nineteenth and early twentieth centuries in the United States opposed their acceptance.

SHIFTING PARADIGMS: PHASE TWO

Wisconsin's Deinstitutionalization Movement (1974–1975)

After spending four years at George Peabody College in Nashville, Tennessee, initially as a postdoctoral fellow receiving training as a clinical child psychologist and later as an assistant professor of psychology, and at the Institute of Mental Retardation and Intellectual Development, which was part of the John F. Kennedy Center on Education and Human Development, I moved to Wisconsin. In 1974 I became director of psychological services, chief psychologist, and unit manager of Crestview, a "normalization-deinstitutionalization" living unit, and of Parkview, a "behavior modification and token economy habilitation-rehabilitation living unit for mild and moderately mentally retarded emotionally disturbed adolescents" at the Northern Wisconsin Developmental Center, Chippewa Falls, Wisconsin. I was there for almost two years. I viewed my major responsibility as preparing our residents to leave the institution and return to the community by giving them the social and educational skills to function adequately in smaller group homes and semi-independent living facilities, programs that the State of Wisconsin was encouraging, rather than living in the large institutional environment.

My role as a psychologist was greatly expanded beyond the role models I had witnessed at the Ladd School in Rhode Island. I could truly carry out the role of a psychologist as envisioned by Witmer and Binet and Simon: clinical service, consultation, training, interdisciplinary and transdisciplinary facilitation among professionals, and research. In addition, I had administrative responsibilities over a large staff of psychologists, educators, social workers, paraprofessionals, and even a physician and a nurse, since I had the Department of Psychology and two living units under my authority. What had caused the paradigm shift regarding the role of the psychologist and attitudes toward persons with disabilities?

The evolution of the paradigm shift could not have occurred without the help of parent groups that formed to promote the general welfare of children and adults with disabilities, starting just before World War II when United Cerebral Palsy was organized. More influential was the organization of the National Association for Retarded Citizens (NARC) in 1950. NARC, almost single-handedly, changed the image of persons with mental retardation and other developmental disabilities from one of social degeneracy and social menace to one of childhood innocence, who required society's aid to grow and prosper.

The National Association for Retarded Citizens served as a model for advocacy and as a catalyst for political change at the local, state, and national levels to provide more educational programming, community residential alternatives, and backup social services. NARC modified public attitudes and stimulated professional attention to an extent virtually without parallel among previous parent groups. The association prepared the way for the return to more optimistic attitudes regarding the education, training, and empowerment of persons with disabilities (and their families) that is characteristic of the present Zeitgeist (which took root earlier in the socially more progressive upper Midwestern states such as Wisconsin and Minnesota).

As fallout from this radical shift in attitude toward persons with disabilities, the training of psychologists slowly began to change. Sarason (1953) argued persuasively that psychologists needed to deal more with the education and training of "mentally defective children" and conduct more basic research with them. In 1953 George Peabody College developed the first doctoral training program in psychology that specifically concentrated in medical, psychological, and sociological aspects of mental retardation. In 1958 a joint conference was held by the American Association on Mental Deficiency (AAMD) and the American Psychological Association (APA), in order to stimulate psychologists' interest in research, program development, and training in the area of mental retardation. In 1972 APA formed Division 33, the Mental Retardation/Developmental Disabilities Division. In 1963 the federal government established the University Affiliated Facilities (UAF) program to train professionals and technical personnel in the area of developmental disabilities and to (a) provide comprehensive multidisciplinary inpatient and outpatient services, (b) train specialized personnel in biomedical, behavioral, and special education, and (c) demonstrate new techniques of specialized services.

The 1960 election to the presidency of John F. Kennedy, who had a sister with mental retardation, Rosemary, and the 1964 election to the vice presidency of Hubert H. Humphrey, who had a granddaughter with mental retardation, Vicki, also helped change public attitude toward persons with mental retardation and other developmental disabilities. These persons were being increasingly seen as worthy human beings who had become injured due to forces beyond their control, yet who could benefit from society's help. People began to understand better that these persons have the *same feelings and rights* as other human beings.

During Kennedy's administration (1961–1963), increasing amounts of federal resources were devoted to the problems of individuals with disabilities and their families. Throughout the mid-1960s and into the 1970s, the large state institutions came under the scrutiny of advocates for individuals with disabilities and legislators who rejected the medical–custodial model of residential services contained within a central, all-purpose institution. The inferior custodial care received by residents of these large institutions was seen as "dehumanizing" and destructive (Blatt and Kaplan, 1966; Vail, 1967; Wolfensberger, 1976), and the institutions themselves were seen as vast wastelands and warehouses of humanity. Much scientific research had been accumulated that showed that residing in an institutional setting limits and decreases intellectual development (Butterfield, 1976; Crissey, 1970; Dennis, 1973; Skeels, 1966). Also, new philosophies were evolving. The medical model was being replaced by the developmental model (Roos, 1974; Switzky et al., 1979), and the principle of normalization (Bank-Mikkelsen, 1969; Grunewald, 1969; Nirje, 1969, 1976; Wolfensberger, 1972, 1980, 1983).

The developmental model conceived of persons with disabilities as individuals who could benefit from training and educational instruction. Within this framework most disabilities can be viewed as conditions that can be improved, not incurable diseases, and individuals with disabilities can grow and develop like other people. The developmental model emphasized the essential humanity of persons with disabilities, and the same principles of learning and development applied to those both with and without disabilities (Switzky, in press). The developmental model functioned as an antidote to dehumanizing conceptions of persons with disabilities.

The principle of normalization originated in the 1950s in Norway, Sweden, and Denmark. N.E. Bank-Mikkelson, a lawyer and director of the Department of Care and Rehabilitation of the Handicapped of Denmark's National Board of Social Welfare, expressed the principle of normalization as allowing individuals with disabilities to obtain an existence *as close as possible to the normal.* Bengt Nirje (1969, 1976), former executive director of the Swedish Parents' Association for Mentally Retarded Children, summarized the normalization principle: making available to persons with disabilities the patterns and conditions of everyday life that are as close as possible to the norms and patterns of mainstream society. Nirje believed that the normalization principle should serve as a guide for decisions and actions for all service providers (psychologists, teachers, social workers, state representatives, lawyers, and members of Congress) who served persons with disabilities. The legal and philosophical commitment to the normalization principle beginning in the 1970s provided the energizing force leading to the legal principles of the deinstitutionalization movement, the least restrictive environment, and civil and vocational rights for citizens with disabilities.

The principle of normalization and the developmental model provided impetus to my role as a psychologist at Northern Wisconsin Developmental Center. The Department of Psychology I pretty much left alone in terms of its role of evaluating intellectual and adaptive behavioral functioning through the use of commercial individualized intelligence tests and tests of adaptive behavior. Some changes were made: I required department psychologists to visit the residents in their living units so as to view them in the social ecology in which they lived.

Parkview, the behavior-modification and token economy habilitation-rehabilitation living unit for adolescents with dual diagnoses, was headed by a psychologist who functioned as both a psychologist and an educator for this population (Reiss, McKinney, and Napolitan, 1990). A combination of behavioral techniques using a remedial approach to strengthening skills was adopted (Matson, 1990; Switzky et al., 1979) as the model used for active behavioral programming. (What a contrast with the models of interventions, or lack of interventions, I had witnessed at the Ladd School.)

I was the first director of Crestview, the normalization-deinstitutionalization living unit. I had a free hand in developing models of active educational/psychological programming based on the theories of normalization and social, ecological, and ecobehavioral analysis (Schroeder, 1990; Switzky, Rotatori, and Cohen, 1978).

At Crestview, residents were being prepared to live in the community, usually in group homes. The unit was organized into thirteen clusters of eight people, which simulated the group home environment. These groups were organized as "families" (Switzky, Rotatori, and Cohen, 1978) since they were going to live together in the same community living facility. I tried to give the "families" as much freedom and responsibility over their lives as they could handle, so that they could obtain an existence as close as possible to the normal flow of life outside the institution. I also allowed our residents total freedom to explore the grounds and to visit the neighboring towns of Chippewa Falls and Eau Claire.

Each cluster had a living room and four bedrooms. Also provided were kitchen facilities, where residents could experiment with making their own group or individual meals, and laundry facilities, where residents could experiment with washing and drying their own clothes. There were two large common halls and a large cafeteria where residents had to tell the food servers what they wished to eat as they lined up before the hot tables. We also had "family-style" meals, where food items were presented in bowls and the members of the family had to learn to communicate with each other in the sharing of food.

I also implemented a program of sexual liberation: any public sexual behavior that was appropriate in the community was appropriate in the public environments of Crestview. Caretakers could not barge into the private bedrooms of residents; they had to knock first. What went on behind closed doors of adult residents was their own business as long as no one was being hurt or abused and appropriate precautions were being observed. Wisconsin was a most progressive state. I had the full backing of the local superintendent and the head of the Division of Mental Retardation and Developmental Disabilities in Madison to carry out the program.

What impressed me the most were the incredible changes in the residents' behavior when they were given so much responsibility and freedom. Many of the residents grew in sophistication, wisdom, and practical intelligence right before our eyes. I expect the staff also saw these wondrous changes and that is why they went along with me as I drastically changed the way things had been done before. We dealt with all levels of functioning residents, from profound to mild, and all ages as well, from elementary-aged to residents in their seventies. We saw women with severe mental retardation who had spent all day staring at strings and carrying dolls give up these infantile and nonfunctional behaviors and learn some advanced self-help skills. They even learned how to feed themselves and to prepare simple meals.

What was even more impressive was that there was no external, explicit, behavioral programming going on. Learning appeared to be based on social learning principles (Bandura, 1993) and Vygotskian-historical contextualist operations based on models of apprenticeship and the zone of proximal development (Bronfenbrenner, 1989; Rogoff, 1990; Vygotsky, 1978). In these models, a more competent person collaborates with an individual to help her move from where she is now to where she can be with help. This more competent person (staff member or peer) accomplishes this feat by means of prompts, modeling, verbal explanations, leading questions, and joint discussions. I can only assume that this was happening at Crestview. I must mention that some residents could not adapt to all this new freedom and responsibility. I saw a few instances of complete withdrawal, sometimes bordering on catatonia.

During my two years in Wisconsin, I saw the role of the psychologist expand from mere test giver to educator, interdisciplinary and transdisciplinary facilitator, consultant to other programs and professionals, administrator, and researcher (we did some research in trying to understand the process of deinstitutionalization). Psychologists could indeed carry out the role envisioned by Witmer and Binet and Simon.

SHIFTING PARADIGMS: PHASE THREE

Working at an Illinois ICF/MR (1981–1986)

I took a position at Northern Illinois University in 1975 and am still currently employed there. I was initially a professor of special education and then became a professor of educational psychology. I developed a rather long-term relationship as a psychological consultant with two local intermediate-care living facilities. The models of service delivery in Illinois for people with disabilities were not as well developed as I had seen in Wisconsin. The role of the psychologist both in the schools and in the community-living facilities was much more traditional: essentially diagnostic testing, a little staff development and training, and consultation. One component of my role did increase substantially, that of counselor and psychotherapist.

Issues of counseling and psychotherapy with populations with cognitive disabilities have had a long history of discussion (Sternlicht, 1977; Sternlicht and Bialer, 1977a, 1977b), with the consensus being that these populations did not have the cognitive capacity or verbal skills necessary for personality change, or so claimed by the Freudians and the Rogerians. More recently, practitioners and theorists (Borthwick-Duffy, 1992; Goode, 1990; Heshusius, 1988; Mercer, 1992) more interested in phenomenology and more humanistic, holistic models and increasing the independence and quality of life of persons with disabilities have argued that personality changes due to psychotherapeutic/educational technologies are possible (Matson, 1990; Reiss, McKinney, and Napolitan, 1990; Stark and Menolascino, 1992; Vanderheiden, 1992).

I spent a great deal of my time listening to the worldviews of persons with disabilities, an area I had not really paid much attention to, and realized that they were real persons too. I witnessed over the years that Illinois was starting to catch up with Wisconsin in allowing persons with disabilities more freedom and responsibility over their lives. They were being treated like real human beings, with dreams, hopes, and fantasies, and were being allowed to take over critical aspects of their lives and plan for the future. I saw people move out of the ICF/MRs into smaller facilities (adult group homes) with community supports, and some moved into small apartments that had been specifically built for people with disabilities and actually began to participate in community activities.

CONCLUSION

The role of the psychologist has moved ever closer to the ideal roles defined by Binet and Simon and Witmer. Psychologists have gone beyond being mere test givers and diagnosticians. The Zeitgeist in the United States has changed most radically for the better. Though often the role of the psychologist working with persons with disabilities is ambiguous (because of the rise of the guild system fostered by the clinical psychologists that dominate the American Psychological Association and their preoccupation with licensure), the role of the psychologist has expanded greatly, as my own personal experiences have documented. The future presents some unprecedented opportunities for those of us in the profession who are willing and prepared to accept the challenge.

REFERENCES

Anderson, V.V. (1922). Feeblemindedness as seen in court. *Boston Medical and Surgical Journal, 76,* 429–431.

Bandura, A. (1993). Perceived self-efficacy in cognitive development and functioning. *Educational Psychologist, 28*(2), 117–148.

Bank-Mikkelsen, N. (1969). Metropolitan area in Denmark-Copenhagen. In R.B. Kugel and W. Wolfensberger (Eds.), *Changing patterns in residential services for the mentally retarded* (pp. 227–254). Washington, DC: President's Committee on Mental Retardation.

Binet, A. (1908a). Un livre recent de W. James sur l'education [A recent book by W. James on education]. *Bulletin de la Societe Libre pour l'Etude Psycholigique de l'Enfant,* No. 46, April, 114–120.

Binet, A. (1908b). Un livre recent de W. James sur l'education (suite): Causerie pedagogique [A recent book by W. James on education (continued): Pedagogical dialogue]. *Bulletin de la Societe Libre pour l'Etude Psychologique de l'Enfant,* No. 48, June, 167–168.

Binet, A. (1911). *Les idees modernes sur les enfants* [Contemporary ideas on children]. Paris: Flammarion.

Binet, A., and Henri, V. (1895). La psychologie individuelle [The psychology of individual differences]. *Annee Psychologique, 2,* 411–465.

Binet, A., and Simon, T. (1905a). Sur la necessite d'etablir un diagnostic scientifique des estats inferieurs de l'intelligence [On the necessity of establishing a scientific diagnosis of low levels of intelligence]. *Annee Psychologique, 11,* 163–190.

Binet, A., and Simon, T. (1905b). Methode nouvelle pour le diagnostic du niveau intellectuel des anormaux [A new method for the diagnosis of intellectual level of abnormal persons]. *Annee Psychologique, 11,* 191–244.

Binet, A., and Simon, T. (1905c). Application des methodes nouvelles au diagnostic du niveau intellectuel des anormaux d'hospice et d'êcole primaire [Application of new methods to the diagnosis of intellectual level of abnormal persons in institutions and elementary schools]. *Annee Psychologique, 11,* 245–336.

Blatt, B., and Kaplan, F. (1966). *Christmas in purgatory: A photographic essay in mental retardation.* Newton, MA: Allyn and Bacon.

Borkowski, J.G., Carr, M., Rellinger, E., and Pressley, M. (1990). Self-regulated cognition: Interdependence of metacognition, attributions, and self-esteem. In B.F. Jones and L. Idol (Eds.), *Dimensions of thinking and cognitive instruction* (pp. 53–92). Hillsdale, NJ: Erlbaum.

Borkowski, J.G., Day, J.D., Saenz, D., Dietmeyer, D., Estrada, T.M., and Groteluschen, A. (1992). Expanding the boundaries of cognitive interventions. In B.Y.L. Wong (Ed.), *Contemporary intervention research in learning disabilities* (pp. 1–21). New York: Springer-Verlag.

Borthwick-Duffy, S. (1992). Quality of life and quality of care in mental retardation. In L. Rowitz (Ed.), *Mental retardation in the year 2000* (pp. 52–66). New York: Springer-Verlag.

Bower, G.H., and Hilgard, E.R. (1981). *Theories of learning* (5th ed.). Englewood Cliffs, NJ: Prentice-Hall.

Bradley, V.J., and Knoll, J. (1995). Shifting paradigms in services to people with diasbilities. In O.C. Karan and S. Greenspan (Eds.), *Community rehabilitation services for people with disabilities.* Boston: Butterworth–Heinemann.

Bronfenbrenner, U. (1989). Ecological systems theory. In R. Vasta (Ed.), *Annals of child development.* Vol. 6. Greenwich, CT: JAI Press.

Butterfield, E. (1976). Some basic changes in residential facilities. In R.B. Kugel and A. Shearer (Eds.), *Changing patterns in residential services for the mentally retarded* (pp. 15–34). Washington, DC: President's Committee on Mental Retardation.

Crissey, M.S. (1970). Harold Manville Skeels. *American Journal of Mental Deficiency, 75,* 1–3.

Davenport, C.B. (1911). *Heredity in relation to genetics.* New York: Holt.

Dennis, W. (1973). *Children of the creche.* New York: Appleton-Century-Crofts.

Denzin. N.K., and Lincoln, Y.S. (Eds.) (1994). *Handbook of qualitative research.* Thousand Oaks, CA: Sage Publications.

Education of All Handicapped Children Act (1975). 20 U.S.C., sections 1400 et seq. and amendments.

Fernald, W.E. (1912). The burden of feeble-mindedness. *Journal of Psycho-Asthenia, 17,* 87–111.

Fernald, W.E. (1915). What is practical in the way of prevention of mental defect? *Proceedings of the National Conference of Charities and Correction,* 289–297.

Fernald, W.E. (1919). A state program for the care of the mentally defective. *Mental Hygiene, 3,* 566–574.

Fernald, W.E. (1924). Thirty years' progress in the care of the feebleminded. *Journal of Psycho-Asthenics, 29,* 206–219.

Galton, F. (1883). *Inquiries into human faculty and its development.* London: Macmillan.

Galton, F. (1892). *Hereditary genius* (2nd ed.). London: Macmillan.

Gardner, J.M. (1968). Lightner Witmer—a neglected pioneer. *American Journal of Mental Deficiency, 72,* 719–720.

Goddard, H.H. (1910). Four hundred feeble-minded children classified by the Binet Method. *Journal of Psycho-Asthenics, 15*(1), 17–30.

Goddard, H.H. (1912). *The Kallikak family.* New York: Macmillian.

Goddard, H.H. (1915). The possibilities of research as applied to the prevention of feeble-mindedness. *Proceedings of the National Conference of Charities and Correction,* 307–312.

Goode, D.A. (1990). Thinking about and discussing quality of life. In R.L. Schalock (Ed.), *Quality of life: Perspectives and issues* (pp. 41–57). Washington, DC: American Association on Mental Retardation.

Greenspan, S., Switzky, H., and Granfield, J. (In press). Everyday intelligence and adaptive behavior: A theoretical framework. In J. Jacobson and J. Mulick (Eds.), *Manual on diagnosis and professional practice in mental retardation.* Washington, DC: American Psychological Association.

Grunewald, K. (1969). A rural county in Sweden: Malmohus County. In R.B. Kugel and W. Wolfensberger (Eds.), *Changing patterns in residential services for the mentally retarded* (pp. 255–285). Washington, DC: President's Committee on Mental Retardation.

Haywood, H.C., and Paour, J. (1992). Alfred Binet (1857–1922): Multifaceted pioneer. *Psychology in Mental Retardation and Developmental Disabilities, 18*(1), 1–4.

Herrnstein, R.J., and Boring, E.G. (1966a). James McKeen Cattell (1860-1944) on mental testing, 1890. In R.J. Herrnstein and E.G. Boring (Eds.), *A source book in the history of psychology* (pp. 423–427). Cambridge: Harvard University Press.

Herrnstein, R.J., and Boring, E.G. (1966b). Hermann Ebbinghaus (1850-1909) on the completion test. In R.J. Herrnstein and E.G. Boring (Eds.), *A source book in the history of psychology* (pp. 434–437). Cambridge: Harvard University Press.

Herrnstein, R.J., and Boring, E.G. (1966c). Alfred Binet (1857-1911) and Victor Henri (1872-1940) on the psychology of individual differences, 1895. In R.J. Herrnstein and E.G. Boring (Eds.), *A source book in the history of psychology* (pp. 428–433). Cambridge: Harvard University Press.

Heshusius, L. (1988). The arts, science and the study of exceptionality. *Exceptional Children, 55*(1), 60–65.

Holland, J.G., and Skinner, B.F. (1961). *The analysis of behavior.* New York: McGraw-Hill.

Irvine, P. (1969). Lightner Witmer (1867–1956). *Journal of Special Education, 3,* 229.

Itard, J.M.G. (1801/1932). *The wild boy of Aveyron* (trans. by G.E.M. Humphrey). New York: Appleton-Century-Crofts.

Jefferis, B.G., and Nichols, J.L. (1921). *Searchlights on health: The science of eugenics.* Naperville, IL: J.L. Nichols.

Kuhlmann, F. (1940). One hundred years of special care and training. *American Journal of Mental Deficiency, 45,* 1–24.

Man and Abnormal Man (1905). Senate Document No. 187, Fifty-Eighth Congress, Third Session. Washington, DC: U.S. Government Printing Office.

Matson, J.L. (Ed.)(1990). *Handbook of behavior modification with the mentally retarded* (2nd ed.). New York: Plenum.

Mercer, J.R. (1992). The impact of changing paradigms of disability on mental retardation in the year 2000. In L. Rowitz (Ed.), *Mental retardation in the year 2000* (pp. 15–38). New York: Springer-Verlag.

Nirje, B. (1969). The normalization principle and its human management implications. In R. Kugel and W. Wolfensberger (Eds.), *Changing patterns in residential services for the mentally retarded* (pp. 179–195). Washington, DC: President's Committee on Mental Retardation.

Nirje, B. (1976). The normalization principle and its human management implications. In R.B. Kugel and A. Shearer (Eds.), *Changing patterns in residential services for the mentally retarded* (pp. 231–240). Washington, DC: President's Committee on Mental Retardation.

Pollack, R.H., and Brenner, M.J. (1969). *The experimental psychology of Alfred Binet.* New York: Springer-Verlag.

Reiss, S., McKinney, B.E., and Napolitan, J.T. (1990). Three new mental retardation service models: Implications for behavior modification. In J.L. Matson (Ed.),

Handbook of behavior modification with the mentally retarded (2nd ed.) (pp. 51–70). New York: Plenum.

Report of the Royal Commission on the Care and Control of the Feebleminded (1908). London: Wyman and Sons.

Rogoff, B. (1990). *Apprenticeship in thinking: Cognitive development in social contexts.* New York: Oxford University Press.

Roos, P. (1974). Human rights and behavior modification. *Mental Retardation, 12*(3), 3–6.

Sarason, S.B. (1953). *Psychological problems in mental deficiency* (2nd ed.). New York: Harper & Row.

Sarason, S.B., and Doris, J. (1969). *Psychological problems in mental deficiency* (4th ed.). New York: Harper & Row.

Schroeder, S.R. (Ed.)(1990). *Ecobehavioral analysis and developmental disabilities: The twenty-first century.* New York: Springer-Verlag.

Seguin, E. (1846). *Traitement moral, hygiene et education des idiots et des autres enfants arrieres* [Moral treatment, hygiene, and education of idiots and other backward children]. Paris: Bailliere.

Seguin, E. (1866). *Idiocy and its treatment by the physiological method.* New York: Wood.

Shannon, T.W. (1917). *Eugenics.* Marietta, OH: S.A. Mulliken.

Skeels, H.M. (1966). Adult status of children with contrasting early life experiences. *Monographs of the Society for Research in Child Development, 31*(3), 1–65.

Skinner, B.F. (1953). *Science and human behavior.* New York: Macmillan.

Stark, J., and Menolascino, F. (1992). Mental retardation and mental illness in the year 2000: Issues and trends. In L. Rowitz (Ed.), *Mental retardation in the year 2000* (pp. 149–162). New York: Springer-Verlag.

Sternlicht, M. (1977). Issues in counseling and psychotherapy with mentally retarded individuals. In I. Bialer and M. Sternlicht (Eds.), *The psychology of mental retardation: Issues and approaches* (pp. 453–490). New York: Psychological Dimensions.

Sternlicht, M., and Bialer, I. (1977a). Psychological issues in mental retardation: An overview. In I. Bialer and M. Sternlicht (Eds.), *The psychology of mental retardation: Issues and approaches* (pp. 3–30). New York: Psychological Dimensions.

Sternlicht, M., and Bialer, I. (1977b). The role of the psychologist in mental retardation. In I. Bialer and M. Sternlicht (Eds.), *The psychology of mental retardation: Issues and approaches* (pp. 33–64). New York: Psychological Dimensions.

Stoddard, L. (1992). The revolt against civilization: The menace of the under man. New York: C. Scribner's Sons.

Switzky, H.N. (1988). *The mainstreaming dilemma.* Dekalb, IL: Northern Illinois University, Department of Educational Psychology, Counseling, and Special Education.

Switzky, H.N. (In press). Individual differences in personality and motivational systems in persons with mental retardation. In W.E. MacLean, Jr. (Ed.), *Handbook of mental deficiency, psychological theory and research* (3rd ed.). Hillsdale, NJ: Erlbaum.

Switzky, H.N., Dudzinski, M., Van Acker, R., and Gambro, J. (1988). Historical foundations of out-of-home residential alternatives for mentally retarded persons. In L.W. Heal, J.I. Haney, and A.R.N. Amado (Eds.), *Integration of developmentally disabled individuals into the community* (2nd ed.) (pp. 19–35). Baltimore: Paul H. Brookes.

Switzky, H.N., Rotatori, A.F., and Cohen, H. (1978). The Community Living Skills Assessment Inventory: An instrument to facilitate the deinstitutionalization of the severely developmentally disabled. *Psychological Reports, 43,* 1335–1342.

Switzky, H.N., Rotatori, A.F., Miller, T., and Freagon, S. (1979). The developmental model and its implication for assessment and instruction for the severely/profoundly handicapped. *Mental Retardation, 17,* 167–170.

Turnbull, A.P., and Turnbull, H.R. (Eds.) (1986). *Families, professionals and exceptionality: A special partnership.* Columbus, OH: Merrill.

Vail, D.J. (1967). *Dehumanization and the institutional career.* Springfield, IL: Charles C Thomas.

Vanderheiden, G.C. (1992). A brief look at technology and mental retardation in the 21st century. In L. Rowitz (Ed.), *Mental retardation in the year 2000* (pp. 268–278). New York: Springer-Verlag.

Vygotsky, L. (1978). *Mind in society.* Cambridge: Harvard University Press.

Wallace, G.L. (1929). Are the feebleminded criminals? *Mental Hygiene, 13,* 93–98.

Wallin, J.E.W. (1924). *The education of handicapped children (Part III).* Boston: Houghton Mifflin.

Wolfensberger, W. (1972). *The principle of normalization in human services.* Toronto: National Institute on Mental Retardation.

Wolfensberger, W. (1976). On the origin of our institutional models. In R. Kugel and A. Shearer (Eds.), *Changing patterns in residential services for the mentally retarded* (pp. 35–82). Washington, DC: President's Committee on Mental Retardation.

Wolfensberger, W. (1980). A brief overview of the principle of normalization. In R.J. Flynn and K.E. Nitsch (Eds.), *Normalization, social integration, and community services* (pp. 71–115). Baltimore: University Park Press.

Wolfensberger, W. (1983). Social role valorization: A proposed new term for the principle of normalization. *Mental Retardation, 21*(6), 234–239.

Yin, R.K. (1989). *Case study research* (rev. ed.). Newbury Park, CA: Sage Publications.

19

Physical Therapy

Ronnie Leavitt

INTRODUCTION

The profession of physical therapy is concerned with the restoration of function and the prevention of disability following disease, injury, or loss of a body part. Physical therapists evaluate and treat individuals through the utilization of physical agents such as heat, light, electricity, water, exercise, massage, and other manual techniques, as well as train people in the use of adaptive equipment, prosthetics, and orthotics. Physical therapists may practice in a wide variety of settings, including hospitals, long-term-care institutions, a consumer's home, schools, private offices, sports medicine clinics, industry, academic institutions, and others. A vast majority of therapists are primarily clinicians, but administration, education, and research are additional professional activities of emphasis.

As a profession, physical therapy is continually evolving and remains in a state of transition, partly in response to the new paradigm and partly in reaction to its ties to the traditional health care system, with its strong medical-model orientation. It has "matured" greatly since its inception and many would claim that it has moved into full adulthood. Nevertheless, if physical therapists are to maximize their potential and remain leaders in the field of rehabilitation, the profession must proactively confront many barriers and issues still before them. Some of these issues are intimately connected to the health care delivery system at large, such as quality assurance, cost control, accountability, and the need to work more effectively with other team members. Other issues are more directly associated with our particular professional enrichment, such as how to maintain relevant and ideal physical therapy education, and how to gain status as a "direct access" profession, whereby consumers may enter the health care system by accessing a physical therapist.

This chapter discusses these and other major issues facing the profession in light of the emerging paradigm shifts that are responsible for contemporary practices. To lay the groundwork for this discussion, the section that follows provides an overview of the historical development of physical therapy.

HISTORICAL EVOLUTION OF PHYSICAL THERAPY

Concepts of rehabilitation and the presence of rehabilitation services, such as physical therapy, vary immensely (Leavitt, 1988). Although an extensive review of the literature reveals little historical information on the subject, it is apparent that rehabilitation, in some form or another, has existed for centuries. In contrast to mechanisms of curing or healing (restoring a sense of normalcy), forms of rehabilitation have allowed for individuals to be maintained within societies with the presence of a disability. Paleontologists have found skeletal remains of hominids presenting with healed fractures, bone diseases, amputations, evidence of muscle atrophy, and other debilitating conditions. The "Old Man of La Chappelle-aux-Saints" was reported to have had a broken rib, severe hip arthritis, diseased vertebrae, and gum disease resulting in his having no teeth. He couldn't hunt or chew well, yet he lived until the age of forty (National Geographic, 1985). Although it is not known what special role this man may have played within his community, it is unlikely that he could have lived so long had some form of rehabilitation not been implemented.

Physical modalities have always been a major contributor to the rehabilitation process. Specific modalities that are used in modern rehabilitation programs, such as massage, hydrotherapy, electrotherapy, and therapeutic exercise, are known to have existed in some form for centuries (Granger, 1976). Although these modalities have been closely associated with magical and religious healing powers, they were also used for their ability to alleviate an impairment in cases where cure was not possible, so that a resulting handicap could be minimized.

Therapeutic massage was used by the Chinese in 3000 B.C., and Hippocrates wrote of it in 460 B.C. The Romans further refined the technique. In 1812 the scientific basis of massage was developed. According to Granger, along with the development of massage came the development of reeducation, or training, of muscle (Granger, 1976; Tappan, 1968).

Hydrotherapy has presumably existed since humans first began to bathe. Homer sings of bathing, citing water as a cure of the wounded Hector. Temples in Greece dedicated to Askelepios (the god of medicine) and his daughter Hygeia (goddess of health) were visited by the infirm. The Roman baths and more modern spas rely on the healing and rehabilitative powers of water. The Nile and the Ganges, worshiped by millions, are also visited by the sick (Granger, 1976).

Minimizing disease with electricity has been done in early civilizations. Shock-producing elements of the environment, such as electric fish and rubbed amber, have been prescribed to minimize ills ranging from headaches to hemorrhage. In 1600 the foundation of modern electrotherapy was laid with the publication of "De Magnete." Benjamin Franklin developed the static machine. In 1791 Galvani discovered the current that bears his name, and in 1831 likewise for Faraday. High frequency was developed in 1890. These methods of localized electrization over muscle motor points were promoted to do many things, from extracting poison from the body to strengthening the generative organs and restoring manly vigor. Not long after, incandescent lights were introduced for radiant baking, and the value of ultraviolet light was recognized (Benton et al., 1981; Granger, 1976).

Historical evidence also reveals that surgical amputations and the subsequent use of prosthetic devices have been prevalent throughout the ages. The first recorded instance of such rehabilitation and physical therapy practice is from the Vedas of ancient India. The Rig-Veda, composed between 2500 and 1800 B.C., contains the account of Queen Vishpla, whose leg was amputated in battle. She was then fitted with an iron leg that enabled her to walk and return to the battlefield (Sanders, 1986).

The oldest prosthesis ever displayed in a museum was unearthed in Italy in 1858. This artificial leg, constructed of bronze and iron with a wooden core, was dated about 300 B.C. More modern eras have witnessed a continuation of the development of prostheses. Today, this area of subspecialty within rehabilitation is quite developed, especially computerized prosthetics.

There is also evidence that traditional cultures use some "modern" rehabilitation techniques. For example, the Eskimos and the Chippewa amputate frozen fingers. The Dama and the Masai also amputate limbs and provide prostheses where appendages are considered useless. The Chippewa, Nez Perce, Hottentot, Tahitians, and Eskimos are known to use splints. Musculoskeletal problems are often treated by massage, and the Leberian Manos use traction (Ackerknecht, 1971).

Although some physical means of rehabilitation have a long history, the concept of comprehensive rehabilitation, including the art and science of physical therapy, has developed very late in time. In the United States there were no comprehensive programs for persons with disabilities prior to World War I, although such programs did exist in Europe. Through the efforts of two orthopedic surgeons, the Division of Special Hospitals and Physical Reconstruction was established in the Surgeon General's office in 1917. Within this division was the department of Women's Auxiliary Medical Aides. Later the department title was changed to Reconstruction Aides (Hazenhyer, 1946).

In March 1918, Mary McMillan, an American-born woman who grew up in England and was trained at the College of Physical Culture in Liverpool, arrived at Walter Reed General Hospital to serve as head reconstruction aide. There she founded the first organized physical therapy department in the U.S. Army. McMillan was also instrumental in training other reconstruction aides. Fourteen institutions were established to meet the requirements outlined by the Surgeon General's office, the largest being Reed College in Eugene, Oregon, which was headed by McMillan. Most of the almost two thousand trainees were physical education teachers (Hazenhyer, 1946).

In 1919, as World War I ended, Mary McMillan and a group of reconstruction aides at Walter Reed Hospital conceived the idea of a national organization to build the profession of physical therapy. In March 1921 the first edition of *The P.T. Review* was published. In that same year McMillan wrote the first American textbook of physical therapy, entitled *Massage and Therapeutic Exercise*, and in 1924 the first bibliography on physical therapy literature was listed (Hazenhyer, 1946).

The American Women's Physical Therapeutic Association (now known as the American Physical Therapy Association, or APTA) was formed in 1922. Johnson (1985, p. 1691) wrote that the stated purpose of the organization was

> to establish and maintain a professional and scientific standard for those engaged in the profession of physical therapeutics; to increase efficiency among its members by encouraging them in advanced study; to disseminate information by the distribution of medical literature and articles of professional interest; to make available efficiently trained women to the medical profession; and to sustain social fellowship and intercourse upon grounds of mutual interest.

Mary McMillan was elected the association's first president.

During the early and mid-1920s, isolated private and public reconstruction programs were initiated for injured persons in either military or civilian life. As early as 1927, it was apparent that physical therapy leaders envisioned a rapidly expanding future. The fledgling organization, whose name was changed to the American Physiotherapy Association, began to establish new physical therapy educational programs as well as mechanisms for approving and improving existing programs; establish a central registry of qualified therapists; develop a national publication; organize local chapters as components of the organization; facilitate a recruitment program; and hold national scientific and organizational meetings (Johnson, 1985).

Two actions undertaken during this period are of historical significance with regard to issues facing the profession of physical therapy today. One was the APTA's request to the Council on Medical Education and Hospitals of the American Medical Association for assistance in overseeing the development and maintenance of standards for educational programs. The second was the inclusion in the APTA bylaws of the notion that physical therapists will "practice under the prescription, direction and supervision of licenced physicians" (Johnson, 1985, p. 1692).

After World War II, when large numbers of war-wounded were surviving their injuries and returning home, the demand for rehabilitation services increased tremendously. The response was a further development of public and private organizations and programs. The polio epidemic in the late 1940s and early 1950s also increased the demand for physical therapy services.

Since that time, rehabilitation facilities, personnel, and programs have continued to expand in quantity and improve in quality. The following decades witnessed continued dramatic changes. During the 1950s and 1960s, the field of physical therapy burgeoned. Most significantly, in 1954 the APTA moved to "divest itself from the bondage of the medical specialty of physical medicine and rehabilitation" (Magistro, 1987, p. 1727). This began the process of developing increased self-esteem, increased opportunities for growth, and the establishment of physical therapy as a distinct profession apart from medicine.

From 1954 to 1964 membership in the APTA grew 78 percent. The establishment of state physical therapy practice acts, the expansion of physical therapy education programs, and the diversification of practice settings began. Thirty-five institutions offered educational programs in 1955. In 1965, forty-five institutions offered sixty-two educational programs: thirty-five at the bachelor's degree level, one at the master's degree level, and twenty-six at the certificate level (Johnson, 1985).

Another significant action taken during this period was the formation of sections within the APTA. In 1955 the APTA board of directors approved and the House of Delegates endorsed the formation of the "self-employed" section, thus beginning the recognition of special interest groups and facilitating the move away from a large majority of therapists practicing in hospitals (Magistro, 1987). Sections "may be organized to provide a means by which members having a common interest in special areas of physical therapy may meet, confer, and promote the interests of respective sections" (APTA, 1989). There are now eighteen sections. Many are defined according to an area of clinical interest, such as pediatrics, geriatrics, oncology, obstetrics and gynecology, and neurology. Others are oriented toward an employment setting, such as veterans affairs, or an area of professional interest, such as community health or education.

Another example of the professional evolution witnessed in the field of physical therapy is that of clinical specialist certification. In 1978 the special interest sections of the APTA established the goal of providing "formal recognition for physical therapists who have acquired advanced clinical knowledge, experience, and skills in a special area of practice" (Ferrier, 1991, p. 66). The first specialists were certified in 1985 by the American Board of Physical Therapy Specialists. Thus far approximately two hundred individuals have completed the rigorous application and examination process in six specialty areas: cardiopulmonary, clinical electrophysiologic, neurologic, orthopedic, pediatric, and sports. The first examination for those wishing to pursue geriatric specialization was offered in 1992.

The physical therapy generalist and noncertified specialist are clearly the norm. According to the director of the Office of Specialist Certification at the APTA, "The specialist certification program itself does not seek to change the natural evolution of the profession. . . . It does not limit the professional activities of a therapist or prohibit a therapist from practicing in a specified arena" (Ferrier, 1991, p. 71).

Nevertheless, specialization is expected to further the advancement of the profession. The technological advancements expanding the scope of professional practice seemingly call for the emergence of clinical specialists. The process provides the consumer with verification that the clinician is expert in a particular field of practice, and it offers the clinician an employment advantage. Hopefully, specialists will be used increasingly as consultants who cross professional and institutional boundaries.

CURRENT PRACTICE

Today, although modern physical therapy services arrived on the scene only during the early to mid-twentieth century, physical therapy is prevalent and firmly entrenched within our health care system. Physical therapy, having originally been conceived in narrow terms (for example, to provide someone an artificial limb), now considers the many facets of rehabilitation for individuals having a broad range of ills such as those within the neuromuscular, musculoskeletal, or cardiopulmonary system; developmental delay; mental retardation; and acute and chronic disease. The role of the physical therapist has evolved and may be described as fluid, as therapists continue to expand their function in increasingly multiple capacities. Physical therapists function not only as clinicians but more often have additional roles as teacher, supervisor, researcher, advocate, and administrator. Practice sites have changed considerably, as more therapists work outside of the acute hospital setting. Although more than 42 percent of the APTA membership reported practicing in a hospital setting in a 1987 survey (Mathews, 1989b, p. 166), therapists are working increasingly in the home setting, independent private practice, other forms of outpatient clinics, school systems, community agencies, industry, and at sports facilities.

To a great extent, the last decades' momentous changes within the profession have paralleled those of the health care system, which has grown increasingly complex, specialized, competitive, and highly technical. Although considerable exceptions exist, the traditional health, rehabilitation, and, hence, physical therapy model has been characterized by its strong medical emphasis. Physician-directed rehabilitation, focusing on the medical management of physical disability, is primarily institution based. The rehabilitation process, defined by a team of highly trained health professionals who for the most part work independently, includes a needs assessment, treatment plan, and treatment program. The team is headed by a physician who makes the referral for care and defines the treatment orders. At its best, this model allows for coordinated care by a team of professionals. However, the person with a disability is a "patient" within a specialized institution, for whom "treatment" is required. The health professionals are often primarily responsible for all decision making on behalf of the patient (Hasselkus, 1989). This system is very expensive, and it is not necessarily conducive to societal integration on the part of the person with a disability.

As the traditional medical model has been criticized for its philosophy and mode of delivery, an alternative physical therapy model has been in the process of evolving concurrent with broader based societal changes. Physical therapy has broadened its scope to focus less on a medically centered approach and more on a person-centered approach. More recently an increasing number of leaders within the profession have begun to identify with the new paradigm focusing on improved quality of life. Arguably those therapists specializing in geriatrics or pediatrics have best modeled their practice on the newer theories. For example, as the profession recognized the continuing increase in the proportion of the aged population, literature is beginning to emerge that documents functional ability as a focus for treatment planning and geriatric health care (Hasselkus, 1989).

Within the subspecialty of pediatrics, there is a longer history of practice that has evolved into a well-defined model in support of many of the features of the newer paradigm. This is particularly so with regard to physical therapy within the educational environment. Hence it is described as an example.

The physical therapist working within the school system must implement the assurances and intent of P.L. 94-142 (the Education of All Handicapped Children Act, now called the Individuals with Disabilities Education Act). Specifically, the physical therapy provisions are addressed under the term "related services," that is, those required to assist a child in benefiting from special education services. Models of structure and function of physical therapy services within the public school environment have been developed by professional organizations and state departments of education. Historically, these have consisted of alternative dichotomous models of practice that include a medically oriented vs. educational model, a direct service treatment vs. an indirect service consultation model, and an isolated therapy vs. an integrated therapy model (Roberts, 1995).

At present the APTA Section on Pediatrics has adopted a policy that supports integrated related service models of practice as the best practice model for therapeutic intervention with persons with disabilities. The characteristics of such a model include multiple setting assessments, multidisciplinary planning, functional program designs, comprehensive and collaborative programming, and evaluation based on individual student attainment of behavioral objectives with design changes occurring if success does not occur (Roberts, 1995).

The following explicit examples are ways in which a physical therapist can function as a support within the educational system and reinforce a best practice model that recognizes the need to work in partnership with other health care professionals and the family members of children with special health care needs.

- The physical therapist can provide the special needs student with screening and individual assessments, and direct and consultative service to address specific areas of need such as functional motor skills within the educational environment, safe mobility, use of assertive/adaptive equipment, positioning for optimal learning, and others.
- The physical therapist can provide the educational staff and other team members with input for the development of individual education plans,

individual programming for students both in therapy and in the school environment, establishment of coordinated physical management plans and consultation, and/or in-service education on a variety of subjects.
- The physical therapist can provide the parent with consultation and strategies that maximize motor potential in school and home, environmental adaptation, and identification of resources for obtaining appropriate equipment and obtaining medical and therapeutic services, as well as serve in an advocacy role.
- The physical therapist can provide the school system administration with assistance and information regarding the best way to develop an effective service delivery system and a framework for utilizing their expertise (Section on Pediatrics of the APTA, 1989).

From this list it should be presumed that physical therapy can be a part of the therapeutic system in a way that maximizes a person's potential for individualization and community integration. In reality, the integrated service model proposed by Roberts and others is often hampered by limited human and financial resources, as well as a lack of knowledge and/or support of school administrators regarding the role of physical therapy. As such, integrating physical therapy services into the natural life environments of persons with disabilities remains as a continuing challenge to the profession.

CRITICAL ISSUES FACING THE PROFESSION

The outlook for the continued growth and professionalization of physical therapy as the twenty-first century draws near is excellent. Disease prevention and health promotion are beginning to take hold, but the rates of disability continue to rise as people survive illnesses and accidents that were once fatal. More individuals are living longer and more babies with developmental problems are surviving. Thus, today we see a still further increase in the demand for services. Physical therapy has been listed among the occupational specialties that will be in the highest demand during the 1990s (Fuchsberg, 1991).

The most recent Bureau of Labor estimates suggest that there are between 73,000 and 75,000 physical therapy practice opportunities currently available within the United States. The APTA estimates that approximately 66,000 therapists are engaged in practice, some only part-time. Thus, a major shortfall exists. By the year 2000, this shortfall is expected to almost triple (Moffat, 1991). Of special concern is the dearth of physical therapy services to those living in rural areas and to historically underserved ethnically diverse individuals with disabilities. For the physical therapist, there are a growing number of customized, flexible, and exciting options available.

The following practice issues have been chosen as items of special attention because they are examples of what is paramount in the minds of the profession's leadership and are indicative of the kind of challenges that lie ahead. Each must be considered within the framework of the current best practice models that will fit within the new paradigm.

Physical Therapy Education

Current issues in physical therapy education primarily stem from the changing definition of our professional identity and our expanding role as we function within this paradigm. Physical therapists can be generalist clinicians, specialist clinicians, managers, researchers, educators, or consultants. The expanding scope and practice of the profession within a new environmental framework entails a reevaluation of past educational practices so that a professional who is both caring and scientifically well versed may be educated. Of particular importance are the level and quality of education, availability and qualifications of faculty, educational standards, and curriculum content. If one reflects back to the history and recent changes within the profession, it is easy to appreciate the difficulties in maintaining a relevant educational system through which to pursue excellence.

A particularly momentous debate resulted in 1979 when the APTA House of Delegates adopted a policy that entry-level education for physical therapy must be at the post-baccalaureate degree level by December 1, 1990. Although this policy has been argued, and it has become clear that the proposed mandate was not realistic, the level of education required for entry-level physical therapy remains a crucial issue.

Currently there are 128 accredited physical therapy programs: 73 at the baccalaureate level and 55 at the master's level. The proliferation of institutions offering physical therapy appears to be continuing as the unprecedented demand for physical therapists has continued to grow and a critical shortage of clinicians has been identified.

Jane Mathews, in her 1989 Presidential Address, "Preparation for the Twenty-first Century: The Educational Challenge" (Mathews, 1989a), has defined eleven goals. A brief review of these will serve as a means of describing the critical issues regarding physical therapy education:

1. Reexamine the accreditation process in order to develop explicit criteria upon which educational programs may be rated.

2. Reexamine the admission process. The profession must reconsider what it believes to be the values and characteristics of an individual who would be a "good" physical therapist. Academic achievement, albeit important, does not necessarily equate with problem-solving skills, independent thinking, or clinical reasoning. A more culturally diverse application pool should be sought.

3. Reexamine the educational environment and the relationship between faculty and students. Faculty must "nurture the development of self-responsibility and accountability in students as active participants in their learning processes. Otherwise, we risk socializing students into subservient behavioral responses that may carry over into their clinical practice relationships with perceived authority figures such as physicians and administrators" (p. 982).

4. Facilitate educational programs' involvement in the professional socialization process so that a greater proportion of therapists become actively involved in professional organizations.

5. Prepare graduates to be reflective practitioners. Mathews refers to the required "mental concentration and considerations experienced by professional practitioners in each client encounter" (p. 984).

6. Evaluate the use of clinicians as didactic faculty resources. They should be highly valued and appreciated and afforded commensurate benefits.

7. Increase the opportunities for physical therapy assistant (PTA) development. Understand our responsibility to delegate appropriate activities and be accountable for effective supervision of the PTA.

8. Contribute to relieving the physical therapy human resource shortage by providing career renewal and reentry opportunities. As the newest APTA data indicate, it is known that 73 percent of the profession is female and that the average physical therapist remains in the field for about twelve years. Many women enter and reenter practice settings up to eight times (Moffat, 1991). The educational system must help to foster flexibility desired by some of these individuals.

9. Reexamine ways to recruit and retain faculty. The shortage of doctorally trained physical therapy faculty remains a substantial problem. Recognize the difficulties of service in the academic environment with its research, education, and service demands while attempting to maintain clinical competence.

10. Continue to strive for the previously proposed "physical therapy campus" composed of a school of physical therapy; a clinical practice center; a center for research, technological development, professional development and career renewal; a day care center; and a residential community for the ill and well.

11. Scrutinize the professional education curricula. A curriculum is easy to add to, but it is often difficult to remove obsolete information. Content and instructional strategies must be reexamined. There needs to be a better fit between content area emphasis and potential frequency of encounters.

For example, to expand on Mathews's ideas regarding curricula development, there needs to be greater emphasis on a curriculum that prepares the student to work with an increasingly diverse population in a wider variety of real-world settings. Recognizing that increasingly greater numbers of consumers will be coming from sociocultural environments that may differ from their own, students must be taught to recognize their own values and biases and how to incorporate the complexities of the consumer's values and health beliefs into their treatment program. Specifically, it is expected that a greater proportion of consumers will be elderly, and a greater number will be Hispanic, African American, Asian American, or from other culturally diverse groups. More direct health care services will be provided within the consumer's home, and physical therapists will be working in relatively new arenas, such as in the area of health promotion and disease prevention. The ability to function well within interdisciplinary collaborative practice models is fundamental. Students must receive far more classroom experience in how to be effective communicators and educators when interacting with consumers and their families, direct service providers, and other interdisciplinary team members.

The introduction of technology along with the professionalization and need for accountability within the field has led to a tremendous increase in the need for the student to have improved research skills. The need for clinically based applied research is particularly urgent.

Realizing that it is desirable for the student to learn more information than can be realistically taught within the confines of a professional education, there needs to be greater emphasis on self-directed learning and problem-solving/decision-making skills.

Of great significance is the idea that post-baccalaureate-level education is essential. In particular Mathews strongly urges the acknowledgment of the link between entry-level programs and direct access (see discussion of direct access below). This can be assured if "our curricula provides graduates with a strong and thorough foundation in systematic, organized client assessment practices that result in differential *physical therapy* diagnosis" (Mathews, 1989a, p. 984).

In sum, this list of goals offers the profession guidelines for the type of educational system needed for the physical therapy professional to remain relevant and up to date in the delivery of services.

Utilization of Physical Therapy Assistants

The burgeoning demand for physical therapy personnel and the inability of the profession to meet that demand, as well as the increasing professionalization of the physical therapist, necessitates a hard look at alternative means by which to provide physical therapy services. It must be recognized that if voids are left in practice settings, some other worker, possibly a non–physical therapist, will fill them. The utilization of the paraprofessional physical therapy assistant can help to solve the dilemma.

Historically, the use of PTAs has been a source of controversy. Smey (1991) cites historical examples of professional leaders suggesting why this might be so. For example, in 1964 Jacqueline Perry, in an article entitled "Professionalism in Physical Therapy," asserted that physical therapists who must be told by the physician what to do and how to do it accept a role for themselves as a "nonprofessional." She goes on to suggest that this kind of thinking contributes to some of the resistance to training and accepting "nonprofessional" support personnel. Catherine Worthingham, in her 1965 analysis of the use of support personnel, recognized that oftentimes physical therapists go into the field because they want the satisfactions that come from "laying on of the hands" and developing close relationships with their patients. By using PTAs for actual patient care, this contact would be diminished. She also pointed out the real possibility of therapists considering that the PTA is a threat to their own economic security.

In spite of such concerns, it is nevertheless critical that one recognize the advantages of working in concert with paraprofessionals such as PTAs, particularly within the proposed framework for meeting the needs of persons with disabilities. As long as each physical therapy supervisor responsibly evaluates the competence of the PTA and delegates tasks appropriately, the PTA can be a valuable team member who adds to the core of service providers during this critical period of shortages. It is presumed that as more states pass direct-access legislation (see following section), the PTA will be in even greater demand to assist with treatment applications.

Although lack of ethnic diversity within the rehabilitation fields remains a critical concern, more PTAs than physical therapists are from diverse cultural backgrounds. Thus they may be more sensitized to the diverse population in need of services and may enhance the consumer/professional match that can facilitate successful services. PTAs also help to reduce health care costs, as they demand lower salaries than the physical therapist. Finally, the effective use of assistants enables the physical therapist to perform evaluative, administrative, and research functions as well as serve as a consultant and problem solver rather than solely a provider of services.

Direct Access

Direct access to physical therapy services refers to evaluation and treatment of consumers by physical therapists without referral from another health care professional. This concept has previously been referred to as "independent practice," "practice without referral," or "practice independent of practitioner referrals." With direct access, therapists can be the first entry point within the health system for a consumer, and referrals can come from physical therapists to other health care professionals.

Currently, slightly more than half of the states have established direct access. An additional number of states have legislated the right for therapists to evaluate a consumer without a referral. In states without full direct-access legislation, either proponents are planning to introduce such legislation or the state physical therapy associations have already gone through the process and have failed to obtain their goal. Direct-access legislation efforts are usually a very high priority for physical therapy leaders.

Some within the professional and lay communities have expressed reservations about direct access. Concerns focus on the effect of direct access on such things as quality of care, cost of care, malpractice insurance rates, and the relationship between physician and physical therapist. Fears about overutilization of services and increased costs do not, thus far, seem to be well founded (Taylor and Domholdt, 1991). Moreover, direct access underscores the fact that the physical therapist can be a primary, direct service provider. It also can allow for greater service flexibility, better use of professionals as consultants, improved collaboration within the system, and increased likelihood of facilitating consumer empowerment by allowing the individual to make his or her own choice of service provider.

CONCLUSION

The concept of increasing professionalism is intimately related to the present status and future progress of physical therapy. In excerpts from a series of presentations on this concept that has generated so much interest, Mathews (1989c) suggests particular behaviors that characterize professionalism, among which are full accountability, lifelong career commitment, commitment to lifelong learning, high ethical/moral standards, value for objectivity, skill at self-criticism, comfort with ambiguities, respect for other health care professionals, advocacy for the consumer, and participation in professional associations. The physical therapy profession and the individual physical therapist must be cognizant of these characteristics as allied health rehabilitation workers prepare to function in the newly developing paradigm appropriate for the approaching twenty-first century.

To facilitate an optimal professional/environmental match, professionals must respond to changes within the environment and be capable of change within themselves. Physical therapists, as part of a rehabilitation team, must be prepared to relinquish their misguided traditional role whereby they view themselves and other health care professionals as the ones to make decisions for consumers. Physical therapists must move toward a role in which they are consultants and part of a support system within consumers' natural community environments. Within this framework, consumers are elevated to a position of dominance through a process whereby they assume authority and decision-making power.

The profession of physical therapy has matured greatly yet remains in a state of evolution. At this juncture, as new ideals of excellence are fostered, there are a great many challenges and opportunities before us. The professional leaders emphasize the need to be unified in our goals and to educate the consumer about our role within the rehabilitation domain. There is a strong desire to gain further autonomy, as exemplified by the actions taken to gain direct access via amendment of the state licensing practice acts, the transition to internal setting of educational standards, and an increase in the educational requirements for the entry-level physical therapist. At the same time, the profession must not negate the values of interdependent collaborative practice and team relationships nor forget that our primary raison d'être is to provide services in a manner that most befits the consumer.

REFERENCES

Ackerknecht, E. (1971). *Medicine and ethnology: Selected essays.* Baltimore: Johns Hopkins University Press.

American Physical Therapy Association (1989). *Bylaws, standing rules and membership rights.* Fairfax, VA: Author.

Benton, L., et al. (1981). *Functional electrical stimulation: A practical clinical guide.* Downey, CA: Rancho Los Amigos Hospital.

Ferrier, M. (1991). One stage in professional evolution. *Clinical Management, 11*(2), 66–71.

Fuchsberg, G. (1991). Despite layoffs, firms find some jobs hard to fill. *The Wall Street Journal,* January 22, C-3.

Granger, F.B. (1976). The development of physiotherapy. *Physical Therapy, 56*(1), 13–21.

Hasselkus, B. (1989). Occupational and physical therapy in geriatric rehabilitation. *Physical and Occupational Therapy in Geriatrics, 7*(3), 3–20.

Hazenhyer, I.M. (1946). A history of the American Physical Therapy Association. *The Physiotherapy Review, 26*(1), 3–14.

Johnson, G.R. (1985). Twentieth Mary McMillan lecture—Great expectations: A force in growth and change. *Physical Therapy, 65*(11), 1690–1695.

Johnson, G.R. (1989). Issues and trends in physical therapy education. In J. Mathews (Ed.), *Practice issues in physical therapy* (pp, 1–22). Thorofare, NJ: Slack.

Leavitt, R. (1988). Rehabilitation services: An international perspective. Unpublished term paper. Storrs: University of Connecticut.

Magistro, C. (1987). Twenty-second Mary McMillan lecture. *Physical Therapy, 67*(11), 1726–1732.

Mathews, J. (1989a). The 1989 presidential address—Preparation for the twenty-first century: The educational challenge. *Physical Therapy, 69*(11), 981–986.

Mathews, J. (1989b). The future of physical therapy in hospital settings. In J. Mathews (Ed.), *Practice issues in physical therapy* (pp. 159–166). Thorofare, NJ: Slack.

Mathews, J. (1989c). Professionalism in physical therapy. In J. Mathews (Ed.), *Practice issues in physical therapy* (pp. 167–173). Thorofare, NJ: Slack.

Moffat, M. (1991). Shortages abound! President's perspective. *Progress Report,* November, 3.

National Geograpic Society (1985). Early man. *National Geographic, 168*(5), 615.

Roberts, P. (1995). A descriptive correlation study of physical therapy services in school systems. Ph.D. dissertation. Worcester, MA: Clark University.

Sanders, G. (1986). *Lower limb amputations: A guide to rehabilitation.* Philadelphia: F. A. Davis.

Section on Pediatrics of the American Physical Therapy Association. (1989). The physical therapist in the educational environment: Providing services to enhance the educational program. Alexandria, VA.: American Physical Therapy Association.

Smey, J. (1991). Issues in aging: The role of the community college. Storrs: University of Connecticut.

Tappan, F. (1968). *Massage techniques: A case method approach.* New York: Macmillan.

Taylor, T., and Domholdt, E. (1991). Legislative changes to permit direct access to physical therapy services: A study of process and content issues. *Physical Therapy, 71*(5), 382–389.

20

Therapeutic Recreation: Historical Paradigms and a Conundrum for Use in the Future

Robert E. Cipriano

INTRODUCTION

Many concepts of leisure and recreation have been held by people from primitive times to the present. As societies have grown more complex, the interpretations of work, leisure, and recreation have changed as a result of changing values and beliefs. In all societies up to and including the present one, humans have been obligated to perform certain subsistence tasks. However, when the necessary tasks were completed, people sought release from the stresses these tasks created. The type of release depended on the particular culture and the individual's own desires. In the twenty-first century, very little time may need to be devoted to subsistence work, and people may have many more hours of free time.

Today, leisure is viewed as a growing component of each human's everyday life. There are few people who do not anticipate using their leisure time. Leisure is free time, a good feeling. Leisure provides experiences that allow for self-expression. It also allows for a re-creation of one's lifestyle. Within the "norm" of society, approximately one-quarter of a person's life is spent in unorganized use of leisure time.

BRIEF HISTORY OF LEISURE AND RECREATION

The Industrial Revolution

By the middle of the eighteenth and continuing into the nineteenth century, the Industrial Revolution brought about changes in life both in Europe and in the United States. The invention of machines, such as the cotton gin, the spinning and weaving machines, and the steam engine, affected work by mechanizing industry.

Home industries were no longer the mode of work; mechanization centralized work. Factories brought about the growth of cities and the uprooting of people from small towns and villages. This pattern was seen in all of western Europe and in the United States. It gave rise to overcrowding in urban areas and the concomitant evils of poor housing, inadequate food, increased crime, and desire to produce as much as possible with the least capital outlay. Further, people were forced to work long hours for mere subsistence because of meager pay.

As working conditions became intolerable in the cities of Europe, people emigrated to the United States. Many of the same conditions existed in America, but because the country was new and growing, the opportunity seemed greater for better living.

The people who came, particularly to the northern states, brought with them basic beliefs about leisure and recreation. Work was the most important element of their lives, and the Protestant ethic that play was sinful conditioned the early leisure and recreation patterns in the United States. In the cities, recreation had the same forms as in Europe. There was theater, music, drama, and other kinds of spectator activities, such as vaudeville and burlesque, gambling, all forms of racing, boxing, wrestling, and others.

As urbanization and slums developed in Europe and the United States, the social reform movement also developed to counteract these conditions. The result was the beginning of the agencies known today as the Ys and settlement houses. Other similar agencies developed. They were committed to the idea of helping people to help themselves find a better life. The founding of the Boston Sand Gardens, started in 1886 to care for children of industrial laborers, is considered the beginning of organized recreation in the United States.

As the United States' frontier expanded westward, work continued to be the single most important part of living. However, there was some relaxation of the strict Puritan ethic, and greater permissiveness in regard to recreation resulted. In addition, people from many parts of the country settled in new areas, and the plurality of lifestyle that is so predominant today had some of its beginnings.

The Early Twentieth Century

Greater and greater industrialization in the United States and the continued expansion on the western frontier brought continuously changing patterns of leisure and recreation. One of the new developments that continues to exert a strong influence on leisure patterns was the invention of the automobile. People became more mobile and were able to enjoy many recreational pursuits that previously had not been available to them. The single most dominant theme in the advent of recreation and leisure services in the United States is the fact that this field has always responded to social needs.

In 1906 the Playground Association of America was formed for the purpose of promoting better recreational opportunities for children. This organization has gone through several changes, and today it is called the National Recreation and Park Association (NRPA). Although the focus of the organization has developed as society in the United States has changed, its purpose remains essentially the promotion and development of leisure services that will bring a better quality of life not only for children but also for all people. A separate branch of the NRPA is the Therapeutic Recreation Section, which provides recreation experiences to all individuals with disabilities.

One of the first changes in focus of the Playground Association was the establishment of War Camp Services during World War I. Services were provided for military men both in the United States and Europe. These services were heavily sports oriented but also provided shows, music, crafts, and other activities. This exposure to a variety of recreation activities was the first for many of the men. Returning to their own communities, these men began to seek the same kinds of services at home. Thus, a real emphasis on the need for community recreation programs began.

In 1918 "The Seven Cardinal Principles of Education" was published by the Commission on Secondary Education. One of these articulated principles was "the worthy use of leisure time." This principle has not been implemented in the schools in general. However, because of many social forces at play in the twentieth-century United States, the schools now may recognize the need to educate for leisure as well as for work.

As the United States moved into the Great Depression, totally different patterns of living were found to exist. The most profound change was the extent of unemployment and its attendant ills: idleness, poverty, and low morale. Programs to alleviate unemployment influenced the development of leisure services.

One major program—the Works Progress Administration (WPA)—included construction of outdoor and indoor facilities for recreation. In addition, program services were introduced into communities, including many leisure pursuits for all ages. Unemployed people worked in these programs, and extensive in-service training programs were conducted to give them the necessary skills to lead programs. Out of these activities grew many community programs and professional preparation programs in recreation education in colleges and universities. As communities began to enjoy their community recreation programs, they began to ask for trained leaders.

During World War II many advances were made in the delivery of leisure services. The armed forces provided extensive services for all personnel both at home and abroad. These services were extended to dependents at home during the war and overseas at war's end. The services demonstrated the advantages of giving people leisure programs. The armed forces also provided recreation services in hospitals. Medical technology had advanced significantly during the early and late 1940s. Men fighting in World War II who would have previously perished were now being saved. They were no longer dying; however, they were maimed and disabled. The soldiers who returned home after their victory in World War II were embraced on their return. The Veterans Administration provided a wealth of recreation services to servicemen returning from the war. These services sparked the development of therapeutic recreation services for all individuals with disabilities, which have been and are continuing to be developed and refined.

Communities provided recreation services for all kinds of war workers. Some of these were in-plant services, others were conducted by community departments. Many times these services were conducted around the clock in order to care for the recreational needs and interests of shift workers. At the close of the war, many leisure service programs were continued as people in communities demanded more such programs that they were exposed to during the war.

Since the 1960s

After World War II, society in the United States experienced profound changes in cultural patterns. As a result of war experiences and the development of the atomic bomb, people began to question the older values. A desire for immediate gratification developed, particularly among young people. They believed that they might not be alive in the future to enjoy the satisfaction of their desire because nuclear war would destroy the world. Many new lifestyles evolved and there was, and is, a relaxation of mores.

The past three decades have witnessed tremendous discord in the United States. The relaxed times of the 1950s have given way to the following anxiety-provoking social issues:

1. Race riots in cities across the country
2. Assassinations of three of the most influential and charismatic political leaders (John F. Kennedy, Martin Luther King, Robert Kennedy) all within five years of each other
3. Continual conflict between various ethnic groups
4. Precarious employment future for many people
5. A breakdown of many social institutions
6. A high illiteracy rate, which continues to grow
7. Conflicts associated with the protracted Vietnam conflict
8. Random violence, along with an escalating crime rate
9. Less time in which to pursue one's leisure interests
10. AIDS
11. Crack cocaine
12. Homelessness
13. Unresponsiveness of political leaders to stop waste and corruption
14. A general feeling of hopelessness
15. Concern for the environment
16. Acting as a "global cop" to police the world
17. An instantaneous graphic depiction, through the media, that presents events in sensational detail

This list is presented as illustrative rather than as an exhaustive hierarchy of events leading to the U.S. malaise. All of these developments had, and still have, an influence on leisure services. Some have been fulfilling, others destructive. The following are examples of such developments.

1. Creation of the Land Water Conservation Fund in 1965 and the establishment of the Bureau of Outdoor Recreation will affect leisure services for many years.

2. Automation has brought increased free time to many people who have begun to try to find satisfying ways to fill that free time. Automation has alienated workers, for work no longer challenges them.

3. As outdoor facilities have been developed by local, state, and federal governments and by private enterprise, there has been an increased interest in outdoor sports and camping. There has been a great increase in use of all kinds of recreational vehicles, from snowmobiles to luxurious homes on wheels.

4. Health care has improved, and people are living longer. Many live for years on retirement from work, during which time they seek increased services.

5. A youth culture has developed that challenges traditional values and no longer accepts traditional leisure pursuits.

6. The challenge given to the leisure services programs has caused professionals to continually reexamine the programs that are being offered and to involve users in the planning and organizing of those services.

7. Changes in sexual morals have affected leisure services programs.

8. The prevalence of drug addiction among many segments of society has caused many changes in societal patterns. Among them is the increase in crime and changed patterns of leisure participation because of crime.

9. With the rise of television, people satisfy their leisure needs by *watching* programs rather than participating in them. People would rather passively watch highly skilled athletes perform than actively participate themselves.

10. Family structure has changed from the extended family to the nuclear family, bringing with it a failure in cross-generation understanding and a failure in transmission of cultural patterns from one generation to the next.

Trends for the Future

As the United States looks toward the twenty-first century, certain developments seem inevitable:

1. Fewer hours of work will be required to satisfy subsistence needs.
2. There will be a greater emphasis on both paid and volunteer work in service types of jobs.
3. People will seek challenges in their free time; they will not be satisfied with busywork.
4. There will be gradual recognition that education for the "worthy use of leisure time" is as important as education for work.
5. Education will become a lifelong endeavor.
6. Having more than one career will become a pattern for many people.
7. New patterns of funding of leisure activities will be introduced as economic pressures affect the delivery of services.
8. There will be an outcry to provide quality recreative experiences to all segments of society.

In the final analysis, the challenge of the future is the need for leisure services personnel to be constantly alert to the changing needs of society.

RECREATION AND LEISURE OPERATIONALIZED

Ball and Cipriano (1978) offer four definitions regarding the term *recreation.* The authors quoted here are five of the early leaders in the recreation field. Therefore, their theories were followed closely by others in the field.

> Recreation may be considered as any form of leisure-time experience or activity in which an individual engages from choice because of the enjoyment and satisfaction which it brings directly to him (Butler, 1967, p. 17).

> Recreation is . . . any activity, either individual or collective, pursued during one's leisure time. Being relatively free and pleasurable, it has its own appeal (Neameyer, 1964, p. 41).

> Recreation is actively voluntarily engaged in during leisure time and primarily motivated by the satisfaction or pleasure derived from it (Meyer and Brightbill, 1961, p. 67).

> Recreation is the natural expression during leisure of human interests seeking satisfaction. . . . (Fitzgerald, 1964, p. 114).

Ellis (1973) provided an early concept of the term *recreation.* This author interpreted recreation according to individual behavior:

> Play is that behavior that is motivated by the need to elevate the level of arousal towards the optimal. . . . Its corollary, work, is the behavior emitted to reduce the level of stimulation, and fits nicely the concept of drive-reduction theories of behavior (p. 110).

Gray and Greben (1973) proposed a theory of recreation that had as its theme feelings of self-satisfaction. They indicated that this theory held promise concerning the future of the recreation profession:

> Recreation is an emotional condition within an individual human being that flows from a feeling of well-being and self-satisfaction. It is characterized by feelings of mastery, achievement, exhilaration, acceptance, success, personal worth, and pleasure. It reinforces a positive self-image. Recreation is a response to aesthetic experience, achievement of personal goals, or positive feedback

from others. It is independent of activity, leisure [time], or social acceptance (p. 42).

These theories dominated the thinking up to the 1980s. Since that time, a new way of thinking has emerged. At present, this thinking has as its major focus the following concept: Because "recreation" is constantly changing, ever evolving, and highly personal, the term cannot be defined. The dynamic nature of this term enables people to characterize its salient components. Major characteristics composing major components of the term *recreation* are listed below:

1. Free
2. Fun
3. Highly individual
4. Personally satisfying
5. Activity-based (passive and/or active)
6. Intrinsically motivating
7. Can take place anywhere
8. Voluntary
9. Educational
10. Self-rewarding
11. Freely chosen
12. Personally pleasurable
13. Personally stimulating
14. Challenging
15. Restorative (i.e., refreshes a person)
16. Can be work or work-related
17. Does not have to be "socially acceptable"
18. Can take place individually or in a group
19. Should elicit positive feelings
20. Other (as expressed by individual preferences and personal choices)

Musings on Leisure

Edginton and Ford (1985) succinctly defined the term *leisure* to include one of the following three concepts: (1) as a block of time, (2) as a state of mind, or (3) as an activity. They freely acknowledge that there is no universally accepted conceptual framework that operationally defines the term *leisure*. Each of these concepts is briefly discussed in the next sections.

Leisure as a Block of Time
When thinking of leisure as a block of time, we think of it as a time when individuals are free to pursue those things that are of interest

to them. Within this block of time, people may select what they want to do; these activities may be active or passive. This concept presupposes that one's life routine can be divided into three concentric circles, namely, existence, subsistence, and leisure or discretionary time.

Leisure as a State of Mind

Viewing leisure as a state of mind strongly suggests that the individual's perception of what constitutes a leisure experience is the central determinant of whether or not a leisure experience has occurred. Therefore, according to this theory, if individuals feel or think that they are experiencing leisure, then in fact they are. Consequently, there is the possibility for leisure to occur at various times and places and in a variety of circumstances.

Leisure as Activities

This theory depends on an analysis of the types of activities in which individuals engage. Therefore, leisure is described or defined in terms of activities such as arts, sports, games, volunteering, reading, writing, ice skating, and so on.

Leisure as a State of Mind

The current thinking in the field overwhelmingly suggests that leisure should be conceptualized as a state of mind. If we subscribe to this popular theory, there are criteria that can be used in order to measure and define it. Three specific criteria have been identified by social psychologists: (1) perceived freedom, (2) intrinsic motivation, and (3) perceived competence.

Perceived Freedom

The belief that people must feel that they have independence and latitude in order for the leisure experience to occur. Simply stated, an individual who does not feel forced or constrained to participate has a higher degree of perceived freedom than one who is compelled to participate. People who perceive that they have control over their own behavior, as opposed to those who attribute events in their lives to chance, fate, or luck, also have a higher degree of perceived freedom.

Intrinsically Motivated

People who are intrinsically motivated are driven from within. They are able to reward themselves and are not dependent on external rewards. These people have a greater sense of perceived freedom, hence, a greater opportunity to experience leisure. Individuals who are intrinsically motivated achieve feelings of satisfaction, enjoyment, and gratification that are inwardly defined and controlled.

Perceived Competence

The perception an individual has of his or her competence while participating in an activity will affect the leisure experience. People must have a perception of competence in order to attain a leisure "state of mind." People do not have to *be* competent, they need only *perceive* themselves as such.

The Nature of Therapeutic Recreation: Process Models

Over the years a variety of terms have been used to operationally define the nature of therapeutic recreation. O'Morrow and Reynolds (1989) wrote that the term "initially used to describe recreation services to the ill and disabled was hospital recreation, with emphasis on the recreation experience within hospitals or institutional settings" (p. 77). *Recreation therapy* was a term used throughout the mid-1960s. This perspective considered those recreation activities or experiences as treatment tools that were prescribed as part of therapy. According to this term, the concern was with illness and treatment of disease. The terms *recreation to the ill and handicapped* and later *recreation for special populations* have been used to describe recreation services to individuals with limited impairments or disabilities in community settings. More recently the terms *community-based programs for special populations* and *special recreation* have been applied. Since 1966 the term *therapeutic recreation* replaced the older terms except for those terms related specifically to the community setting.

Many authors (Ball, 1978; Berryman, 1972; Frye and Peters, 1972; Gunn and Peterson, 1984) have written that the term *therapeutic recreation* is a process to describe the series of steps that the therapeutic recreation specialist takes to meet the needs and interests of special population members through recreative experiences. The implication inherent within all of these models is that the therapeutic recreation process is concerned with moving members from a particular point in the environment, where they are involved in activity as a result of unconscious needs or interests or are unable to participate because of a variety of circumstances, to a point where they are able to fulfill their responsibility for meeting their own recreation needs and interests at a conscious level—or short of this, participating in recreative experiences to the extent possible within the limitations imposed by the circumstances.

O'Morrow and Reynolds (1989) indicate that "Dividing the process into phases is an artificial separation of actions that cannot be separated in actual practice since the basic concept of the process suggests it is a unified whole" (p. 79). Therefore, the entire process is dynamic in view of the fact that data from one phase can alter or support the other phases. However, in spite of these cautions, the therapeutic recreation process is divided into the following phases or steps.

1. *Assessment* of the focus individuals' therapeutic recreation needs and interests
2. *Development* (planning) of goals for therapeutic recreation action
3. *Implementation* of therapeutic recreation action to meet goals
4. *Evaluation* of the effectiveness of therapeutic recreation action

IMPORTANCE OF LEISURE AND RECREATION

The literature indicates that positive attitudes toward leisure have a positive impact on an individual's social and psychological adjustment in life (Cheseldine and Jeffree, 1981). Awareness of the role leisure plays in one's life as well as participation in recreation activities are key components in the development of social and psychological well-being and positively affect an individual's life satisfaction (Certo, Schleien, and Hunter, 1983; Fardig, 1986; Wuerch and Voeltz, 1982).

Play participation and play training are related to increases in skill level in a variety of academic areas (Voeltz and Wuerch, 1981); and knowledge of leisure skills and attitudes is related to decreases in negative and inappropriate behavior (Adkins and Matson, 1980; Flavell, 1973; Schleien, Kiernan, and Wehman, 1981). Further, constructive use of leisure and free time is related to the successful maintenance of persons in community settings (Barrett, 1987, Ray et al., 1986; Schleien and Ray, 1988; Wehman, 1977; Wuerch and Voeltz, 1982). From these and other studies, it is clear that there is a growing body of evidence about the importance of the leisure experience to the lives of people.

For individuals with disabilities, free (nonwork) time is of special importance in part because as they grow up, there may be diminished opportunities for participation in the workforce. Even with the current focus on transition and increased effectiveness in job training, placement, and supported employment, full participation may not be achieved or desired by all persons with handicapping conditions. Thus, it may be through leisure alone that the opportunity will exist to enhance the quality of their lives and bring greater meaning to their days. Unfortunately, in contemporary U.S. society, persons with disabilities are often unaware of or are ill-prepared to participate in the numerous and varied recreation pursuits available, or they are unable to make sound recreation choices.

Satisfying and productive use of leisure time is an important factor contributing to the quality of life of all persons. Americans spend billions of dollars annually on recreation and leisure pursuits. For the population at large, one eighth or 12.5 percent of the average family's expenditures are recreation related.

Recreation and leisure pursuits are major components of any individual's life. Approximately two thirds of an individual's life is spent in the nonschool/nonwork environment. Self-perception during that time greatly affects how one functions during the total course of one's life. Research strongly indicates direct relationships between leisure satisfaction and enhanced social skills, self-concept, competence, and so on (Baumgaart et al., 1982; Schleien and Wehman, 1986; Shevin and Klein, 1984). Successful participation in recreation activities encourages feelings of control and competence (Iso-Ahola, 1980), which enhance self-concept and independence. All of these factors positively affect an individual's quality of life.

Many nonhandicapped citizens already have the requisite attitudes, skills, and opportunities necessary to allow them satisfying and independent leisure functioning. The same statement simply is not true for the nation's individuals who are handicapped. Persons with disabilities often do not have the requisite leisure attitudes and recreation skills or opportunities necessary to enable participation in recreation in the least restrictive environment. Thus, they may have diminished social integration (Bullock, 1993).

Attitudes must be developed and recreation skills need to be taught to remediate deficits and better prepare people with disabilities for full involvement in life. This intervention must occur early in a person's life, as research suggests that a lack of self-esteem, self-confidence, and independent functioning when manifested by secondary school-aged students is highly resistant to change. These problems are frequently related to difficulty in making a successful transition from school to work and community living in later years (Schleien and Ray, 1988; Schleien and Werder, 1985; Wehman and Schleien, 1981).

A NEW INTERPRETATION OF
THERAPEUTIC RECREATION

When one conceptualizes the term *therapeutic recreation* and superimposes both the historical perspective of this term and the generic term *recreation*, it becomes clear that a new interpretation is needed. We are dominated by a way of thinking that suggests that all individuals wish to be in control of their destiny. This new self-determination is becoming the engine that fuels the rehabilitation train as we move forward into the twenty-first century.

Recreation, with its dominant themes of freedom of choice, individual satisfaction, intrinsic motivation, voluntary participation, self-reward, and so on, should be thought of in new and more encompassing terms. Recreation services for individuals with disabilities can play a major role in enhancing their quality of life. It appears that therapeutic recreation personnel will be called on to modify their roles to meet the diverse needs of individuals with disabilities. Traditionally, therapeutic recreation specialists served as providers of a variety of recreation activities that they planned and implemented for individuals with disabilities.

It is logical to assume that in the not-so-distant future, therapeutic recreation specialists will be enablers and facilitators rather than leaders and programmers. They will be knowledgeable concerning the myriad human and facility resources available in the community where individuals with disabilities live, work, and recreate. They will facilitate the active participation of people with disabilities by identifying key people to work with each focus individual to enable that person to utilize the generic recreation resources distinct and unique to each local community. What follows is an interpretation of this concept, that is, a person-centered therapeutic recreation program designed to enhance the quality of life of individuals with disabilities.

Therapeutic Recreation: A Person-Centered Approach

In the last fifteen years, there has been a dramatic change in recreation services offered to individuals with disabilities. Over this period of time the value of providing both chronologically age-appropriate and inappropriate recreation activities in specially designed "segregated facilities" has been seriously questioned. In its place, recreation services that support chronologically age-appropriate activities in typical school, community, and home environments have flourished. Many policy, fiscal, and programmatic changes have been made in order to promote recreation activities that allow individuals with disabilities to participate in integrated environments. These more recent services and models have focused on changing the locations in which services are available, moving service to people rather than people to services. Decentralized school services, supported employment, community-based integrated recreation programs, semidependent group homes, and supported living are all examples of a reorganization and redistribution of resources that focus on services within integrated community environments. This programmatic and philosophical switch has dramatically increased the likelihood of people with all disabilities functioning in integrated environments.

The sophistication of therapeutic recreation service delivery is constantly expanding. Advances in the "science" of leisure preference/assessment have facilitated the development of major changes in the overall approach to therapeutic recreation. These new approaches draw much more heavily on an individualized system of planning, supporting, and expanding the number of people involved in designing and providing a wealth of recreative opportunities and experiences. Such approaches require generic recreation agencies to develop service delivery models that provide a great deal of flexibility in how services are provided, what they encompass, and who will provide them.

A holistic, person-centered planning approach to the field of therapeutic recreation appears to warrant significantly further study. Each consumer will be supported to develop, expand and involve a group of family, friends, coworkers, and recreation staff to establish and continually re-evaluate an individualized leisure plan. The person centered goal refers to a comprehensive array of objectives, including "futures planning," informed consumer decision making, relationship building, functional assessment, ongoing problem solving, individualized recreation choices, and development of natural supports.

Many conversion efforts have been criticized as being primarily directed by providers' needs. In such models, the consumer becomes the recipient of the planning process (i.e., "Have we got a recreation activity for you!"). It is suggested that a better alternative is that the plan be directed by the needs and interests of the consumer. In this model, the agency now becomes the recipient of the plan (i.e., "These are the support services I need from the agency!").

Historically, the recreation and leisure service delivery system has offered consumers choices by organizing and providing the consumer with *program* options. Recently, however, a new way of thinking about how we plan *with* people rather than *for* them has emerged. Planning that is directed and driven *by* the individual who will be utilizing the services has been called "person-centered planning." The traditional notion of offering "program options" in a segregated setting becomes replaced with the responsibility of responding to individualized "support service needs."

Person-centered planning is a highly individualized process that focuses on a person's strengths, capacities, and specific needs. It is designed to result in connecting that person to the community and workplace where he or she lives. The process encourages the individual, as well as those closest to him or her, to express dreams, aspirations, and concerns. This may involve a somewhat formal "circle of friends" or may simply include gatherings of family members, significant others, friends, coworkers, neighbors, employers, and support providers for the purpose of celebrating a person's successes, building his or her future, and problem solving. Therapeutic recreation can be a synergistic agent to connect an individual with a disability to his or her community. Planning team members come together creatively and collaboratively to decide which problem-solving ideas make sense and who will be responsible for which actions.

It is important to note that, in this process, the roles of recreation professionals shift significantly. Traditionally, these professionals have been viewed as controllers and providers of services, whereas a person-centered approach requires that professional recreators assume more subtle roles as facilitators, "connectors," and community resource locators. The change from program providers to members of a support team is not only a significant role change for the community recreation agency, but also includes expectations that family and friends consider active new roles in transportation, problem solving, leisure education, accessibility, and other newly emerging support areas.

THE FUTURE

The field of therapeutic recreation had its inception in response to meeting a specific social need; that is, the veterans with disabilities returning from World War II were provided with a variety of recreation activities in Veterans' Administration facilities across the country. Since this rather unstructured beginning, the discipline of therapeutic recreation has undergone significant changes. Each of the changes has reflected an attempt to be responsive to the more global concerns of society—for example, unemployment, gang violence, changing values in society, issues of empowerment for groups of people who have been traditionally underrepresented, and so on. What conceptual framework will be the synergistic agent that will drive the field as we move into the twenty-first century?

Rationale/Importance

In 1955 the U.S. Supreme Court, the highest legal authority in the land, held that a system of "separate but equal" public education for blacks and whites was counter to the spirit and the letter of the Constitution. Since that time, a steady stream of legislation and litigation has consistently reaffirmed the concept of "equal opportunity" for all U.S. citizens in virtually every area of public life. The principle has stood and continues to stand as a national sociological ideal. The concept of "separate but equal" has all but disappeared as a rationale for segregating lifestyles.

In 1977 the U.S. Congress signed into law Section 504 of the Rehabilitation Act of 1973, which states, in part:

> No otherwise qualified handicapped individual in the United States . . . shall, solely by reason of his [or her] handicap, be excluded from the participation in, be denied the benefits of, or be subjected to discrimination under any program or activity receiving federal financial assistance.

Section 504 was one of the last two significant pieces of civil rights legislation to come out of Washington. The Americans with Disabilities Act (ADA) was passed into law in 1990 and has far-reaching implications to enhance the quality of life of many individuals with disabilities. It took Congress a long time to realize that people with disabilities were a minority group that was being denied equal opportunity as much as or more than any other—in public education, transportation, employment, and recreation.

Prior to 1977, the concept of "separate but equal" was often used as a rationalization for providing "special," segregated opportunities for persons with disabilities. We told ourselves that such opportunities were best for people with disabilities because they have "special" capabilities, "special" needs, "special" goals, "special" means, "special" bodies, "special" personalities, "special" minds. "Special but equal" took the place of "separate but equal," but the segregation was just as real.

In spite of Section 504, as well as P.L. 94-142 (IDEA) and ADA, equal opportunity for people with disabilities to participate in recreation programs and activities is still the exception rather than the rule. The concept of "special but equal" has become a standard for providing leisure opportunities to people with disabilities. "Special populations" programs abound in public/community recreation departments and agencies. The natural focus on "specialness" in these programs has nurtured stereotypical attitudes regarding individuals with disabilities. It has encouraged the recreation community to be overly attentive to the ways in which people with disabilities seem different from "us" and like each other, rather than the ways in which we are all alike.

It is the right of *all* of us to choose the ways in which we will participate in public life. This right is embedded in our law and our heritage. Providing only segregated recreation opportunities for people with disabilities violates this basic right of choice. It is our responsibility as recreation service providers to be sure that *all* people, whatever their disabilities, are afforded an equal opportunity to participate in all recreation opportunities and programs and to be as "unspecial" as anyone else.

A recent Carnegie Council on Children report condemns the psychology–medicine–special education community for contributing to the damaging misconception that people with disabilities are "sick," thus offering a "rationalization for excluding" them from normal life. Many associations supporting the legal rights of individuals with disabilities assume assertive advocacy postures and lobby for "generic services" for their clientele. The federal government, through various funding agencies, supports personnel training demonstration projects and other efforts designed to facilitate the inclusion of persons with disabilities in community-based leisure settings. Colleges and universities are reorienting and refocusing professional curricula to emphasize coursework and practicum experiences relating to the involvement of children and adults with disabilities in public education, employment, and generic leisure service agencies. This constitutes a growing commitment of human service personnel to accept and embrace the principle of person-centered program planning and utilize this philosophy as a guiding force in their interactions with individuals with disabilities, thereby providing equal opportunities for all.

For equal opportunity to become a reality in recreation service provision, full accessibility must be accomplished, both physical/environmental and programmatic. This means that every reasonable attempt should be made to enable participants with disabilities to get into buildings and facilities and, once there, to receive the same benefits, services, and information provided to all other participants.

To achieve full accessibility, we have to look at people with disabilities the same way we look at everyone else. There are differences between any two people—they look different, they act different, they can do different things at different levels of ability. We accept these differences as part of the diversity of humankind, and we proceed with the task of providing them with recreational services, not according to how they are different but according to how they are alike.

People with disabilities have the right to be accepted and served in the same way, to be included in the diversity of humankind. They have the same variety of needs, wants, desires, expectations, and abilities as other people. The only course to full accessibility is programming by abilities rather than disabilities, and then attending to whatever barriers may stand in the way of including any potential participant who has those abilities. Individuals with disabilities should be taught to assess their abilities, gain access to recreation programs where they live, work, and play, and obtain the myriad benefits of a person-centered recreation approach.

Operationalization between Person-Centered
Planning and Leisure and Recreation Services

Although the philosophical and legislative impetus for person-centered planning has been articulated (see Wehman and Schleien, 1981), the following eight concepts provide an interrelationship and operational ideology concerning person-centered planning and the leisure and recreation field.

1. *Person-centered planning is a multifaceted process designed to involve individuals with disabilities in everyday life experiences (including recreation opportunities) to the maximum extent possible.*

Adherence to the principle involves a variety of practices designed to reduce both the "differences" in appearance and performance of persons with disabilities while simultaneously expanding the public's degree of acceptance for differences. Key leadership and programming responsibilities for recreators include utilizing "culturally normative" techniques that facilitate acceptance on the part of the public with whom the person will be interacting. Recent leadership techniques, including task analysis, behavior modification, skill sequence, procedural, and facility modifications, have the combined effects of developing leisure skills that may generalize to other community settings and of enabling the public to observe persons with disabilities participating successfully in normal leisure pursuits.

2. *The integration process inherent in person-centered planning, which stresses the interaction of individuals with disabilities and their nondisabled peers in natural environments of everyday living, is an important corollary of this approach and as such is applicable to a wide range of disabilities.*

Person-centered planning has been found to be a sound principle for guiding the interactions of a variety of persons with special needs. The "best practices" leadership intervention strategies (i.e., behavioral programming techniques) are applicable to many individuals needing leisure skills enhancement.

3. *Being "integrated" in certain leisure settings does not preclude involvement in "special or separate" programs.*

Because person-centered program planning may be perceived as both a process and a goal, segregated recreation programs may play an *initial* role in the reinvolvement of individuals with disabilities in community-based recreation experiences. However, special programs, catering only to persons with disabilities, should be viewed merely as "stepping-stones" to mainstream participation.

4. *Successful integration in recreation settings depends on the involvement of small groups or individuals in existing programs or services.*

Individuals with disabilities will be accepted more readily by their nondisabled counterparts if their numbers in a specific setting do not exceed a proportion that could reasonably be expected to occur through normal interactions.

5. *Person-centered planning does not mean grouping people with different disabilities together.*

Successful involvement of persons with disabilities with nondisabled individuals, not those of other disability groups, is the primary aim of the person-centered process. Therefore, instructional or purely recreative pursuits such as handicapped riding programs, special event days catering exclusively to members with disabilities of a community, and leagues and tournaments for individuals with disabilities do not achieve the ultimate goal of providing individual, normal recreational environments.

6. *The person-centered process requires careful planning; it is not synonymous with "dumping."*

The process inherent within person-centered planning comprises a number of critical components designed to ensure that individuals with disabilities are assimilated socially as well as physically into the mainstream of society. Therefore, meaningful participation in leisure settings demands that attention be paid to various barriers that may prevent the inclusion of persons with disabilities in community-based programs. Attitudes of other staff and participants, transportation, lack of personnel, and building accessibility must be considered thoroughly and in conjunction with efforts designed to upgrade the skills level of persons with disabilities.

7. *Person-centered planning implies involvement in appropriate activities in community-based services.*

Recreation and leisure activities and experiences should be presented that are consistent with a range of chronological ages and interests of individuals with disabilities. Also, recreation and leisure activities should be conducted in settings and time frames typical of society at large.

8. *The involvement of persons with disabilities in community settings can best be achieved by a cooperative approach.*

A major advantage of person-centered planning is that any and all resources are called upon to actively interact with the focus individual to eliminate barriers to enhance the quality of life of this person. Potential resource persons who can exert a significant influence on the leisure lifestyle of a person with a disability include family members, education and recreation personnel, volunteers and staff of advocacy associations, college, university, or high school personnel, and municipal recreation and social service personnel.

CONCLUSION

Being sure that every person has equal opportunity to participate in a specific recreation activity can be a simple task. The first step is
thoroughly looking at the specific activity as it is currently being offered
by a particular recreation agency and determining what kinds and levels
of skills and capabilities are required to participate successfully. The
second step is looking at the specific individual who wants to participate
and determining if that individual has the kinds and levels of skills and
capabilities identified as necessary for participation. If so, the activity is
already programmatically accessible.

If a person clearly does not have the requisite skills to participate, it
may be possible to make the activity accessible through some form of
adaptation—either by the specific participant to compensate for a skill or
capability deficit, or by the activity itself in a manner that does not significantly affect the enjoyment and satisfaction of other participants.

Making programs accessible to people with disabilities has both social
and practical benefits. It encourages the assimilation of people with disabilities into the mainstream of society. It also may reduce the need for
dedicating resources to special, segregated programs and can increase participation in (and possibly revenue of) regular programs without additional
expenses.

However, the primary reason for making recreation programs fully
accessible is the basic right of all people to be judged according to their
capabilities, not their disabilities; their right to be included in all aspects
of public life; their right to have fun like everybody else. After all, that is
what rehabilitation is really all about.

REFERENCES

Adkins, J., and Matson, L. (1980). Teaching institutionalized mentally retarded
    adults socially appropriate leisure skills. *Mental Retardation, 18,* 249–252.

Ball, E.L. (1978). The meaning of therapeutic recreation. *Therapeutic Recreation
    Journal, 4*(1), 17–18.

Ball, E.L., and Cipriano, R.E. (1978). *Leisure services preparation: A competency
    based approach.* Englewood Cliffs, NJ: Prentice-Hall.

Barrett, S. (1987). Trends and issues in developing community living programs for young adults who are deaf-blind and profoundly handicapped. In A. Covert and H. Fredericks (Eds.), *Transition for persons with deaf-blindness and other profound handicaps: State of the art* (pp. 39–49). Monmouth, OR: Teaching Research.

Baumgaart, D., et al. (1982). Principle of partial participation and individual adaptations in educational programs for severely handicapped students. *Journal of the Association for the Severely Handicapped, 7*, 17–27.

Berryman, D. (1972). In V. Frye and M. Peters, *Therapeutic recreation: Its theory, philosophy, and practice* (p. 41). Harrisburg, PA: Stackpole Books.

Bullock, C.C. (1993). Personal correspondence, Madison, CT.

Butler, G.D. (1967). *Introduction to community recreation.* New York: McGraw-Hill.

Certo, N., Schleien, S., and Hunter, D. (1983). An ecological assessment inventory to facilitate community recreation participation by severely disabled individuals. *Therapeutic Recreation Journal, 17*(3), 29–38.

Cheseldine, S., and Jeffrey, D. (1981). Mentally handicapped adolescents: Their use of leisure. *Journal of Mental Deficiency Research, 25,* 49–59.

Edginton, C., and Ford, P.M. (1985). *Leadership in recreation and leisure service organizations.* New York: John Wiley and Sons.

Ellis, M.J. (1973). *Why people play* (p. 110). Englewood Cliffs, NJ: Prentice-Hall.

Fardig, D. (1986). Informal assessment for the severely handicapped. Sec. II: Special issues. *Pointer, 30*(2), 47–49.

Fitzgerald, G. (1964). *Recreation: Pertinent readings.* Dubuque, IA: W.C. Brown.

Flavell, J. (1973). Reduction of stereotypes by reinforcement of toy play. *Mental Retardation, II*(4), 21–23.

Frye, V., and Peters, M. (1972). *Therapeutic recreation: Its theory, philosophy, and practice.* Harrisburg, PA: Stackpole Books.

Gray, D., and Greben, S. (1973). Future perspectives. *1973 work program, building professionalism* (p. 42). Arlington, VA: National Recreation and Park Association.

Gunn, S.L., and Peterson, C.A. (1984). *Therapeutic recreation program design: Principles and procedures* (2nd ed.) (pp. 53–62). Englewood Cliffs, NJ: Prentice-Hall.

Iso-Ahola, S.E. (1980). *The social psychology of leisure and recreation.* Dubuque, IA: W. C. Brown.

Meyer, H.D., and Brightbill, C. (1961). *The theory of play and recreation* (3rd ed.). New York: The Ronald Press Company.

Neumeyer, M. (1964). *Recreation.* Dubuque, IA: W.C. Brown.

O'Morrow, G.S., and Reynolds, R.P. (1989). *Therapeutic recreation: A helping profession* (3rd ed.). Englewood Cliffs, NJ: Prentice-Hall.

Ray, T., et al. (1986). Integrating persons with disabilities into community leisure environments. *Journal of Expanding Horizons in Therapeutic Recreation*, *I*(1), 49–55.

Schleien, S., Kiernan, J., and Wehman, P. (1981). Evaluation of an age-appropriate leisure skills program for moderately retarded adults. *Education and Training of the Mentally Retarded*, *16*, 13–19.

Schleien, S., and Ray, T. (1988). *Community recreation and persons with disabilities: Strategies for integration*. Baltimore: Paul H. Brookes.

Schleien, S., and Wehman, P. (1986). Severely handicapped children: Social skills development through leisure skills programming. In G. Cartledge and J. Milburn (Eds.), *Teaching social skills to children: Innovative approaches* (2nd ed.) (pp. 219–245). Elmsford, NY: Pergamon Press.

Schleien, S., and Werder, J. (1985). Perceived responsibilities of special recreation services in Minnesota. *Therapeutic Recreation Journal*, *19*(3), 51–62.

Shevin, L., and Klein, N.K. (1984). The importance of choice-making skills for students with severe disabilities. *Journal of the Association for Persons with Severe Handicaps*, *9*(3), 159–166.

Voeltz, L., and Wuerch, B. (1981). Monitoring multiple behavioral effects of leisure activities training upon severely handicapped adolescents. In L. Voelta et al. (Eds.), *Leisure activities training for severely handicapped students: Instructional and evaluational strategies*. Honolulu: University of Hawaii, Department of Special Education.

Wehman, P. (1977). *Helping the mentally retarded acquire play skills: A behavioral approach*. Springfield, IL: Charles C Thomas.

Wehman, P., and Schleien, S. (1981). *Leisure programs for handicapped persons: Adaptations, techniques, and curriculum*. Austin, TX: Pro-Ed.

Wuerch, B., and Voeltz, L. (1982). *Longitudinal leisure skills for severely handicapped learners: The Ho'onanea curriculum*. Baltimore: Paul H. Brookes.

Index

Violence, training program on client, 106-107
Vocational Education Act (1914), 45-46
Vocational rehabilitation, 25, 42-43, 255
   brief history of, 256-258
   legislation on, 44-50, 256-258
   See also Rehabilitation counseling
Vocational Rehabilitation Act (1920), 46, 48-49
Vocational Rehabilitation Act (1973). *See* Rehabilitation Act (1973)
Vocational Rehabilitation Amendments. *See* Rehabilitation Act, Amendments
Vocational Rehabilitation Law (1918), 46

Vocational Rehabilitation Program, 47, 48, 49-50, 51, 64
Vois Shapes, 279

Wagner-O'Day Act (1938), 49
Walter Reed General Hospital, 423
Whistle-blowers, 99
Willowbrook study, 73
Workers' compensation laws, 44
Works Progress Administration (WPA), 439
World Health Organization, 32
Worldview, 193, 196-197, 198
   and cultural identity, 194-196
   defined, 194
World War I, 42, 423, 439
World War II, 424, 440, 451
Wyatt v. *Stickney*, 7